Medical Education in Geriatrics

Andrea Wershof Schwartz
Editor

Medical Education in Geriatrics

Strategies for Teaching the Care of Older Adults

Springer

Editor
Andrea Wershof Schwartz
Harvard Medical School
Harvard T.H. Chan School of Public Health
Brigham and Women's Hospital
New England Geriatric Research Education and Clinical Center
at VA Boston Healthcare System
Boston, MA, USA

Disclaimer: The content available in this textbook is not an attempt to provide specific medical advice, and although attempts have been made to provide up to date medical information, users should always consult with medical professionals for medical advice. Use of this textbook does not establish a doctor-patient relationship. Always consult with a physician or healthcare professional for any health-related questions.

ISBN 978-3-031-32498-7 ISBN 978-3-031-32499-4 (eBook)
https://doi.org/10.1007/978-3-031-32499-4

This Springer imprint is published by the registered company Springer Nature Switzerland AG
The registered company address is: Gewerbestrasse 11, 6330 Cham, Switzerland

Foreword

Medical Education in Geriatrics: Strategies for teaching the care of older adults is a gift to those charged with training medical practitioners to care for older adults. Teaching in medicine has long been considered a matter of "*see one, do one, teach one*," with little attention paid to who is being taught, how content and effective teaching methods may need to differ depending on the site of practice, and what "success" looks like, particularly in those specialties that are primarily cognitive. Within geriatrics, we have defined "minimal competencies" for medical students, residents in internal, family, and emergency medicine, and geriatric fellows (see Chaps. 3, 5, and 6). These can be used to guide the content to be taught, but still leaves often busy clinicians and researchers on their own to make sure their material is up to date and evidence-based, and to figure out ways to effectively engage learners, to teach them how to approach clinical reasoning and the care of older adults, and to evaluate their learners' success while simultaneously seeing and caring for their own patients.

Through generous funding from the government's Health Resources and Service Administration and the Donald W. Reynolds and John A. Hartford Foundations, among others, we in geriatrics have been able to develop several creative methods for teaching geriatrics to health professionals. These can be found in the literature, including in the *Journal of the American Geriatrics Society* online Geri Corner, on *MedEdPortal*, and many more (see Chap. 24 for many examples). *Medical Education in Geriatrics*, however, provides a single place to look, replete with tables describing many of these high-quality resources, allowing educators to avoid reinventing the wheel and instead spend their limited time and energy adapting these materials to their learners and site of practice. Similarly, the book provides a course in the principles of Adult Learning with tips for how to best teach and evaluate the current generation of healthcare learners.

There are too few geriatricians to teach all who will be caring for older adults. Faculty in all fields will need to step up to fill this gap. *Medical Education in Geriatrics* is the first place geriatricians and these faculty should look for the keys to assuring that their teaching results in graduates who are able to provide high-quality care to their older patients. Thanks to all those who contributed to writing this incredibly helpful book.

Rosanne M. Leipzig
Brookdale Department of Geriatrics and Palliative Medicine,
Icahn School of Medicine at Mount Sinai,
New York, NY, USA

Introduction: The Importance and Urgency of Geriatrics Medical Education

Nearly every doctor will care for older adults during their career; from internists and family medicine doctors for whom older adults make up a growing portion of outpatient and inpatient care, to pediatricians who care for an increasing number of children being raised by or living with grandparents, to surgeons and other specialists adapting to meet the unique needs of the many older adults under their care. Yet, Geriatrics is not a required course or clerkship in most medical schools, creating a tremendous need and important opportunity to integrate Geriatrics into other aspects of medical education to ensure all doctors are prepared to provide truly excellent care to their older patients. This book fills an important gap by providing a guide for how to teach Geriatrics to medical trainees.

As our population ages, medical education in the principles of geriatric medicine is indeed critical to prepare physicians to provide evidence-based person-centered care for older adults. The COVID-19 pandemic demonstrated the vulnerability and unique needs of older adults, who have borne 80% of the mortality burden in the US, increasing the urgency of geriatric education to prepare providers. Given the small number of specialty-trained physicians in Geriatrics, each physician with Geriatrics expertise must learn to teach effectively and efficiently, and be familiar with key educational techniques to effectively engage learners. Additionally, many medical educators who have not had formal Geriatrics training must learn to teach principles of Geriatric Medicine in order to prepare every physician to improve the care of older adults in their specific specialty or setting.

Medical Education in Geriatrics: Strategies for teaching the care of older adults provides an overview of evidence-based strategies for teaching Geriatrics and applying these strategies to the many settings in which Geriatric medical education occurs. We hope this book will close a gap in the literature by creating a resource both for those with Geriatrics expertise seeking to increase their knowledge and skill in education, and for those medical educators seeking to expand their knowledge of how to teach geriatric principles to their learners.

Through chapters written by experts in both Geriatric Medicine and medical education from the United States and Canada, this book provides approaches for creating effective educational experiences in Geriatrics. The book is divided into **four sections**:

1. The first section focuses on the **landscape of Geriatrics education**, and frameworks for teaching the care of older adults.
2. The second section describes strategies for **teaching Geriatrics to learners of different levels**, ranging from preclinical medical students, through residency, fellowship, and continuing medical education, as well as interprofessional education, with an emphasis on diagnosing the learner to build on their prior knowledge in Geriatrics.
3. The third section discusses **educational strategies for teaching Geriatrics in a variety of classroom and clinical settings**, including the hospital, outpatient settings, nursing home, home care, and telemedicine.
4. The fourth section considers **issues of special importance in teaching Geriatrics**, including diversity, equity and inclusion; feedback; assessment and evaluation, and communication.

A common thread throughout the book is the **Geriatrics 5Ms** [1], discussed in Chap. 1, a framework that aligns with the **Age Friendly Health Systems initiative** [2], and focuses on key domains in the health of older adults: Mobility, Mind, Medications, Multicomplexity, and What Matters. These domains help clarify the areas of focus in Geriatric Medicine and provide a shared language and learning scaffold for the areas that the medical educator ought to teach well and emphasize to their trainees.

Medical Education in Geriatrics: Strategies for teaching the care of older adults aims to provide practical and evidence-based strategies for teaching principles of Geriatrics in a variety of settings and we hope it will be a valuable resource for clinicians, educators, and trainees seeking to learn strategies to improve the care of older adults through education. All material was current and up to date at the time of printing, though may no longer be current by the time you read this book: we encourage readers to consult the ever-growing medical literature in Geriatrics education. While this book is focused on medical education of physicians, we hope principles discussed here may be useful for other professionals and trainees involved in the care of older adults, as collaborative interprofessional care is the bedrock of Geriatric Medicine. Ultimately, we hope this book will help clinicians learn and teach the care of older adults to promote Age-Friendly person-centered medical care in every setting.

References

1. Tinetti M, Huang A, Molnar F. The Geriatrics 5M's: a new way of communicating what we do. J Am Geriatr Soc. 2017;65(9):2115.
2. Mate KS, Berman A, Laderman M, Kabcenell A, Fulmer T. Creating age-friendly health systems—a vision for better care of older adults. Healthc (Amst). 2018;6(1):4–6.

Harvard Medical School
Harvard T.H. Chan School of Public Health
Brigham and Women's Hospital
New England Geriatric Research Education and Clinical Center at VA Boston Healthcare System
Boston, MA, USA

Andrea Wershof Schwartz

Gratitude and Acknowledgments

When I started off as faculty in Geriatrics at Harvard Medical School and VA Boston, I was struck by the incredible opportunities to contribute in Geriatrics education, and the tremendous need to train others to do so as well. Geriatricians are a small and mighty group, and as our population ages there is an increasing recognition and desire for medical education in Geriatrics at all levels. As I delved into the literature in Geriatrics education and was inspired by many colleagues nationally and beyond, I was motivated to create this book as a resource to share with trainees and colleagues that could help us all teach principles of Geriatrics, build on one another's work, and collaborate to improve the care of older adults in every setting.

This book, which I wish had existed when I was starting out in my career, is a result of the collaboration of more than 50 talented colleagues from across the United States and Canada, who share a passion for teaching Geriatrics and ultimately for delivering Age-Friendly person-centered care to older adults. I am grateful to each and every one of them for their expertise and outstanding contributions to this volume, and in particular to the time and thoughtfulness they devoted to this project during the years of the COVID-19 pandemic, which both demanded more of each of us personally and professionally and highlighted the urgency of improving care for older adults. I am indebted to Dr. Rosanne Leipzig for contributing the preface to this volume; many of the chapter authors, myself included, have benefitted from her incredible leadership and mentorship in Geriatrics education and continue to learn so much from her inspiring example.

I am grateful to the wonderful role models and educators who inspired me to make Geriatrics the focus of my career. I have learned from and attempted to build on the impactful work of my incredible teachers, mentors, and colleagues in Geriatric Medicine and beyond, including many of the chapter authors, as well as many others at Mount Sinai School of Medicine, Hebrew University of Jerusalem, Brigham and Women's Hospital, The Harvard Multicampus Geriatrics Fellowship, Hebrew Senior Life, VA Boston, Harvard Medical School (HMS), Harvard T.H. Chan School of Public Health and beyond. I am especially grateful to my earliest mentors in Geriatrics, including Dr. Shelley Sternberg, Dr. Mark Clarfield, Dr. Sarah Berry, Dr. Lara Michal Skarf, Dr. Jenny Driver, Dr. Lew Lipsitz, Dr. Ariela

Orkaby, Dr. Serena Chao, Dr. Sharon Levine, Dr. Louise Aronson and Dr. Anne Fabiny. To the dedicated faculty, staff, and students at HMS with whom I am privileged to work: thank you for the opportunity to collaborate with such thoughtful educators and learners on the HMS Aging and End of Life Theme and the Medical Education course. I also gratefully acknowledge the support of the Harvard Medical School Dean's Innovation award for Medical Education.

Thank you to the many incredible trainees, mentees, and students with whom I have had the pleasure to work: I hope this book will help you and your colleagues grow as teachers in Geriatrics, or as clinicians who deliver Age-Friendly care, which ever field you enter. I have been fortunate to be a part of inspiring teams dedicated to improving care for older adults including at the VA, The Institute for Healthcare Improvement's Age Friendly Health Systems Initiative, the AGS/ADGAP Tideswell Leadership program, and committees through the American Geriatrics Society and AAMC, and am grateful for all their wisdom and dedication. Thank you to the professional staff at Springer who helped usher this book through to publication.

A special thank you to my wonderful colleagues at the VA, including the Geriatrics team at VA Boston and the New England Geriatrics Research Education and Clinical Center, who are phenomenal role models dedicated to serving older veterans, for whom I am constantly grateful and from whom I am always learning. Though I worked on this book "off tour" and not as a part of my official VA responsibilities, I should note that the views expressed in this book are those of the authors and do not necessarily reflect the position or policy of the Department of Veterans Affairs or the United States government.

My family serves as a source of inspiration for me, and I learned the importance of honoring our elders from my dedicated parents, Minda and Peter Wershof, who always showed devotion to my beloved grandparents of blessed memory, Miriam and Abe Rudy, and Miriam and Max Wershof. My parents, as well as my in-laws, Barbara and Jack Schwartz, are incredible role models and sources of support and wisdom, as are my dear brother Stu, and my amazing brothers- and sisters-in-law. My wonderful husband Rabbi Charlie Schwartz provided unwavering support and insight as I worked on this book and throughout my medical training, and our delightful children Maayan, Aviv, and Noa remind me of the better world we are working towards as they fill our lives with joy and meaning.

My deepest appreciation goes to my patients who have helped me learn over the years the diversity of ways people experience aging, and have been generously shared their stories, vulnerabilities, and resilience with me. I hope that this work enables us to aspire to "rise before the aged and show honor to elders."

Contents

Editor and Contributors

About the Editor

Andrea Wershof Schwartz, MD, MPH, AGSF, a national leader in Geriatrics education, is a geriatrician at Harvard Medical School (HMS), where she co-directs the Aging and End of Life Theme, integrating principles of geriatrics and palliative care into the longitudinal medical school curriculum. Dr. Schwartz co-directs the Medical Education course for Medical Students and serves as Associate Director of the Harvard Multicampus Geriatrics Fellowship and Associate Director of the New England Geriatrics Research Education and Clinical Center at VA Boston Healthcare System. A Fellow of the American Geriatrics Society, Dr. Schwartz completed her undergraduate degrees at Columbia University and the Jewish Theological Seminary, MPH at The Hebrew University of Jerusalem, medical training at the Mount Sinai School of Medicine, residency at Brigham and Women's Hospital, and the Harvard Multicampus Geriatrics Fellowship. She is on faculty at the Harvard T.H. Chan School of Public Health and the Division of Aging at Brigham and Women's Hospital, and is a recipient of numerous teaching and mentoring awards, including the American Geriatrics Society Outstanding Junior Clinician Educator award.

Contributors

Louise Aronson, MD, MFA University of California, San Francisco School of Medicine, San Francisco, CA, USA

Steven Barczi, MD Madison VA Geriatric Research, Education, and Clinical Center, William S. Middleton Memorial Veterans Hospital, University of Wisconsin-Madison School of Medicine and Public Health, Madison, WI, USA

Laura K. Byerly, MD Oregon Health and Science University, Portland, OR, USA

Angela G. Catic, MD, MEd Michael E. DeBakey VA Medical Center, Baylor College of Medicine, Houston, TX, USA

Emily Cetrone, MD University of North Carolina, Chapel Hill, School of Medicine, Chapel Hill, NC, USA

Karen J. Chahal, MD Beth Israel Deaconess Medical Center, Harvard Medical School, Boston, MA, USA

Anna Chang, MD University of California, San Francisco School of Medicine, San Francisco, CA, USA

Serena Hsiou-Ling Chao, MD Cambridge Health Alliance, Harvard Medical School, Boston, MA, USA

Elizabeth N. Chapman, MD Madison VA Geriatric Research, Education, and Clinical Center, William S. Middleton Memorial Veterans Hospital, University of Wisconsin-Madison School of Medicine and Public Health, Madison, WI, USA

Ryan Z. Chippendale, MD Boston University Chobanian & Avedisian School of Medicine, Boston, MA, USA

Colleen Christmas, MD The Johns Hopkins University School of Medicine, Baltimore, MD, USA

Jade Connor, MD Harvard Medical School, Massachusetts General Hospital, Boston, MA, USA

Travis W. Crook, MD Vanderbilt University School of Medicine, Nashville, TN, USA

Catherine M.P. Dawson, MD New England Geriatric Research Education and Clinical Center at Veterans Affairs Bedford Healthcare System, Boston University Chobanian & Avedisian School of Medicine, Bedford, MA, USA

Mariu C. Duggan, MD, MPH Tennessee Valley Veterans Affairs Geriatric Research, Education and Clinical Center, Vanderbilt University School of Medicine, Nashville, TN, USA

Helen M. Fernandez, MD Icahn School of Medicine at Mount Sinai, New York, NY, USA

Carolina Fonseca Valencia, MD Beth Israel Deaconess Medical Center, Harvard Medical School, Boston, MA, USA

Lauren J. Gleason, MD, MPH University of Chicago School of Medicine, Chicago, IL, USA

Kady Goldlist, MD Mount Auburn Hospital, Harvard Medical School, Boston, MA, USA

Lisa J. Granville, MD Florida State University College of Medicine, Tallahassee, FL, USA

Alison M. Holliday, MD, MPH Harvard Medical School, Brigham and Women's Hospital, Boston, MA, USA

Reena Karani, MD, MHPE Icahn School of Medicine at Mount Sinai, New York, NY, USA

Ilona Kopits, MD, MPH Boston University Chobanian & Avedisian School of Medicine, Boston, MA, USA

Judy Kwok, MD Cambridge Health Alliance, Harvard Medical School, Boston, MA, USA

Helene R. Labonte, DO Mayo Clinic, Scottsdale, AZ, USA

Andrea Justine Landi, MD University of Chicago School of Medicine, Chicago, IL, USA

Deborah S. Lee, MD Massachusetts General Hospital, Harvard Medical School, Boston, MA, USA

Rosanne Leipzig, MD, PhD Brookdale Department of Geriatrics and Palliative Medicine, Icahn School of Medicine at Mount Sinai, New York, NY, USA

Simone Lescott, MBBS Yale School of Medicine, New Haven, CT, USA

Sharon Levine, MD Massachusetts General Hospital, Harvard Medical School, Boston, MA, USA

Julia V. Loewenthal, MD Brigham and Women's Hospital, Harvard Medical School, Boston, MA, USA

Songprod Jonathan Lorgunpai, MD Mount Auburn Hospital, Harvard Medical School, Boston, MA, USA

Rebecca Masutani, MD Icahn School of Medicine at Mount Sinai, New York, NY, USA

Alyson R. Michener, MD Perelman School of Medicine, University of Pennsylvania, Philadelphia, PA, USA

Rachel K. Miller, MD Corporal Michael J. Crescenz Veterans Philadelphia Healthcare System, Perelman School of Medicine, University of Pennsylvania, Philadelphia, PA, USA

Frank Molnar, MSc, MDCM, FRCPC University of Ottawa, The Ottawa Hospital, Ottawa, ON, Canada

Lauren R. Moo, MD New England Geriatric Research Education and Clinical Center at Veterans Affairs Bedford Healthcare System, Massachusetts General Hospital, Harvard Medical School, Boston, MA, USA

Susan Nathan, MD VA Boston Healthcare System, Harvard Medical School, Boston, MA, USA

Daniele D. Ölveczky, MD Beth Israel Deaconess Medical Center, Harvard Medical School, Boston, MA, USA

Alexandra E. Petrakos, MD Vanderbilt University School of Medicine, Nashville, TN, USA

Feinberg School of Medicine, Northwestern University, Chicago, IL, USA

Becky B. Powers, MD San Antonio Veterans Affairs Geriatric Research Education and Clinical Center, University of Texas Health San Antonio, San Antonio, TX, USA

Ravishankar Ramaswamy, MD Icahn School of Medicine at Mount Sinai, New York, NY, USA

Andrea Wershof Schwartz, MD, MPH New England Geriatric Research Education and Clinical Center at Veterans Affairs Boston Healthcare System, Harvard Medical School and Harvard T.H. Chan School of Public Health, Brigham and Women's Hospital, Boston, MA, USA

Mandi Sehgal, MD Cleveland Clinic Florida, Weston, FL, USA

Amit A. Shah, MD Mayo Clinic, Scottsdale, AZ, USA

Rainier P. Soriano, MD Icahn School of Medicine at Mount Sinai, New York, NY, USA

Rachel Stark, MD, MPH Veterans Affairs Boston Healthcare System, Boston, MA, USA

Lisa A. Strano-Paul, MD Stony Brook School of Medicine, Stony Brook, NY, USA

Shoshana Streiter, MD Brigham and Women's Hospital, Harvard Medical School, Boston, MA, USA

Shaleen Thakur, MD Wake Forest School of Medicine, Winston-Salem, NC, USA

Jeremy D. Whyman, MD Beth Israel Deaconess Medical Center, Harvard Medical School, Boston, MA, USA

Megan E. Young, MD Boston University Chobanian & Avedisian School of Medicine, Boston, MA, USA

Natalie Young, MD University of California, San Francisco School of Medicine, San Francisco, CA, USA

Part I
Introduction: The Importance and Urgency of Medical Education in Geriatrics

Chapter 1
Age-Friendly Health Systems and the Geriatric 5Ms: Frameworks for Teaching Geriatrics

Andrea Wershof Schwartz, Alison M. Holliday, and Frank Molnar

Geriatrics Education: A Growing Need

When we imagine the type of care an older adult (including our families and our future or current selves) would want, we recognize that physicians, and all health care professionals, need appropriate training to be able to deliver it. For trainees who lack sufficient training in delivering geriatrics principles and skills, caring for older adults may be daunting. Gaining skills in geriatrics will help medical trainees, and all clinicians, feel competent and ready to deliver the care older adults deserve.

At every level of medical education, trainees need to develop skills in geriatrics, which are complex and many, by learning from educators skilled in both Geriatrics and teaching. However, many skilled medical educators may not have received sufficient Geriatrics education themselves, and many geriatricians may not have received training in how to teach [1]. Further, given the complexity of Geriatrics, and the lack of required training in many medical training programs, trainees may be exposed to several important areas, such as diseases occurring in older adults, but lack training in other key areas, such as managing multimorbidity. Developing a shared language and framework for teaching Geriatrics can begin to close this gap.

A. W. Schwartz
Harvard Medical School and Harvard T.H. Chan School of Public Health, Brigham and Women's Hospital, New England Geriatric Research Education and Clinical Center at Veterans Affairs Boston Healthcare System, Boston, MA, USA
e-mail: awschwartz@hsph.harvard.edu

A. M. Holliday
Harvard Medical School, Brigham and Women's Hospital, Boston, MA, USA
e-mail: aholliday@partners.org

F. Molnar (✉)
University of Ottawa, The Ottawa Hospital, Ottawa, ON, Canada
e-mail: fmolnar@toh.ca

A. W. Schwartz (ed.), *Medical Education in Geriatrics*,
https://doi.org/10.1007/978-3-031-32499-4_1

The Development of the Geriatric 5Ms: Effectively Focus Learners and Communicate with Care Partners

Geriatricians are considered experts in complexity in patient care; however, simplicity and clarity are required when explaining what we do. Geriatricians are often asked by patients and other health professionals, "what is it you do in geriatrics?" and "when should I think of referring patients to you?" Learners in Geriatrics similarly struggle to identify which topics fit into geriatrics: trainees and teachers alike may by daunted by the huge array of seemingly endless topics relevant to the care of older adults.

A fundamental challenge for Geriatric Medicine is comprehensively defining itself in terms that others outside the specialty find meaningful, readily recall, and support. It is self-evident that a cardiologist deals with cardiac issues, but it is difficult to comprehensively define all that a geriatrician does. Rather than develop the ultimate perfect fully comprehensive definition, geriatricians sought a memorable way to define what we do.

One solution was suggested by Dr. George Heckman in an article titled "*Geriatric Medicine Leadership of Health Care: Transformation: To Be or Not To Be?*" [2] which stated "geriatric medicine is far too multi-faceted to be comprehensively captured by a simple definition. Perhaps a better strategy is for the specialty to highlight key core competencies that match the greatest societal needs." Similarly, Dr. Mary Tinetti suggested that the field ought to distinguish between "Big G" geriatrics which consists of specialty trained Geriatrics health professionals, and "little g" geriatrics which refers to the training all providers who care for older adults need [3]. Defining Geriatrics is a key part of ensuring adequate training for all physicians and healthcare professionals.

A Brief History of the Development of the Geriatrics 5Ms and the 4Ms of Age-Friendly

Over the last decade several specialized Geriatrics teams sought to define Geriatric Medicine by focusing on memory and mobility, with others adding medications. In 2015 in Canada, The University of Ottawa Division of Geriatric Medicine adopted what they named the geriatric 4Ms—Mind, Mobility, Medications, Multicomplexity—into their 2015–2020 strategic plan. At the same time, several groups in the USA, including the then-nascent Age-Friendly Health Systems initiative, developed similar and overlapping 4Ms—What Matters, Mobility, Medication, and Mentation—that were drawn from a study of evidence-based geriatric care models [4, 5] (Figs. 1.1 and 1.2).

This convergence of thinking was recognized, and in early 2017 Dr. Allen Huang, Dr. Mary Tinetti, and Dr. Molnar settled on and published the Geriatrics 5Ms: mind, mobility, medications, multicomplexity, and what matters most [6]. The new 5Ms were launched at the 2017 Canadian Geriatrics Society Annual Scientific Meeting

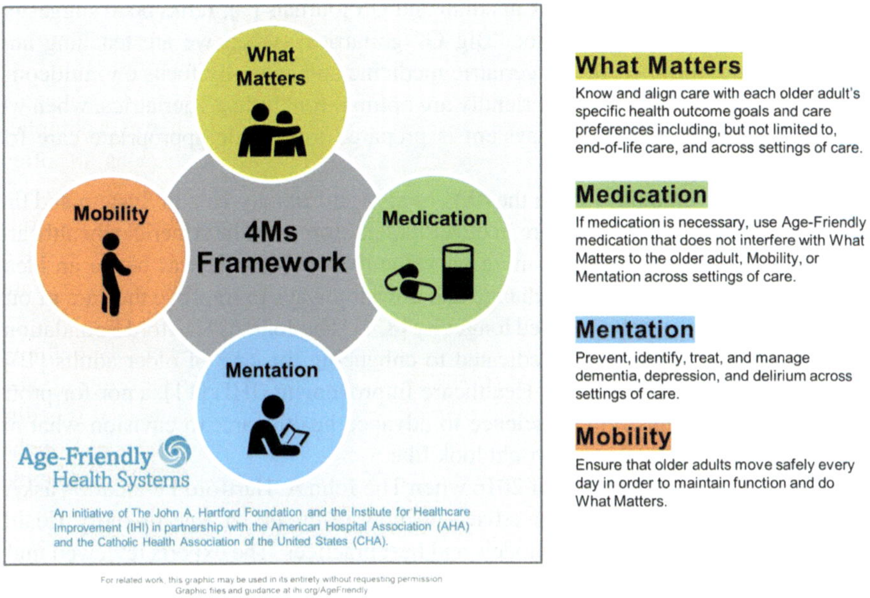

Fig. 1.1 The 4Ms of an Age-Friendly Health System (Source: The Institute for Healthcare Improvement) https://www.ihi.org/Engage/Initiatives/Age-Friendly-Health-Systems/Pages/default.aspx)

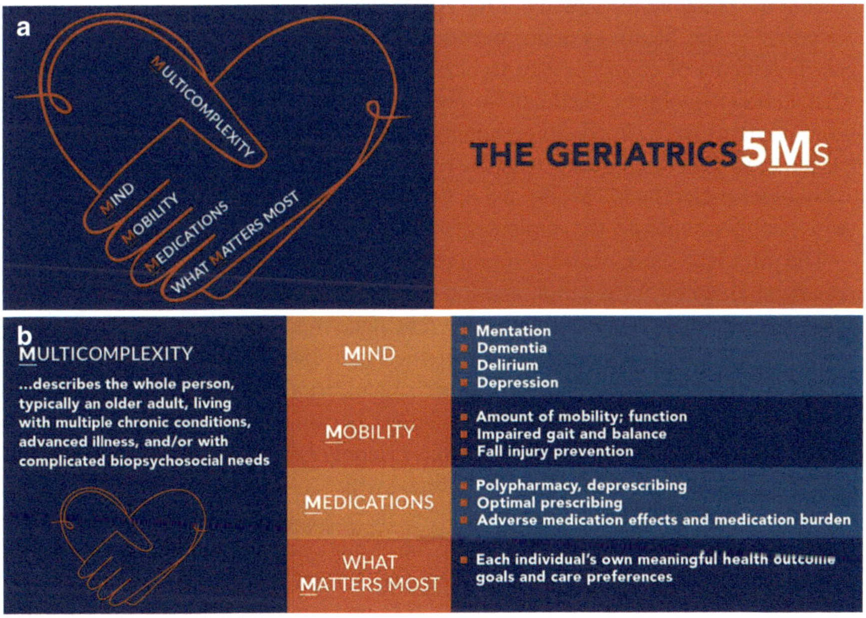

Fig. 1.2 (**a**, **b**) The Geriatrics 5Ms [6] (image source: The American Geriatrics Society, https://www.healthinaging.org/tools-and-tips/tip-sheet-5ms-geriatrics and https://www.healthinaging.org/age-friendly-healthcare-you)

with follow-up publications in Canadian and US journals [7]. It has been suggested that the 5Ms are best suited for "Big G" geriatrics—when we are teaching and learning about the specialty of geriatric medicine and naturally focus on multicomplexity, while the 4Ms of Age-Friendly are optimal for "little g" geriatrics, when we are making sure every health system is prepared to provide appropriate care for older adults in every setting.

Around the same time when the 4Ms of an Age-Friendly Health System and the Geriatrics 5Ms frameworks were in development, forces in the American healthcare system were already focusing more on value over volume. It was hence an ideal time to take advantage of this change and envision ways to improve the care of our aging society with unprecedented longevity [8, 9]. The John A. Hartford Foundation, a philanthropic organization dedicated to enhancing the care of older adults [10], partnered with the Institute for Healthcare Improvement (IHI) [11], a not-for-profit leader in using improvement science to advance health care, to envision what an Age-Friendly Health System would look like.

The work began at the end of 2016 when The John A. Hartford Foundation asked experts around the country for advice on how to create an Age-Friendly Health System using evidence-based models and best practices. The experts reviewed multiple models of care and ultimately arrived on 4 evidence-based domains that these models shared most frequently [11], which became known as the 4Ms: What Matters, Mobility, Medication, and Mentation. The 4Ms were first piloted among several health systems around the USA (including Anne Arundel Medical Center, Ascension, Kaiser Permanente, Providence St. Joseph Health, Trinity Health), pioneering an initiative to implement the Age-Friendly 4Ms across their populations. Specifically, the health systems were charged with reliably providing evidence-based elements of excellent care to older patients by discussing and documenting what matters, mobility, medication, and mentation for all patients. While some health systems were already integrating some of the 4Ms into their care for patients, the purpose was to come up with best practices to reliably integrate all 4Ms for every older patient, and "assess and act on" each M domain. The IHI worked with those health systems on the implementation science of the initiative [12].

The pilot was successful, the moral imperative for the project was clear, and the American Hospital Association and the Catholic Health Association of the United States joined as partners in the initiative. The team made a bold aim to have 20% of US hospitals and medical practices become Age-Friendly Health Systems by the end of 2020. The IHI provided healthcare organizations with quality improvement tools as well as resources on making a business case to become an Age-Friendly Health System [13]. Subsequently, the Age-Friendly Health System initiative spread rapidly across the continuum of care settings, with "action communities" run by the IHI and several other large organizations to increase uptake of the model and provide coaching and support, including the American Hospital Association, the American Geriatrics Society, and the Veterans Affairs Healthcare System [14, 15]. Health systems began implementing the 4Ms and submitting their work to IHI to then be recognized as an *Age-Friendly Health System—Committed to Care Excellence*, with thousands of care settings joining the movement [16].

Not only has the Age-Friendly Health Systems movement taken off, but there is now a growing emphasis on creating an Age-Friendly ecosystems [17], a world where discussions and actions around the cities and towns in which patients live, social determinants of health, and public health systems are all Age-Friendly, meeting a critical need for aging populations, particularly in the wake of the devastation of the COVID-19 pandemic, which disproportionally affected older adults [18].

Future Directions with the Geriatrics 5Ms and the Age-Friendly 4Ms: A Shared Language for Teaching About the Care of Older Adults

In the years since the publication of the Geriatrics 5Ms and the emergence of the Age-Friendly Health Systems initiative, the momentum in the field of Geriatrics around these shared frameworks is clearly evident. The Geriatrics 5Ms and the age-friendly 4Ms are used to frame both clinical work and medical education in the USA, Canada, the UK, New Zealand, and Australia, among other countries. They have been translated into multiple languages, including French and Spanish, and used in multiple different educational contexts, as described in subsequent chapters of this book [19–23]. The American Geriatrics Society adopted the Geriatrics 5Ms and created patient-facing materials [24]. Funders ask applicants to address the 4Ms, such as in the Geriatric Workforce Enhancement Program and Geriatric Academic Career Awards (see Chap. 2) [25], while curricula and resources make use of the Geriatrics 5Ms to communicate shared learning objectives for learners of diverse levels (Chaps. 3–8) and within different settings (Chaps. 9–17). The frameworks are being adapted to a variety of subspecialties [26, 27] and health professions trainees [28, 29]. The utility of a shared framework makes sharing resources easier and more practical, while the memorable Ms allow for easier scaffolding and spaced learning for students of Geriatrics [30].

The Geriatrics 5Ms create context for our learners—helping them understand how individual topics fit into the big picture. The 5Ms create boundaries that make the study of Geriatrics less daunting for new learners. What Matters brings the other 4Ms together to allow learners and clinicians to focus on elders' meaningful values and goals of care. The Geriatrics 5Ms represent our common language, enhancing our ability to effectively focus learners and communicate with care partners with a shared goal of creating an Age-Friendly Health System. The Geriatrics 5Ms has the potential to make us all better educators and teachers of Geriatrics by more easily sharing and building on one another's work and more clearly explaining teaching in Geriatrics for our learners.

The 4Ms of an Age-Friendly Health Systems initiative, which by design is aimed beyond specialists in Geriatrics, is being adopted rapidly as a unifying framework for the many evidence-based geriatric clinical programs such as the Geriatric Surgery Verification Program and Geriatric Emergency Department certification [31]. By focusing on interprofessional teams implementing the 4Ms using quality improvement methods such as Plan-Do-Study-Act (PDSA) cycles, the Age-Friendly Health Systems initiative is building momentum among small clinical settings as well as large health systems such as the VA and CVS Minute Clinic. Ongoing research into the most effective ways to implement and teaching about AFHS will be a priority in the years ahead [32–34].

Leaders within "Big G" geriatrics need to be expert in the Geriatrics 5Ms and more and use this shared language to better build collaborations [35]. Leaders in other fields of medicine and other health professions need to be proficient in the skills of the Geriatrics 5Ms described in subsequent chapters and use this training to be effect participants in and advocates for Age-Friendly Health Systems in their specialties and settings.

As educators, we are responsible for preparing the next generation of providers to deliver evidence-based person-centered care for older adults. Teaching trainees about the Age-Friendly Health System initiative, involving them in related quality improvement projects [36], and inspiring them to create an Age-Friendly ecosystem for patients will be a crucial part of their education to achieve person-centered care. The shared language of these impactful frameworks has the potential to usher in an era of improved Geriatrics education and compassionate and effective clinical care for older adults in every setting.

Disclosures Dr. Molnar, together with Dr. Tinetti and Dr. Huang, is a creator of the Geriatrics 5Ms. Dr. Schwartz serves as a faculty member for the Institute for Healthcare Improvement's Age-Friendly Health Systems initiative and as a leader of the Age-Friendly movement within the VA. The views expressed here are the authors and do not necessarily represent the views of the VA or the US government.

References

1. Rivera V, Yukawa M, Aronson L, Widera E. Teaching geriatric fellows how to teach: a needs assessment targeting geriatrics fellowship program directors. J Am Geriatr Soc. 2014;62(12):2377–82. https://doi.org/10.1111/jgs.13187.
2. Heckman GA, Molnar FJ, Lee L. Geriatric medicine leadership of health care transformation: to be or not to be? Can Geriatr J. 2013;16(4):192–5. https://doi.org/10.5770/cgj.16.89.
3. Tinetti M. Mainstream or extinction: can defining who we are save geriatrics? J Am Geriatr Soc. 2016;64(7):1400–4. https://doi.org/10.1111/jgs.14181.
4. Mate K, Fulmer T, Pelton L, et al. Evidence for the 4Ms: interactions and outcomes across the care continuum. J Aging Health. 2021;2021:898264321991658. https://doi.org/10.1177/0898264321991658.
5. Better Care Playbook. https://bettercareplaybook.org/. Accessed 15 November 2022.
6. Tinetti M, Huang A, Molnar F. The Geriatrics 5M's: a new way of communicating what we do. J Am Geriatr Soc. 2017;65(9):2115. https://doi.org/10.1111/jgs.14979.
7. Molnar F, Frank CC. Optimizing geriatric care with the GERIATRIC 5Ms. Can Fam Physician. 2019;65(1):39. https://www.ncbi.nlm.nih.gov/pubmed/30674512.
8. Fulmer T, Mate KS, Berman A. The age-friendly health system imperative. J Am Geriatr Soc. 2018;66(1):22–4. https://doi.org/10.1111/jgs.15076.

9. Mate KS, Berman A, Laderman M, Kabcenell A, Fulmer T. Creating age-friendly health systems - a vision for better care of older adults. Healthcare. 2018;6(1):4–6. https://doi.org/10.1016/j.hjdsi.2017.05.005.
10. About us. The John A. Hartford Foundation. https://www.johnahartford.org/about. Accessed 15 November 2022.
11. What is an age-friendly health system? https://www.ihi.org/Engage/Initiatives/Age-Friendly-Health-Systems/Pages/default.aspx. Accessed 15 November 2022.
12. Fulmer T, Pelton L. Age-friendly health systems: a guide to using the 4Ms while caring for older adults. Institute for Healthcare Improvement. 2022.
13. https://www.ihi.org/Engage/Initiatives/Age-Friendly-Health-Systems/Documents/IHI_Business_Case_for_Becoming_Age_Friendly_Health_System.pdf.
14. Schwartz AW. No wrong floor on the elevator: A vision for the VA as an Age-Friendly Health System. Fed Pract. 2023;40(03):98–100. https://doi.org/10.12788/fp.0368.
15. Farrell TW, Volden TA, Butler JM, et al. Age-friendly care in the veterans health administration: past, present, and future. J Am Geriatr Soc. 2022. https://doi.org/10.1111/jgs.18070.
16. Health systems recognized by IHI. https://www.ihi.org/Engage/Initiatives/Age-Friendly-Health-Systems/Pages/recognized-systems.aspx. Accessed 15 November 2022.
17. Fulmer T, Patel P, Levy N, et al. Moving toward a global age-friendly ecosystem. J Am Geriatr Soc. 2020;68(9):1936–40. https://doi.org/10.1111/jgs.16675.
18. Aliberti MJR, Szlejf C, Avelino-Silva VI, et al. COVID-19 is not over and age is not enough: using frailty for prognostication in hospitalized patients. J Am Geriatr Soc. 2021;69(5):1116–27. https://doi.org/10.1111/jgs.17146.
19. The geriatric 5Ms. www.geriatric5ms.ca. Accessed 15 November 2022.
20. Holliday AM, Hawley CE, Schwartz AW. Geriatrics 5Ms pocket card for medical and dental students. J Am Geriatr Soc. 2019;67(12):E7–9. https://doi.org/10.1111/jgs.16226.
21. Michener A, Fessler E, Gonzalez M, Miller RK. The 5M's and more: a new geriatric medical student virtual curriculum during the COVID-19 pandemic. J Am Geriatr Soc. 2020;68(11):E61–3. https://doi.org/10.1111/jgs.16855.
22. Phillips SC, Hawley CE, Triantafylidis LK, Wershof SA. Geriatrics 5Ms for primary care workshop. MedEdPORTAL. 2019;15:10814. https://doi.org/10.15766/mep_2374-8265.10814.
23. Wu BJ, Honan L, Tinetti ME, Marottoli RA, Brissette D, Wilkins KM. The virtual 4Ms: a novel curriculum for first year health professional students during COVID-19. J Am Geriatr Soc. 2021;2021:17185. https://doi.org/10.1111/jgs.17185.
24. Age Friendly Health Care and You. The American Geriatrics Society: Health in Aging. Accessed 30 July 2022. https://www.healthinaging.org/age-friendly-healthcare-you.
25. Foley KT, Luz CC, Hanson KV, Hao Y, Ray EM. A national survey on the effect of the geriatric academic career award in advancing academic geriatric medicine. J Am Geriatr Soc. 2017;65(5):896–900. https://doi.org/10.1111/jgs.14884.
26. Liu CK. Mobility and what matters: moving kidney care toward the 4Ms of an age-friendly health system. Kidney Med. 2022;4(6):100481. https://doi.org/10.1016/j.xkme.2022.100481.
27. Kochar B, Ufere NN, Ritchie CS, Lai JC. The 5Ms of geriatrics in gastroenterology: the path to creating age-friendly care for older adults with inflammatory bowel diseases and cirrhosis. Clin Transl Gastroenterol. 2022;13(1):e00445. https://doi.org/10.14309/ctg.0000000000000445.
28. Hawley CE, Doherty K, Moye J, et al. Implementing an interprofessional workshop based on the 4Ms for an age-friendly health system. J Am Geriatr Soc. 2021. https://doi.org/10.1111/jgs.17502.
29. Schwartz AW, Hawley CE, Strong JV, et al. A workshop for interprofessional trainees using the geriatrics 5Ms framework. J Am Geriatr Soc. 2020;68(8):1857–63. https://doi.org/10.1111/jgs.16574.
30. Versteeg M, Hendriks RA, Thomas A, Ommering BWC, Steendijk P. Conceptualising spaced learning in health professions education: a scoping review. Med Educ. 2020;54(3):205–16. https://doi.org/10.1111/medu.14025.
31. Recognition. https://www.ihi.org/Engage/Initiatives/Age-Friendly-Health-Systems/Pages/Recognition.aspx. Accessed 15 November 2022.

32. Burke RE, Ashcraft LE, Manges K, et al. What matters when it comes to measuring age-friendly health system transformation. J Am Geriatr Soc. 2022. https://doi.org/10.1111/jgs.18002.
33. Prusaczyk B, Burke RE. Age-friendly learning health systems: opportunities for model synergy and care improvement. J Am Geriatr Soc. 2022. https://doi.org/10.1111/jgs.17901.
34. Emery-Tiburcio EE, Berg-Weger M, Husser EK, et al. The geriatrics education and care revolution: diverse implementation of age-friendly health systems. J Am Geriatr Soc. 2021. https://doi.org/10.1111/jgs.17497.
35. Callahan KE, Tumosa N, Leipzig RM. Big 'G' and Little 'g' geriatrics education for physicians. J Am Geriatr Soc. 2017;65(10):2313–7. https://doi.org/10.1111/jgs.14996.
36. Severance JJ, Hadley L, Butler Carroll T, Hartos J, Knebl JA. Quality improvement for age-friendly care: an experiential model for instructing medical students in system-based practice. Gerontol Geriatr Educ. 2022;2022:1–7. https://doi.org/10.1080/02701960.2022.2069763.

Chapter 2
The Landscape of Geriatrics Medical Education: Past, Present, and Future

Catherine M. P. Dawson, Lisa J. Granville, and Mandi Sehgal

Advancements in modern medicine have made it possible for people to live longer lives. The number of older adults who will require physicians to care for them is increasing, exposing a critical need to train medical professionals in evidence-based Geriatrics principles.

The upcoming chapters in this book will present strategies for teaching geriatrics and will raise important considerations in shaping the future of Geriatrics medical education. In this introductory chapter, we reflect on how Geriatrics has been incorporated into medical education in the United States from a historical perspective, considering the following questions: Where did we begin? Where are we now? and Where are we going? Though our present scope concerns physician education with a perspective heavily anchored in medicine, Geriatrics care is and must be the synergistic endeavor of a talented, collaborative, interprofessional team.

C. M. P. Dawson
New England Geriatric Research Education and Clinical Center at Veterans Affairs Bedford Healthcare System, Bedford, Massachusetts, USA

Boston University Chobanian & Avedisian School of Medicine, Bedford, Massachusetts, USA
e-mail: catherine.dawson@va.gov

L. J. Granville
Florida State University College of Medicine, Tallahassee, Florida, USA
e-mail: lisa.granville@med.fsu.edu

M. Sehgal (✉)
Cleveland Clinic Florida, Weston, Florida, USA
e-mail: sehgalm@ccf.org

A. W. Schwartz (ed.), *Medical Education in Geriatrics*,
https://doi.org/10.1007/978-3-031-32499-4_2

Geriatrics Medical Education: Where Did We Begin?

Contextual Considerations for Early American Medical Schools

In the 1850s, the average life expectancy at birth was around 40 years, based on estimates from life tables from the Northeast region of the United States [1]. Other estimates from the Antebellum South are even lower, with an average lifespan of 25.5 years for white persons and 21.4 years for black persons [2]. Many died very young: 22% of newborns died before their first birthdays, and almost half of all children (46%) died before age 15 [3]. Only about 4% of the total United States population reached age 60, but, for those who did, life expectancy was estimated to be another 15–17 years, with survival into their mid-70s [1].

Medical schools of the day were largely attended by and presided over by white men, but fledging inroads into the expansion of physician demographics also appeared. Dr. David J. Peck became the first black United States medical school graduate in 1847 (alma mater Rush Medical College in Illinois) [4], Dr. Elizabeth Blackwell became the first female United States medical school graduate in 1849 (alma mater Geneva Medical College in New York) [5], and Dr. Rebecca Lee Crumpler became the first black female United States medical school graduate in 1864 (alma mater New England Female Medical College in Massachusetts) [6]. The late 1800s yielded the establishment of eleven historically black medical schools [7], five women's medical schools [6], and a smattering of medical schools that allowed a small number of black or female students [6, 8].

Medical education in the United States was not standardized in this era. Medical schools of the 1800s had widely varying academic and apprenticeship programs, and physicians entered into practice with heterogenous levels of experience and skill [9].

The Flexner Report of 1910 signposted a paradigm shift for United States medical schools. Robust basic science education prior to clinical training was upheld as a gold standard, and many medical schools failing to meet standards for strong preclinical sciences were shuttered in the wake of the report [10].

Interestingly, Abraham Flexner, the report's primary author, was not a physician at all. Rather, he was a professional educator who had gained recognition for his book *The American College: A Criticism*, which led to his recruitment for a review of United States medical schools [10]. When setting benchmarks to evaluate the quality of medical school curricula, Flexner relied heavily on the counsel of physicians at a prominent local institution (Johns Hopkins), literature review—particularly of the contemporary German system of medical education, his own experiences in nonmedical education, and the direction of the philanthropic organization that had recruited him for the report (the Carnegie Foundation) [10]. The sovereignty of science ideology captured in the Flexner Report is lauded as paving the way for important medical discoveries over the following century and our current emphasis on the evidence-based practice of medicine.

The primacy placed on basic sciences, though, has also garnered criticism for setting in motion a "hidden curriculum" of deconstruction of the whole person into component parts [10]. Devoid of clinical background, Flexner could not appreciate how an overemphasis on the identification and treatment of disease, organ system by organ system, might miss the mark in training physicians to establish trusting therapeutic relationships and achieve patient-centered goals of care. Enchanted by the elixir of scientific discovery, access to research subjects was too often allowed to prevail over access to care—a nefarious harbinger of horrid experiments at the Holmesburg Prison and Tuskegee, as well as myriad other racial injustices and tragic violations of personhood, with which the medical community, and society at large, must now reconcile [10, 11].

Concerningly, school closures also disproportionately affected people already underrepresented in medicine. Instead of growing in numbers, women in the field of medicine declined from 6% of the workforce in 1900 to 4% of the workforce in 1940 [12]. Only two of the seven historically black medical schools operating at the time of the Flexner Report remained open (Howard University College of Medicine and Meharry Medical College) [13]. In 1905, the vast majority of black physicians graduated from historically black medical schools (85.5%) [8]. If the additional five schools had remained open, it is estimated that an additional 35,315 physicians graduating from these schools may have joined the workforce by 2019, significantly broadening physician diversity [7].

Assumptions of Aptitude in Early American Residency Training

In contrast to the basic science focus of the medical school classroom, early postgraduate medical training was intensely focused on the clinical setting. Sir William Osler, a prominent physician and educator at Johns Hopkins, is credited with founding the first United States residency program at the end of the nineteenth century. Its hierarchal structure of interns, residents, chief residents, and overseeing physicians was molded to meet the needs of wards with high clinical volume [9]. Trainees were presumed to develop the ability to practice independently by virtue of their supervised clinical experiences [9]. Absent from this model were rigorous assessments of trainee competence and formalized feedback at each stage of training. The length of training varied by each postgraduate specialty, rather than by the level of achievement of its learners [9].

The Origins of Geriatrics as a Specialty

A contemporary of Flexner and Osler, Dr. Ignatz Nascher, a dual degree pharmacist and physician practicing in New York, first introduced the term "Geriatrics" in 1909 [14]:

Signposts in the Timeline of US Geriatrics Medical Education	
1909	Dr. Ignatz Nascher introduced the term "Geriatrics"
1910	Flexner Report was published
1935	Social Security Act was passed into law
1942	American Geriatrics Society was founded
1945	Gerontological Society of America was founded
1965	Medicare, Medicaid, and the Older Americans Act were all passed into law
1968	Specialized training programs in Geriatrics were started in the US at City Hospital Center in New York
1974	National Institute on Aging was founded
1978	Institute of Medicine published its first Geriatrics workforce report
	Veterans Health Administration established 12 Geriatrics fellowship training programs
1982	First freestanding Geriatrics Department was founded at Mount Sinai in New York
1983	HRSA-funded Geriatric Education Centers program was founded
1988	Geriatric Medicine fellowships of two-year duration became fully accredited by the Accreditation Council for Graduate Medical Education (ACGME)
	The American Boards of Internal Medicine (ABIM) and Family Medicine (ABFM) offered the first 10-year Certificate of Added Qualification (CAQ) in Geriatrics
1989	HRSA-funded Geriatric Training for Physicians, Dentists, and Behavioral and Mental Health Professionals was founded
1990	Association of Directors of Geriatric Academic Programs (ADGAP) was founded
1991	The American Osteopathic Boards of Family Physicians (AOBFP) and Internal Medicine (AOBIM) began offering a 10-year CAQ in Geriatrics
1994	The Practice Pathway for Geriatrics Certificate of Added Qualification was ended by ABFM, ABIM, & AOBIM
1998	Geriatric Medicine Fellowship training was shortened from two years to one year
	HRSA-funded Geriatric Academic Career Awards (GACA) program was founded
2001	The final medicine Practice Pathway for Geriatrics Certificate of Added Qualification was ended by AOBFP

Table 2.1 Boxes shaded in green denote early historical landmarks in Geriatrics medical education, such as the first major Geriatrics professional societies, the first Geriatrics department, and allopathic and osteopathic qualification pathways in geriatrics. Boxes shaded in blue denote education-specific landmarks, including training programs, competencies, milestones, and entrustable professional activities. Boxes shaded in gray denote United States government-related landmarks, including laws, agencies, and funding. *HRSA = Health Resources and Services Administration, an agency of the United States Department of Health and Human Services*

2008	Institute of Medicine report "Retooling for an Aging America" was published
2009	Minimum Competencies in Geriatric Medicine for Medical Students were published[33]
2010	Minimum Geriatric Competencies for multiple resident groups were published: Family Medicine & Internal Medicine[34], Emergency Medicine[35], Psychiatry[36]
2014	Curricular Milestones for Geriatric Medicine Fellowship Programs was published[37]
2015	Entrustable Professional Activities (EPAs) for Geriatric Medicine was published[38]
	HRSA-funded Geriatric Workforce Enhancement Program (GWEP) was founded
2021	Minimum Competencies in Geriatric Medicine for Medical Students was updated[33]
	Curricular Milestones for Geriatric Medicine Fellowship Programs was updated

Table 2.1 (continued)

> Geriatrics, from *geras*, old age, and *iatrikos*, relating to the physician, is a term I would suggest as an addition to our vocabulary, to cover the same field in old age that is covered by the term pediatrics in childhood, to emphasize the necessity of considering senility and its diseases apart from maturity and to assign it a separate place in medicine [15].

Nascher's first textbook, *Geriatrics: The Diseases of Old Age and Their Treatment*, contained many topics that remain relevant in present-day medicine, such as differences between the expected physiology of aging and the pathophysiology of aging, challenges of home care and institutionalized settings, and legal considerations such as decision-making capacity [14, 16].

Subsequent acceptance of Geriatrics as a medical specialty in the United States was gradual, first buoyed by federal legislature and professional societies and then fueled by government grants and the investment of private foundations [17]. The timeline in Table 2.1 delineates many of these important events, which we will now explain further.

In 1929, America was one of the only developed countries lacking a safety net program for elders, so, during the Great Depression, older adults in the United States were thrust into poverty, losing their homes, their savings, and consistent access to food and medical care [17]. The Social Security Act, signed into law in 1935, supported older adults in meeting their basic needs.

Professional societies of Geriatrics, such as the American Geriatrics Society (AGS) and the Gerontological Society of America (GSA), began to be chartered in the 1940s, with missions centering on older adult care and the study of aging [18]. Their affiliated peer-reviewed journals at the time, such as *The Journal of Gerontology* and the *Journal of the American Geriatrics Society*, created a home for new scholarly work in the field [18]. Philanthropic investors, such as the Josiah Macy Jr. Foundation, contributed to the formation of early Geriatrics organizations [17].

In the United Kingdom, Dr. Marjorie Warren, a physician referred to as the mother of Geriatrics, broke ground in creating new Geriatrics models of care in the 1940s and 1950s [19]. Dr. Warren championed optimization and diversification of healthcare settings to meet the needs of older adults, strongly advocating for geriatric care that maximized independence and function [19]. Such care, Dr. Warren asserted, should be provided by an interprofessional team that partnered closely with patients and their families, and her writing still resonates deeply with the goals of Geriatrics today [19].

The 1960s and 1970s welcomed new legislation supporting older adults in the United States with the passing of Medicare, Medicaid, and the Older Americans Act, as well as the establishment of the National Institute on Aging. The Veterans Health Administration promoted Geriatrics in this era by developing inpatient Geriatric Evaluation and Management (GEM) Units in 1974 as well as Geriatric Research, Education, and Clinical Centers (GRECCs) as scholarly hubs devoted to older adult care in 1975 [17, 20]. In 1978, the Institute of Medicine published "Aging and Medical Education," the first in a series of reports focused on the aging of the population and the need for Geriatrics workforce training (1987, 1993, and 2008) [20]. In 1982, the first freestanding Geriatrics department emerged, at Mount Sinai, predating official accreditation in this new specialty [20].

Geriatrics Fellowships, Accreditation, and Certification

Specialized training programs in Geriatrics were started in the United States in 1968 by a physician at City Hospital Center in New York, Dr. Leslie Libow [17]. Dr. Libow created two model programs: (1) a Geriatrics track housed within a pre-existing Internal Medicine residency, in which the third year of residency training was devoted to Geriatrics and (2) a two-year stand-alone Geriatric Medicine fellowship program, entered into after completion of residency [18]. A signature of these new training systems included clinical experiences at "academic nursing homes," which were meant to parallel academic teaching hospitals [18]. In the early years of formalized geriatrics training programs, the Veteran's Health Administration was a significant early adopter of Geriatrics fellowships, establishing 12 nationwide in 1978 [20].

In 1988, Geriatrics fellowships became fully accredited by the Accreditation Council for Graduate Medical Education (ACGME), with a standard two-year training program [20]. That same year, the American Boards of Internal Medicine and Family Medicine (ABIM and ABFM) offered the first 10-year Certificate of Added Qualification in Geriatrics [20]. Two routes existed to achieving certification. The first was completion of a 2-year Geriatrics fellowship, followed by passing the certification examination [21]. The second offered experienced, practicing clinicians the opportunity to sit for the examination without fellowship training, the "practice pathway" [21]. The American Osteopathic Boards of Family Physicians and Internal Medicine (AOBFP and AOBIM) followed suit in offering a Certificate of Added Qualification in Geriatrics through these two pathways in 1991 [21].

Perhaps to honor the value of specialty fellowship training, the practice pathway to the Geriatrics Certificate of Added Qualification was eliminated by multiple medicine boards (ABIM, ABFM, and AOBIM) in 1994, with the American Osteopathic Boards of Family Physicians (AOBFP) closing the final door on this pathway in

2001 [21]. With the extinction of the practice pathway, though, the number of physicians newly certified in Geriatric Medicine each year plummeted from over 2000 in 1994 to under 500 in 2004 [21]. Though controversial [17], a decision was made in 1998 to shorten the length of Geriatric Medicine fellowship training from two years to one year in the hopes of incentivizing more fellowship applications. This intervention did not have its desired effect, and the number of graduating geriatric medicine fellows per year has remained in the 200s–300s for the past two decades [21, 22].

Despite this stagnation in the number of geriatricians, the field has surged ahead. The U.S. Health Resources and Services Administration (HRSA) contributed significant funding to Geriatrics education and workforce efforts (such as Geriatric Education Center Programs, Geriatric Training for Physicians, Dentists, and Behavioral and Mental Health Professionals, the Geriatric Academic Career Awards (GACA), and the Geriatric Workforce Enhancement Program (GWEP)) [21, 23]. Associations centered on Geriatrics education, such as the Association of Directors of Geriatrics Academic Programs (ADGAP) and the National Association for Geriatric Education/Geriatric Education Centers, have enhanced collaboration among educators. Additional professional societies have been founded, such as the American Academy of Home Care Medicine and AMDA—The Society for Post-Acute and Long-Term Care Medicine, and philanthropic organizations, such as the John A. Hartford Foundation, the Donald W. Reynolds Foundation, and the American Federation for Aging Research among others, have backed important Geriatrics initiatives [20]. As a result, tremendous advances in the understanding and management of frailty, falls, delirium, cognitive impairment, social isolation, caregiver burden, patient safety, transitions of care, and models of care (from Acute Care of the Elderly to Program of All-inclusive Care for the Elderly) have been achieved by the Geriatrics community [24].

Geriatrics Medical Education: Where Are We Now?

Big G, Little g Geriatrics

The number of older adults in the United States continues to far outstrip the number of Geriatrics specialty providers trained to care for them [25]. The Geriatrics community has debated the best strategy to fill this gap [26]. Dr. Mary Tinetti, a geriatrician known for her influential work on mobility, the Geriatrics 5Ms Framework [27], and Age-Friendly Health Systems [28], proposed focusing on disseminating Geriatrics principles widely throughout medical training and healthcare systems as little "g" geriatrics, rather than striving to produce a large number of specialized big "G" Geriatricians to care for every older adult [24]. She envisioned big "G" Geriatrics as: "…a small elite workforce that discovers and tests geriatric principles through our research, that teaches these geriatric principles to all health professionals and to the public, and that disseminates and implements these geriatric principles through our health system and health policy leadership" [24].

To educate all health professionals in little "g" geriatrics and to train a small group of health professionals in big "G" Geriatrics, a multipronged approach is needed, guided by clear education targets.

Geriatrics Competencies, Milestones, and Entrustable Professional Activities

Rather than relying on a designated amount of time in training to produce expert clinicians, medical education in the twenty-first century has become increasingly tied to setting specific goals for learners and assessing their progress toward these goals.

Competencies are formalized goals for what a trainee should be able to accomplish at the completion of a designated level of training, such as medical school, residency, or fellowship [29]. Milestones are narrative descriptions of learner knowledge, skills, or attitudes that demonstrate each competency, and educational progress is tracked along levels from novice to expert [30]. Entrustable Professional Activities (EPAs) describe the essential activities that physicians are entrusted to perform safely and effectively without supervision by the end of their training in a given discipline [30].

At the level of Undergraduate Medical Education, the Liaison Committee on Medical Education requests that schools teach care across the life cycle (Standard 7.2) [31], but medical school accrediting bodies do not explicitly require training in geriatrics. Population trends, however, demand a strong foundation in geriatrics for present-day graduating medical students.

Minimum Geriatrics Competencies for Graduating Medical Students were first published in 2009, developed jointly with the American Geriatrics Society, the John A. Hartford Foundation, and the Association of American Medical Colleges [32]. These minimum competencies identified key clinical behaviors that cut across disciplines of medicine, organized into eight domains: (1) medication management, (2) cognitive and behavioral disorders, (3) self-care capacity, (4) falls, balance, and gait disorders, (5) health care planning and promotion, (6) atypical presentation of disease, (7) palliative care, and (8) hospital care for elders [32]. The level of skill to attain targeted that of the day 1 intern, who would be responsible for detecting concerns, initiating care and advising others of the patient's care needs.

The Minimum Geriatrics Competencies for Graduating Medical Students were updated in 2021 [33]. The new competencies are organized into the Geriatrics 5Ms of Mind, Mobility, Medications, Multicomplexity, and Matters Most [27], and they are in alignment with the Age-Friendly Health Systems initiative [28]. Emphasis is given to prioritizing function over disease, addressing social determinants of health and bias, collaborating with interprofessional team members, and individualizing care that aligns with patients' goals.

In Graduate Medical Education, geriatrics competencies for residents build upon the 2009 Minimum Competencies for medical students. For Internal Medicine and

Family Medicine residents, competencies in geriatrics are grouped into seven domains: (1) medication management, (2) cognitive and behavioral health, (3) palliative and end-of-life care, (4) hospital patient safety, (5) chronic illness, (6) transitions of care, and (7) ambulatory care [34]. Other residency programs, such as Emergency Medicine [35] and Psychiatry [36], have also incorporated competencies related to Geriatrics within their training programs; these two specialties also offer geriatrics fellowships.

Focusing in on Geriatric medicine fellowship training programs, fellows are evaluated at specified intervals on their progress from novice to expert in twenty-three milestones [37]. Before the conclusion of training, fellowship directors must decide whether fellows are able to expertly, safely, and independently perform the twelve Entrustable Professional Activities required to practice as a Geriatrics specialist [38].

Geriatrics Medical Education for the Twenty-First Century: Where Are We Going?

Aligning Geriatrics Medical Education with Population Needs

Geriatrics education for physicians must continue to anticipate the older population's needs and promote holistic care across the spectrum from hale to frail. We can feel fairly certain that, unless there is a dramatic, unforeseen change, the population as a whole will continue to grow older. The Age-Friendly Health Systems [28] initiative shows promise as a guiding light down the path toward person-centered, evidence-based care for older adults. Teaching the next generation of clinicians how to routinely employ Geriatrics principles is a crucial step along the way.

For learners to recognize and attain competencies in Geriatrics, training content needs to be clearly identified, offered with repetitive practice, applied to patient care across disciplines, and rigorously assessed. When medical students build a firm foundation in Geriatrics competencies, they can bring this skillset forward as they enter residency. They are then prepared to differentiate into their chosen disciplines, like multipotent stem cells, already equipped with essential skills in older adult care. Residency and fellowship programs can subsequently refine the depth and breadth of these Geriatrics skillsets, as relevant to the specific field.

We urge every training program to ensure their graduates have achieved competence in Geriatrics care. Each program can determine when, where, and how Geriatrics training should occur, as best aligns with their unique resources and priorities. Not all medical schools and academic centers currently have access to geriatricians or faculty with expertise in Geriatrics. Achievement of Geriatrics competencies remains possible, though, independent of availability of geriatricians, through the use of such curricular tools as the Geriatrics for Specialty Residents Toolkit (free, available at: https://geriatricscareonline.org/ProductTypeStore/geriatrics-for-specialty-residents-toolkits/6/) and Aquifer Geriatrics [39] (subscription based), and through the guidance of the expert Geriatrics educators, including those who have contributed chapters to this book.

Possible Future Directions in Geriatrics Medical Education

When considering possible future directions in Geriatrics medical education, interesting questions arise:

- Will Geriatrics one day become, like pediatrics, a core clerkship in almost every medical school?
- Will the rise of telehealth be sustainable for older adults, leading to augmented Geriatrics telehealth skills training in medical schools and residency programs?
- Will medical schools and residency programs prioritize training across transitions of care, requiring clinical experience in skilled nursing facilities in addition to academic hospitals?
- Will overhauls in the fee-for-service physician reimbursement model increasingly reward complex medical decision-making, attracting more qualified trainees to big "G" Geriatrics?

In the upcoming pages of this book, you will find guidance for teaching Geriatrics at your own institution, using current best practices. Our cumulative efforts in teaching Geriatrics principles will define our way forward, as we work together to prepare our workforce to provide excellent care for older adults now and in the years to come.

References

1. The Bureau of the Census. Historical statistics of the United States 1789-1945: a supplement to the statistical abstract of the United States. 1949. https://www.census.gov/library/publications/1949/compendia/hist_stats_1789-1945.html. Accessed 28 December 2021.
2. Stanford School of Medicine. Ethnogeriatrics. 2021. https://geriatrics.stanford.edu/ethnomed/african_american/fund/health_history/longevity.html. Accessed 13 December 2021.
3. Roser M. Mortality in the past – around half died as children. Our world in data. 2019. Accessed 28 December 2021. https://ourworldindata.org/child-mortality-in-the-past.
4. Harris MJ. David Jones Peck, MD: a dream denied. J Natl Med Assoc. 1996;88(9):600–4.
5. Blackwell E. Pioneer work in opening the medical profession to women: autobiographical sketches. London: Longmans, Green, and Co.; 1895. Accessed 30 December 2021. https://digital.library.upenn.edu/women/blackwell/pioneer/pioneer.html#III.
6. Bonner TN. To the ends of the earth: women's search for education in medicine. Cambridge: Harvard University Press; 1992.
7. Campbell KM, Corral I, Infante Linares JL, Tumin D. Projected estimates of African American medical graduates of closed historically black medical schools. JAMA Netw Open. 2020;3(8):e2015220. https://doi.org/10.1001/jamanetworkopen.2020.15220.
8. Duke University Medical Center Library and Archives. Black history month: a medical perspective – education. 2021. https://guides.mclibrary.duke.edu/blackhistorymonth/education. Accessed 30 December 2021.
9. Custers EJFM, Cate OT. The history of medical education in Europe and the United States, with respect to time and proficiency. Acad Med. 2018;93(3):S49–54. https://doi.org/10.1097/ACM.0000000000002079.
10. Duffy TP. The Flexner report–100 years later. Yale J Biol Med. 2011;84(3):269–76.

11. Washington HA. Medical apartheid: the dark history of medical experimentation on Black Americans from colonial times to the present. Doubleday, 2006.
12. Moehling CM, Niemesh GT, Thomasson MA. Shut down and shut out: women physicians in the era of medical education reform. Social Science History Association, 2019 Annual Meeting. 2019. https://ostromworkshop.indiana.edu/pdf/piep2019/moehling-niemesh-thomasson.pdf. Accessed 30 December 2021.
13. Miller LE, Weiss RM. Revisiting black medical school extinctions in the Flexner era. J Hist Med Allied Sci. 2012;67(2):217–43.
14. Cohen AB. Nascher's Geriatrics at 100. J Am Geriatr Soc. 2014;62(12):2428–9. https://doi.org/10.1111/jgs.13155.
15. Nascher IL. Longevity and rejuvenescence. N Y Med J. 1909;89:359.
16. Nascher IL. Geriatrics: the diseases of old age and their treatment. Philadelphia: P. Blackston's Son & Co.; 1914.
17. Morley JE. A brief history of geriatrics. J Gerontol A Biol Sci Med Sci. 2004;59(11):1132–52. https://doi.org/10.1093/gerona/59.11.1132.
18. Libow LS. From Nascher to now-75 years of U.S. geriatrics. J Am Geriatr Soc. 2004;52(9):1594. https://doi.org/10.1111/j.1532-5415.2004.52430_15.x.
19. St John PD, Hogan DB. The relevance of Marjory Warren's writings today. Gerontologist. 2014;54(1):21–9. https://doi.org/10.1093/geront/gnt053.
20. Warshaw GA, Bragg EJ. The training of geriatricians in the United States: three decades of progress. J Am Geriatr Soc. 2003;51(7):S338–45. https://doi.org/10.1046/j.1365-2389.2003.51345.x.
21. Institute of Medicine (US) Committee on the Future Health Care Workforce for Older Americans. Retooling for an aging America: building the health care workforce. Washington: National Academies Press; 2008.
22. Accreditation Council for Graduate Medical Education. ACGME Data Resource Book 2020-2021 (online). https://www.acgme.org/About-Us/Publications-and-Resources/Graduate-Medical-Education-Data-Resource-Book. Accessed 10 December 2021.
23. U.S. Department of Health and Human Services, Health Resources and Services Administration, National Center for Health Workforce Analysis. Geriatrics workforce enhancement program: academic year 2018-2019 (online). https://bhw.hrsa.gov/sites/default/files/bureau-health-workforce/funding/geriatrics-workforce-enhancement-programs-2019.pdf. Accessed 14 December 2021.
24. Tinetti M. Mainstream or extinction: can defining who we are save geriatrics? J Am Geriatr Soc. 2016;64(7):1400–4. https://doi.org/10.1111/jgs.14181.
25. U.S. Department of Health and Human Services. Health resources and services administration, national center for health workforce analysis. National and regional projections of supply and demand for geriatricians: 2013-2025. Rockville, Maryland, 2017.
26. Callahan KE, Tumosa N, Leipzig RM. Big 'G' and Little 'g' geriatrics education for physicians. J Am Geriatr Soc. 2017;65(10):2313–7. https://doi.org/10.1111/jgs.14996.
27. Tinetti M, Huang A, Molnar F. The geriatrics 5M's: a new way of communicating what we do. J Am Geriatr Soc. 2017;65(9):2115. https://doi.org/10.1111/jgs.14979.
28. Age-Friendly Health Systems. Institute for healthcare improvement. http://www.ihi.org/Engage/Initiatives/Age-Friendly-Health-Systems/Pages/default.aspx. Accessed 30 September 2021.
29. Carraccio C, Englander R, Van Melle E, et al. Advancing competency-based medical education: a charter for clinician-educators. Acad Med. 2016;91(5):645–9. https://doi.org/10.1097/ACM.0000000000001048.
30. Wagner SJ, Reeves S. Milestones and entrustable professional activities: the key to practically translating competencies for interprofessional education? J Interprof Care. 2015;29(5):507–8. https://doi.org/10.3109/13561820.2014.1003636.
31. Liaison Committee on Medical Education. Functions and structure of a medical school: standards for accreditation of medical education programs leading to the MD degree. 2021. https://lcme.org/publications/. Accessed 16 August 2021.

32. Leipzig RM, Granville L, Simpson D, et al. Keeping granny safe on July 1: a consensus on minimum geriatrics competencies for graduating medical students. Acad Med. 2009;84(5):604–10. https://doi.org/10.1097/ACM.0b013e31819fab70.
33. American Geriatrics Society Geriatrics Competencies Working Group. Minimum competencies in geriatrics for medical students. 2021. https://adgap.americangeriatrics.org/education-training/competencies/geriatrics-competencies-medical-students. Accessed 15 August 2021.
34. Williams BC, Warshaw G, Fabiny AR, et al. Medicine in the 21st century: recommended essential geriatrics competencies for internal medicine and family medicine residents. J Grad Med Educ. 2010;2(3):373–83.
35. Hogan TM, Losman ED, Carpenter CR, Sauvigne K, Irmiter C, Emanuel L, Leipzig RM. Development of geriatric competencies for emergency medicine residents using an expert consensus process. Acad Emerg Med. 2010;17(3):316–24. https://doi.org/10.1111/j.1553-2712.2010.00684.x. Accessed 15 September 2021.
36. American Association for Geriatric Psychiatry. Geriatric core competencies: adapted from proposed geriatric psychiatry core competencies for subspecialty training. https://www.aagponline.org/index.php?src=gendocs&ref=GeriatricCoreCompetencies&category=Education&link=GeriatricCoreCompetencies. Accessed 13 September 2021.
37. The Accreditation Council for Graduate Medical Education. Geriatric medicine milestones. 2021. https://www.acgme.org/globalassets/PDFs/Milestones/GeriatricMedicineMilestones.pdf. Accessed 30 September 2021.
38. Leipzig RM, Sauvigne K, Granville LJ, et al. What is a geriatrician? American Geriatrics Society and Association of Directors of Geriatric Academic Programs end-of-training entrustable professional activities for geriatric medicine. J Am Geriatr Soc. 2014;62:924–9.
39. Sehgal M, Syed Q, Callahan KE, et al. Introducing aquifer geriatrics, the American Geriatrics Society National Online Curriculum. J Am Geriatr Soc. 2019;67:811–7. https://doi.org/10.1111/jgs.15813.

Part II
Teaching Geriatrics to Different Levels of Medical Learners

Chapter 3
Healthy Aging, Aging Physiology, and Anti-Ageism to Undergraduate Medical Learner

Kady Goldlist, Julia Loewenthal, and Louise Aronson

Healthy Aging, Aging Physiology, and Anti-Ageism

Most of us spend more decades as older adults (65+) than as children. Yet, medical education and training in the USA underrepresent three critical content areas in the care of older adults: healthy aging, aging physiology, and psychology of aging. Many medical students learn geriatrics by caring for frail older adults in inpatient settings. However, this does not capture the majority of older adults who are thriving in the community. In fact, it is estimated that less than 11% of community-dwelling older adults are frail and most older adults are independent and robust [1, 2]. As a result, many medical students underestimate the health and function of older adults living in the community. Although not common in medical education and not well studied, there is evidence that when medical students are taught about normal aging as part of their curriculum, their attitudes toward older adults improve [3, 4]. This chapter will help educators incorporate three key areas of geriatrics into their teaching: (1) the concept of healthy aging, (2) important changes with physiological aging, and (3) opportunities to recognize and address medical ageism and

K. Goldlist (✉)
Mount Auburn Hospital, Harvard Medical School, Boston, MA, USA
e-mail: kady.goldlist@mah.harvard.edu

J. Loewenthal
Brigham and Women's Hospital, Harvard Medical School, Boston, MA, USA
e-mail: jloewenthal@bwh.harvard.edu

L. Aronson
University of California, San Francisco School of Medicine, San Francisco, CA, USA
e-mail: louise.aronson@ucsf.edu

A. W. Schwartz (ed.), *Medical Education in Geriatrics*,
https://doi.org/10.1007/978-3-031-32499-4_3

its consequent health inequities. In each section, we will define core content and provide educational examples and frameworks for how to teach these concepts in the context of medical education.

Healthy Aging

Definitions

The terms healthy aging and successful aging are sometimes used interchangeably. Successful aging is defined as "multidimensional, encompassing the avoidance of disease and disability, the maintenance of high physical and cognitive function, and sustained engagement in social and productive activities" [5]. In contrast, The World Health Organization (WHO) defines healthy aging as the process of developing and maintaining the functional ability that enables well-being in older age. The WHO explains that functional ability includes the ability to meet basic needs, to learn, grow, and make decisions, to be mobile, to building and maintain relationships, and to contribute to society [6]. Healthy aging is preferred because successful aging requires the absence of disease, eventually turning all people into aging "failures." A more constructive conceptual framework posits healthy aging as an individualized approach to optimizing human health and function regardless of disease burden [7]. Although often used in the lay public and for-profit sectors to refer exclusively to primary prevention of disease and disability, medical frameworks of healthy aging include secondary and tertiary prevention as well. For example, the National Prevention Council's Healthy Aging Strategy organizes the concept of healthy aging into five categories: (1) promoting health, preventing injury, and managing chronic conditions, (2) optimizing cognitive health, (3) optimizing physical health, (4) optimizing mental health, and (5) facilitating social engagement [8]. Even using a narrow medical lens, this conceptual framework of healthy aging acknowledges that patients with the same disease process can choose wildly divergent paths based on factors including their tolerance for burdens of medical care, financial resources, religious and/or cultural customs, family and other social supports, and patient perception of a treatment's risks and benefits [9–11].

Healthy Aging in Undergraduate Medical Education

The literature on how healthy aging is incorporated into current medical school curricula is limited. This may be because there is such variable language used to describe healthy aging and no widespread accepted definition. Table 3.1 summarizes models of teaching healthy aging in U.S. medical schools. The outcomes in the table are discussed in the context of the Kirkpatrick Evaluation Model (Level 1:

Table 3.1 Healthy aging curricula in undergraduate medical education

Journal	Learner	Description	Outcome (Kirkpatrick evaluation model)
Batsis et al. [9]	• First, second, third, and fourth year medical students (did not specify number of students)	• Problem based-learning and annual geriatrics-based educational activity • Assigned older adults to conduct a life history and discuss shared experiences	• Level 2—learning • Students had increased awareness and knowledge of geriatrics and more-positive attitudes about geriatric care • Exposure to healthy agers in the community
Mohler et al. [3]	• 37 third-year medical students	• Two 2-hour sessions where medical students were matched with volunteers aged 65 who were in good general health and lived independently • Sessions included a PowerPoint presentation and one-on-one physical interview and counseling between student and mentor. Following the session students and mentors completed an end-of-session evaluation form	• Level 2—learning • Students were taught about physical activity interviewing and counseling in older adults • 92.3% of students rated Health Aging Rounds as excellent or good • All students felt the activity led them to have the same or more-positive attitudes about aging
Rull et al. [12]	• First, second, third, and fourth year medical students (did not outline number of students)	• Designed around an aging couple from age 60 to age 90. One partner representing the healthy aging process and the other partner experiencing multiple health problems • Included patient experiences, small-group encounters, and paper-based learning modules	• Level 1—reaction • Students rated the experience positively • Students reflected on the complexity of issues and impact on other family members
Muniak and Mulhausen [11]	• 34 medical students	• Virtual geriatrics elective that included education on healthy aging and included the 5M Geriatric Framework • Day 9 of the 10-day elective was titled Matters Most and included reading on Healthy Aging and discussion on aging well There was also a patient telephone interview with an older adult	• Level 2—learning • Among students that completed the elective students felt more prepared to care for older adults (96%) • Positive reflections by students outlined on day 9 of the course

reaction or how did the student respond, Level 2: learning or what did the student learn and has their skills improved, Level 3: behavior or have the students applied what they learned, and Level 4: results or has the organization experienced any benefits as a result of the curriculum) [13].

Most medical school curricula focus on geriatric syndromes when teaching geriatric medicine and do not introduce healthy aging concepts. As evident by the outcomes and Kirkpatrick evaluation model in Table 3.1, current curricula teach medical students about healthy aging but do not help learners incorporate healthy aging principles into their clinical skills.

Integrative Medicine and Lifestyle Medicine

The fields of integrative medicine and lifestyle medicine offer approaches and frameworks that are compatible with the aims of healthy aging. Both fields include nonpharmacologic approaches and behavior change as cornerstones of patient management. However, they encompass all age ranges, with variability in how recommendations are tailored for older adults.

Integrative medicine brings together both conventional and complementary approaches to health in a safe, coordinated way, emphasizing a holistic, patient-focused approach to health care and wellness. Practices encompass dietary, psychological, and physical approaches, often in multimodal systems. In the past, these approaches were often termed "complementary and alternative," but there has been a movement toward integrating complementary therapies with conventional care rather than using them in place of this care, so the term "alternative" has been deemphasized. In the literature, the term "complementary and alternative medicine" or "CAM" is still commonly used. Approximately 45% of US medical schools offer some form of CAM education [14]. Data on content are limited, but acupuncture appeared to be the most frequently taught modality. Delivery methods also varied widely, but often included interactive teaching methods such as workshops and case discussions, paired with an immersive clinical activity with a CAM practitioner. Educational outcomes most frequently included student reactions and knowledge (Kirkpatrick Level 1 and 2).

Lifestyle medicine is an evidence-based clinical approach to preventing, treating, and even reversing diseases by replacing unhealthy behaviors with positive ones. Lifestyle medicine focuses on 6 domains: healthful eating of a whole, plant-based diet; avoiding risky substances; improving sleep; forming and maintaining relationships; developing strategies to manage stress; and increasing physical activity [15]. In 2017, the American Medical Association passed a resolution to support the incorporation of lifestyle medicine curricula into medical schools [16]. The American College of Lifestyle Medicine published curriculum implementation standards in 2021, as well as descriptions of implementation in five different medical schools [17, 18].

Table 3.2 offers suggestions to incorporate healthy aging into medical curricula using the healthy aging categories by the National Prevention Council's Healthy Aging Strategy: (1) promoting health, preventing injury, and managing chronic conditions, (2) optimizing cognitive health, (3) optimizing physical health, (4) optimizing mental health, and (5) facilitating social engagement [8].

Table 3.2 Healthy aging and educational integration

Healthy aging framework categories [8]	Healthy aging examples	Example of educational integration
Promoting health, preventing injury, and managing chronic conditions	• Limit polypharmacy by prioritizing essential medications based on patient goals (longevity and/or comfort; toxicity; ease of use) • Deprescribe when possible • Optimize nutrition through diet as much as possible, rather than supplements	• When teaching about medication history include questions about supplements and herbal remedies. Also include deprescribing resources such as medstopper.com • Educate nutrients in a healthy diet and using food as medicine. AN example is emphasis on calcium in diet rather than supplements • Counsel on protein supplementation and evidence-based dietary plans (Mediterranean and MIND diets) [9]
Optimizing cognitive health	• Emphasis on sleep hygiene • Use of meditation • Encouraging intellectual stimulation with books, educational classes, and social engagement • Assess vision/hearing regularly	• Knowledge of sleep hygiene and resources such as meditation apps (example is Headspace, Calm, Sleepio, CBT-i) • Medical students should learn to evaluate patients for hearing and vision impairment
Optimizing physical health	• The four types of exercise include cardio, strength, balance, and stretching	• Have trainees write individualized exercise prescriptions when counseling patients [19] • Educate on the evidence of Tai Chi and fall prevention
Optimizing mental health	• Tie health promotion to social circumstances and goals of care [20] • Limit alcohol consumption • Encourage psychotherapy • Educate and support caregivers	• Catering advance care planning discussions for all older adults • Medical students writing a narrative on an older adults life story [21] • Age appropriate alcohol counseling • Familiarize with local psychotherapy resources and caregiver support groups
Facilitating social engagement	• Intellectual stimulation, social engagement, stress management, exercise that requires executive function • Preserve level of function, reverse disability where possible, and decrease progression of frailty level • Social structures in place to support any level of frailty/comorbidities	• Medical students can familiarize themselves with local senior centers to engage older adults in the community • Collaborate with social workers to learn about local resources [22] • Example: create an interactive jigsaw lesson with medical students on the different sites of care for older adults, including senior centers, assisted living facilities, PACE programs, and home health services. Ask for local examples of each site of care [23] • Example: Use of OSCE to teach aging and functional change over time [12]

Aging Physiology

Definition

Aging physiology is defined as universal, expected changes in the body with particular attention to biological age. In contrast to chronological age which is based on birth date, biological age is determined by function. The rate is influenced by modifiable and non-modifiable factors. Modifiable factors include environmental exposure, cultural beliefs and traditions, and personal behaviors. Non-modifiable factors include genetic predisposition and biological mechanisms. Despite age-related changes, in the absence of disease organ systems continue to maintain function and homeostasis. However, the ability to maintain homeostatic conditions under times of stress diminishes. Homeostenosis is an organ system's inability to maintain homeostasis under stress. As a result, an insult that might be buffered by younger organs can lead to disease or injury in older organs. Frailty is the phenotype that emerges when an individual is unable to recover to their baseline after a stressor because of homeostenosis and loss of reserve. A frail person has increased risk for adverse health outcomes compared to a non-frail person of the same chronological age. Frailty is not a steady state; both progression and reversion are common, offering opportunities for intervention [24].

Aging Physiology and Medical Education

Age-related physiological changes and their pathological correlates should be included throughout the pre-clinical organ system teaching of health professions students. A lifestage approach to each system, noting usual physiology from birth through old age, would better prepare learners for the full age-range of patients they encounter in clinical settings. It would also increase recognition that each individual's aging and old age are shaped by their health and experiences beginning in utero and continuing throughout life. A body system chart of physiological changes with age and their potential pathological sequelae is presented in Table 3.3, which also includes examples of educational integration of this information in teaching in clinical settings.

Anti-Ageism and Why Language Matters

Definition

Healthy aging is an attractive concept because of its positive impact and individualized approach to all human lives. Many times, society associates aging with multimorbidity, functional decline, and dependency. However, most older adults in the

Table 3.3 Physiologic changes in different body systems with aging, and examples of educational integration [24]

Body system	Physiologic change	Example of educational integration
Nervous	• Decrease in number and function of sensory neuron • Decrease in muscle innervation and fine motor control because of decrease in the number of neurons and decrease in action potential speed [25] • Increase in lipofuscin and tangled neurofibrils in neurons in the brain	Setting • A learner is seeing a new patient for memory concerns. Generalized parenchymal volume loss is noted on an MRI of the brain Teaching point • With aging there is generalized volume loss seen on brain imaging. This finding is non-specific and does not indicate memory loss. There are other important pieces in a memory work up aside from imaging including history and subjective concerns
Skin, hair, and nails	• Decrease in elasticity and decrease in thickness. There is an increase in collagen cross-links. Loss of skin elasticity leading to skin sagging and wrinkling • Hair density and color decrease. Hair follicles atrophy and hair turns gray • Eyebrow, ear, and nasal hair increase in length and coarseness especially in men • Nail thickness and strength decrease. Increase in dull, brittle, and yellowish nails	Setting • An older adult presents to the resident clinic interested in learning about vitamins that can fix her hair loss Teaching point • Hair density decreases with age • There are no FDA approved vitamins that treat hair loss • Counseling is usually based on cosmetic options once metabolic etiology is ruled out (such as thyroid disease)
Eyes	• Decrease accommodation and dark adaptation and decrease in ability to focus on near objects because of decrease in pupil diameter and increase in thickening of lens	Setting • In the trauma bay an older adult is evaluated after a motor vehicle accident at night Teaching point • Older adults have a diminished ability to adapt to dark • Some older adults should be counseled to avoid driving at nighttime
Ears	• Increase in conductive deafness (low-frequency range) because of decrease of elasticity and efficiency of ossicular articulation in the middle ear • Increase in sensorineural hearing loss (high-frequency sounds) • Increase in ear wax volume and hardening. Decrease in the size and number of otoliths and decrease in cochlear neurons. Increase in the thickening of the tympanic membrane and organ atrophy	Setting • An audiologist is evaluating a patient for hearing loss and notes cerumen impaction bilaterally, obstructing view of the tympanic membrane Teaching point • Ear wax volume increases as a result of cerumen gland atrophy and decreased function of the cilia in the ear. Gland atrophy increases cerumen dryness and decrease function of cilia leads to cerumen buildup [26] • Students should be taught to always check the ears of older adults on physical exam. They can also learn about ear wax removal in the office or at bedside

(continued)

Table 3.3 (continued)

Body system	Physiologic change	Example of educational integration
Cardiovascular (heart and vasculature)	• Increase in left ventricular wall thickness and myocardium thickening from fat deposition and fibrosis. Increase in heart size and weight • Increase in vessel rigidity • Decrease in responsiveness to agents • Decrease in baroreceptors and pacemaker cells (10% decrease per decade)	Setting: Teaching about orthostatic hypotension in the inpatient setting. Teaching point: • Baroreflex impairments result in decreased ability to mount a robust heart rate response to preload reduction (due to defects in the beta-receptor response to sympathetic stimulation) • Hypovolemia leads to orthostasis when compensate by cardio-acceleration is blunted • Counsel on changing positions slowly • Knowing when and how to do orthostatic vital signs
Pulmonary	• Decrease in exercise tolerance and pulmonary reserve because of decreased vital capacity, forced expiratory volume, and forced vital capacity (decrease by 30% by age 80) • Decreased elastic recoil of the lung • Increase in collagen cross-links and residual volume	Setting: Medical students rotating through the intensive care unit and seeing older adults with difficulty to wean off the ventilator Teaching point • Lung reserve diminishes with age leading to lower likelihood of recovery from intubation. For patients aged 65–74, only 31% will survive intubation. For older adults 80–84 years old, only 19% will survive intubation and for those over 90 years old, only 14% survive intubation. Post-intubation, 40% of older adults will have a severe functional disability at hospital discharge unless their baseline functional status was completely independent [27] • When discussing do not resuscitate with older adults, students should be able to relay the survival likelihood to their patients • Using non-invasive means to support breathing and optimize lung volume such as incentive spirometry, chest physiotherapy, and encouraging patients to be mobile and out of bed
Gastrointestinal	• Decreased absorption of iron, B_{12}, and calcium because of increased mucosal cell atrophy and altered intestinal absorption • Decrease in saliva production • Increase in constipation, diverticula, transit time, and dysphagia	Setting: A dental student is examining an older adult and notes multiple cavities Teaching point • Decreased saliva in older adults can lead to increase in frequency of dental caries • Since older adults are at increased risk for dry mouth, learners can appreciate an additional risk with prescribing anticholinergic medications

Table 3.3 (continued)

Body system	Physiologic change	Example of educational integration
Renal	• Decrease in kidney size and weight. Decreased number of functional glomeruli leading to decreased renal concentrating ability and glomerular filtration rate • Decrease in renal blood flow	Setting: In the emergency department, a patient presents with fatigue and is found to have acute renal injury after he took NSAIDs for 2 weeks for a knee injury Teaching point • Kidneys are more susceptible to injury from renally metabolized medications in the older adult • Consideration of renally dosed medications and adjustments
Urinary	• Increase in prolapse, diverticula, and urethral mucosal atrophy	Setting: At the obstetrics office, an older female is embarrassed to go out for dinner with her friends because of her urinary incontinence that has been worsening over 2 years Teaching point • Pelvic floor muscles weaken in older adult increasing the frequency of urinary incontinence • Students should ask about urinary symptoms and episodes of nocturia
Endocrine	• Decrease in growth hormone, prolactin, melatonin, total serum calcitonin, aldosterone, serum cortisol, renin, testosterone, estrogen, and progesterone • Increase in parathyroid hormone, baseline cortisol, norepinephrine, and erythropoietin • Increase in atrophy of pituitary, thyroid, and thymus • Decrease in insulin receptors and cellular glucose transporters	Setting • A resident sees a patient in the endocrinology clinic and his diabetes is no longer controlled with oral antihyperglycemics. The preceptor, who has treated the patient for decades, suggests starting insulin Teaching point • Insulin receptors decrease with age and type 2 diabetes can require insulin for control • Students should learn about different diabetes clinics that their institution offers. If not then what other supports providers can offer new insulin users
Bone	• Increase in joint stiffness and decrease in bone density and flexibility • Decrease in bone mass especially in postmenopausal women • Decrease in bone height as intervertebral discs lose fluid and become thinner	Setting • A nurse helps set up an infusion for an older adult's annual antiresorptive therapy after she broke her hip last year secondary to a ground level fall Teaching point • here is a decrease in bone mass in postmenopausal women because of decrease in estrogen. The prevalence of low bone mass, a precursor of osteoporosis, in women over the age of 50 is 51.5% compared to 33.5% in men over 50 [28] • Students can counsel on dietary calcium and vitamin D3 recommendations and weight bearing exercises

(continued)

Table 3.3 (continued)

Body system	Physiologic change	Example of educational integration
Muscle	• Decrease strength and tone and contractility • Fibers shrink • Increase in lipofuscin and fat deposits • Decrease in type II (fast twitch) fibers • Decrease in muscle tissue and lean body mass (30% muscle mass decline after age 60)	Setting • In clinic, a geriatrician asks a patient to stand from a seated position without using their arms and the patient is unable to rise from the chair without using hands Teaching point • Older adults are at risk of sarcopenia and are at risk for decreased proximal muscle strength • Using the chair stand as a diagnostic and therapeutic technique during a patient visit
Immune	• Decrease in immune functioning and response to new pathogens • Decrease in T lymphocytes, natural killer cells, and cytokines needed for growth and maturation of B cells • Increase in autoimmune abnormal antibodies	Setting • An older adult gets the high dose influenza vaccine from a pharmacist Teaching point • Older adults have a decrease in immune response to new pathogens • Recommending the high dose flu shot to older adults

twenty-first century describe themselves as in good to excellent health whether they have medical issues or not [7]. Despite abundant evidence to the contrary, society often continues to frame aging in a negative way. Discrimination based on stereotypes and prejudices about age is termed ageism [29]. When ageism is directed at older people, it often involves assumptions that older people are less competent, less attractive, and less vigorous than younger people, rather than at a different developmental stage in the human lifespan. Ageism has a significant negative impact on older people's health and well-being, throughout all areas of life [30]. One example of ageism is when a highly qualified candidate is not hired for a job because of their age [30]. In medicine, ageism manifests when older patients are excluded from clinical trials based on their age or comorbidities but their treatment is guided by the results of those same trials. Research has shown a connection between ageism and negative physical and mental health outcomes [31]. Internalized ageism increases cortisol levels, decreases health-promotion behaviors, and leads to earlier and more severe disease presentations and higher healthcare costs [32]. Addressing ageism is a way society can promote healthy aging for everyone [33].

Health care providers at all levels and in all settings can help address ageism through word choice. The online resource FrameWorks Institute provides guidance on how to use language to shift perspective [30]. Oftentimes, people are not aware of their own prejudices and hold implicit bias toward older adults because of the society they are raised in. For example, movies and the news often portray old people as forgetful, or frail, and these stereotypes can translate to everyday encounters with older adults. These cultural norms are reinforced in medicine because health care professionals are often exposed to the most frail and ill older. However, the small selection of older adults in hospitals is not representative of the larger group of people who are living healthy and functional lives into their 8th, 9th, or even 10th decade of life. Lundebjerg et al. suggest alternative language for common phrases society uses to describe older adults that lead to implicit bias and ageism. For example, instead of using the words "tidal wave, tsunami or epidemic" to describe aging adults in the United States, use the phrase "as Americans live long and healthier lives…". The authors suggest viewing aging as a dynamic process with opportunities for people of all ages instead of labeling aging as a struggle, battle, or fight [34]. If society swaps ageist language for more positive language, it can create a shift to a more positive outlook on growing older.

Anti-Ageism and Medical Education

On an individual level and as health professionals, we can adapt anti-ageism tools to improve the way we address older adults in any work environment and in the community at large. On a societal level, campaigns are being launched to combat ageism. For example, the World Health Organization launched a campaign on ageism in 2016 and dedicates funding to changing the way public health addresses ageism. On an educational level, models such as the PEACE Model (Positive Education about Aging and Contact Experiences) have shown benefit to shift students' attitudes toward older adults. This model was created for many settings including education, employment, health care, and in the home and can be applied to learners at any age. The PEACE model has two parts. The first part focuses on aging education in a positive light including providing positive older role models. The purpose of this first part is to decrease negative associations with older adults. The second part includes individualized cooperative encounters and involves sharing personal information with older adults so that they can be seen as equal status. The purpose of the model is to bridge gaps between older adults and other generations to reduce negative stereotypes and discrimination associated with aging [35]. Another publication directed at healthcare professionals discusses a term, Elderspeak. Elderspeak is a kind of speech used by medical professionals that is characterized by simplifying sentences, more repetitions, a lower speech rate, a louder voice, and a patronizing tone, often the one they use with children and pets. These speech modifications have shown to have a negative effect on the recipient including lower self-esteem [36]. As already mentioned, implicit bias can lead to health care professionals using Elderspeak without being aware of it. Teaching and talking about Elderspeak can increase awareness and hopefully decrease the prevalence of Elderspeak.

In summary, by understanding the physiology of aging, the spectrum of function and ability in aging and the impact of approach to older adults through how we practice medicine, lifestyle medicine, and addressing ageism, we can ultimately provide better care for older adults and make the world a better place for all of us to grow old.

References

1. Collard RM, Boter H, Schoevers RA, Oude RC, Voshaar. Prevalence of frailty in community-dwelling older persons: a systematic review. J Am Geriatr Soc. 2012;60(8):1487–92.
2. Kojima G. Prevalence of frailty in nursing homes: a systematic review and meta-analysis. J Am Med Dir Assoc. 2015;16(11):940–5.
3. Mohler MJ, D'Huyvetter K, Tomasa L, O'Neill L, Fain MJ. Healthy aging rounds: using healthy-aging mentors to teach medical students about physical activity and social support assessment, interviewing, and prescription. J Am Geriatr Soc. 2010;58(12):2407–11.
4. Shue CK, McNeley K, Arnold L. Changing medical students' attitudes about older adults and future older patients. Acad Med. 2005;80(10):6–9.
5. Rowe JW, Kahn RL. Successful aging. Aging. 1998;10(2):142–4.
6. Rudnicka E, Napierała P, Podfigurna A, Męczekalski B, Smolarczyk R, Grymowicz M. The World Health Organization (WHO) approach to healthy ageing. Maturitas. 2020;139:6–11.
7. Aronson L. Healthy aging across the stages of old age. Clin Geriatr Med. 2020;36(4):549–58.
8. National Prevention Council (U.S.). Healthy aging in action: advancing the national prevention strategy. Washington: U.S. Department of Health and Human Services; 2016.
9. Batsis JA, Daniel K, Eckstrom E, Goldlist K, Kusz H, Lane D, Loewenthal J, Coll PP, Friedman SM. Promoting healthy aging during COVID-19. J Am Geriatr Soc. 2021;69(3):572–80.
10. Friedman SM, Mulhausen P, Cleveland ML, Coll PP, Daniel KM, Hayward AD, Shah K, Skudlarska B, White HK. Healthy aging: american geriatrics society white paper executive summary. J Am Geriatr Soc. 2019;67(1):17–20.
11. Muniak JD, Mulhausen P. How do geriatric principles inform healthy aging? Clin Geriatr Med. 2020;36(4):559–67.
12. Rull G, Rosher RB, McCann-Stone N, Robinson SB. A simulated couple aging across the four years of medical school. Teach Learn Med. 2006;18(3):261–6.
13. The Kirkpatrick Evaluation Model: How to Measure Training Effectiveness. 2019. https://www.lucidchart.com/blog/how-to-use-the-kirkpatrick-evaluation-model.
14. Soliman M, Bilszta J. Teaching complementary and alternative medicine in undergraduate medical education: a scoping review. J Int Assoc Med Sci Educ. 2021;12(July):140–9.
15. American College of Lifestyle Medicine. 2021. https://www.lifestylemedicine.org/ACLM/About/What_is_Lifestyle_Medicine_/Lifestyle_Medicine.aspx.
16. American Medical Association. H-425.972 Healthy Lifestyles. 2017. https://policysearch.ama-assn.org/policyfinder/detail/lifestyle%20medicine?uri=%2FAMADoc%2FHOD.xml-0-3746.xml.
17. Rea B, Worthman S, Shetty P, Alexander M, Trilk JL. Medical education transformation: lifestyle medicine in undergraduate and graduate medical education, fellowship, and continuing medical education. Am J Lifestyle Med. 2021;15(5):514–25.
18. Trilk JL, Worthman S, Shetty P, Studer KR, Wilson A, Wetherill M, Whelan L, et al. Undergraduate medical education: lifestyle medicine curriculum implementation standards. Am J Lifestyle Med. 2021;15(5):526–30.
19. Jadczak AD, Tam KL, Solomon Y, Visvanathan R. Medical students' perceptions of the importance of exercise and their perceived competence in prescribing exercise to older people. Australas J Ageing. 2017;36(3):E7–13.
20. Tinetti ME, Naik AD, Dindo L, Costello DM, Esterson J, Geda M, Rosen J, et al. Association of patient priorities–aligned decision-making with patient outcomes and ambulatory health care burden among older adults with multiple chronic conditions. JAMA Intern Med. 2019;179(12):1688–97. https://doi.org/10.1001/jamainternmed.2019.4235.
21. Nathan S, Fiore LL, Saunders S, Vilbrun-Bruno SO, Hinrichs KL, Ruopp MD, Schwartz AW, Moye J. My life, my story: teaching patient centered care competencies for older adults through life story work. September: Gerontology Geriatrics Education; 2019. p. 1–14.

22. Miller RK, Michener J, Yang P, Goldstein K, Groce-Martin J, True G, Johnson J. Effect of a community-based service learning experience in geriatrics on internal medicine residents and community participants. J Am Geriatr Soc. 2017;65(9):130–4.
23. Goreshnik A, Corey MT, Rhodes Kropf J, Schwartz AW. Learning about sites of care for older adults: a jigsaw educational session for medical students. Age Ageing. 2022;51(3):afac032. https://doi.org/10.1093/ageing/afac032. PMID: 35231089; PMCID: PMC9383527.
24. Medina-Walpole A, Pacala JT, Potter JF. GRS. New York: American Geriatrics Society; 2016.
25. Sleimen-Malkoun R, Temprado J-J, Lee Hong S. Aging induced loss of complexity and dedifferentiation: consequences for coordination dynamics within and between brain, muscular and behavioral levels. Front Aging Neurosci. 2014;6(June):140.
26. Meador JA. Cerumen impaction in the elderly. J Gerontol Nurs. 1995;21(12):43–5.
27. Ouchi K, Jambaulikar GD, Hohmann S, George NR, Aaronson EL, Sudore R, Schonberg MA, Tulsky JA, Schuur JD, Pallin DJ. Prognosis after emergency department intubation to inform shared decision-making. J Am Geriatr Soc. 2018;66(7):1377–81.
28. Sarafrazi N, Wambogo EA, Shepherd JA. Osteoporosis or low bone mass in older adults: United States, 2017-2018. NCHS Data Brief. 2021;405:1–8.
29. Officer A, de la Fuente-Núñez V. A global campaign to combat ageism. Bull World Health Organ. 2018;96(4):295–6.
30. Sweetland J, Volmert A, O'Neil M. Finding the frame: an empirical approach to reframing aging and ageism. Washington: FrameWorks Institute; 2017.
31. Solway E. Policy series: the impact of ageism on health and efforts to address it through reframing aging. Innov Aging. 2020;4:722. https://doi.org/10.1093/geroni/igaa057.2556.
32. Levy BR, Moffat S, Resnick SM, Slade MD, Ferrucci L. Buffer against cumulative stress. GeroPsych. 2016;29:141–6. https://doi.org/10.1024/1662-9647/a000149.
33. Inouye SK. Creating an anti-ageist healthcare system to improve care for our current and future selves. Nat Aging. 2021;1(2):150–2.
34. Lundebjerg NE, Trucil DE, Hammond EC, Applegate WB. When it comes to older adults, language matters: Journal of the American Geriatrics Society Adopts Modified American Medical Association Style. J Am Geriatr Soc. 2017;65(7):1386–8.
35. Levy SR. Toward reducing ageism: PEACE (positive education about aging and contact experiences) model. The Gerontologist. 2016;58(2):226–32. https://doi.org/10.1093/geront/gnw116.
36. Schroyen S, Adam S, Marquet M, Jerusalem G, Thiel S, Giraudet A-L, Missotten P. Communication of healthcare professionals: is there ageism? Eur J Cancer Care. 2018;27(1):12780. https://doi.org/10.1111/ecc.12780.

Chapter 4
Teaching Geriatrics to Clinical Medical Students: Introducing Complexity and Subtlety and Teaching Clinical Reasoning

Amit A. Shah and Helene Labonte

A geriatrician is, "by definition, an expert in subtlety and complexity" [1]. How best to teach a medical student to develop expertise in handling the complexity and recognize the subtle presentations of illness we often see in older patients? Early trainees can quickly become overwhelmed by the complexity of many older patients, especially when lacking a framework for dealing with this complexity. These often overwhelming early clinical experiences can result in negative attitudes about caring for older patients [2, 3]. Students become intimidated by long problem lists and lengthy medication lists and can become frustrated when their patient does not "read the textbook" and presents with disease presentations that do not match the illness scripts learned in their preclinical courses.

In this chapter, we discuss three ways to teach medical students about complexity and break open the "black box" of the geriatrician's clinical reasoning. One way is to broaden the illness scripts that students learn by explicitly teaching different illness scripts applicable to older patients. Another is to teach about multicomplexity by modifying plans of care based on integrative approaches, including a focus on goals of care and functional status. The final method is to teach about the differences and nuances in clinical reasoning with older patients and how this may result in diagnostic errors.

Geriatricize the Students' Illness Scripts

An important part of developing clinical expertise is assembling illness scripts which are a type of "mental cue card" used to represent individual diseases [4, 5]. This non-analytic, pattern-recognition approach is how practicing physicians think most often, drawing from a large number of well-developed illness scripts from

A. A. Shah (✉) · H. Labonte
Mayo Clinic, Scottsdale, AZ, USA
e-mail: Shah.Amit@mayo.edu; Labonte.Helene@mayo.edu

A. W. Schwartz (ed.), *Medical Education in Geriatrics*,
https://doi.org/10.1007/978-3-031-32499-4_4

their experiences to develop a differential diagnosis [6]. Illness scripts combine what is learned in basic sciences such as epidemiology and pathophysiology with the presenting symptoms and physical exam findings, which then lead to diagnosis and treatment plans. In geriatric medicine, we tend to encounter "atypical" presentations, which is a way of saying that the typical illness scripts often fall short, especially when superimposed with multiple chronic illnesses. This is due to the variability of changes that occur during aging from the accumulation of chronic diseases, physical disabilities, and physiologic deterioration that is not linear with chronological age and results in heterogeneity [7]. Therefore, the heterogeneity of aging makes illness scripts much less straightforward. One approach is to teach different "geriatricized" illness scripts that incorporate geriatric patients and these "atypical" presentations. For example, a student may have an illness script around urinary tract infections which includes dysuria and a positive urinalysis. The educator can explicitly teach other illness scripts, for example, that a "positive urinalysis" may be difficult to interpret due to increased incidence of pyuria and bacteriuria in older patients who do not have an infection [8]. Using compare/contrast to the "typical" illness script the student would have learned early in their training can be valuable, especially when connected to epidemiological or pathophysiological principles of aging. For example, for a patient with possible pyelonephritis, the educator would teach that for a healthy younger patient, this would more likely present with dysuria, fever, and flank pain (an illness script the early clinical student would likely have learned), but that the frail older patient is much more likely to present without fever or flank pain (due to immunosenescence and other factors) and may instead present with delirium or more severe illness such as urosepsis.

Other geroscience principles, such as sarcopenia and frailty, aging-related inflammation, cellular senescence, and homeostenosis/loss of physiological reserves can be worked into illness scripts that teach how these aging-associated changes impact each organ system to result in a different set of illness scripts for the older patient. For example, one could teach how reduced motility of the large bowel due to reduction of myenteric plexus cells and other factors results in a higher incidence of constipation and increased susceptibility to constipation from medications [9]. This teaching can then be used to modify and add to the student's illness scripts of abdominal pain. Another example is cellular senescence and age-related loss of nephrons in the kidneys. The teacher can explain that due to these changes, the older patient may have a reduction in functional glomeruli by up to 50% by age 75 and explain how this affects the ability to maximally concentrate urine, resulting in a higher likelihood of dehydration when under stress. This same pathophysiology can also be used to explain why medication doses of renally cleared medications must be adjusted. The learner can use this information to enhance their treatment scripts.

Teach About Multicomplexity and Approaches to Address Multicomplexity

Occam's Razor: "Pluralitas non est ponenda sine necessitate" (Plurality ought never be posited without necessity)—*attributed to fourteenth century logician William of Ockham*

versus

Hickam's Dictum: "Patients can have as many diseases as they damn well please."—*Dr. John Hickam, Chair of Medicine, Indiana University 1958–1970*

In addition to teaching students about broadening and adding nuance to their illness scripts, the geriatric medicine educator must teach students about how to manage patients with multiple concurrent illnesses. A geriatric syndrome generally refers to a clinical presentation that is the accumulation of multiple insults or illnesses such as is common with the geriatric syndrome of delirium. This is in contrast to a medical syndrome in which multiple symptoms are the result of a single illness such as Cushing's syndrome [10]. Early on, students are taught to search for a unifying diagnosis with the principle that a singular unifying diagnosis is more likely to be correct than separate explanations of concurrent illnesses (*Occam's Razor* vs *Hickam's Dictum* above) [11]. The classic Oslerian approach to clinical reasoning is useful at times but it often falls short, especially in older patients [12].

The geriatric medicine educator must help students to think about multiple concurrent illnesses and the impact of these illnesses on each other, as this is the norm in geriatric medicine. According to the National Institute on Aging, approximately 85% of Medicare beneficiaries have at least one chronic illness, 68% have two or more, and 36% have 4 or more, with prevalence increasing for lower economic status adults [13]. By 2030, twenty percent of the US population will be over age 65 and those of age 80 will reach 20 million, so regardless of specialty choice, physicians must possess the skills to evaluate and manage this older demographic with multiple concurrent chronic illnesses. Goals of care in younger populations may focus more on treatment or cure of episodic illness, while the focus of geriatrics is often driven toward the maintenance of independence and quality of life. For learners, this requires a shift of their learning process from solely relying on illness scripts to instead focusing on goals of care to help individualize care plans.

The geriatric medicine educator must also be able to teach trainees about clinical reasoning in the face of uncertainty. Medical uncertainty, or not knowing the best way to approach an illness or complaint, will occur in our learners just as it occurs with seasoned physicians. Uncertainty is best addressed using a systematic process and open communication with our patients in order to lead us to patient-centered recommendations that reflect the older patients' goals of care [14, 15]. Although diagnostic and therapeutic decision-making uncertainty is present in all parts of medicine, it can be particularly prevalent in geriatric medicine due to various clinical reasoning challenges discussed below including multicomplexity and the historical underrepresentation of older patients with multiple comorbidities in clinical trials. The geriatric medicine educator can role model that this uncertainty is not a deficit of the trainee or their knowledge base or efforts to provide good care but is an inherent (and enjoyable!) part of caring for complex older patients [14].

The American Geriatrics Society has published the Minimum Competencies in Geriatrics for Medical Students divided into the Geriatrics 5Ms (Mind, Mobility, Medications, Multicomplexity, and Matters Most) (see Chap. 1) [16]. Multicomplexity in Geriatrics incorporates medical illnesses and aging physiology with the domains of cognition, functional status, mental health, social situation, and availability of resources. The Geriatric Medicine educator can help teach the student not to become overwhelmed by this complexity by teaching core principles of geriatric assessment, interprofessional approaches to care, and how to incorporate goals of care into care plans. One of the ways this can be taught is by using some geriatrics clinical reasoning pearls and aphorisms that have been passed down by generations of geriatricians [17] and can be a helpful and memorable way to teach some of these principles [18] as described in Table 4.1 [18].

Table 4.1 Aphorisms to help teach geriatric clinic reasoning

Geriatric principle/5M	Teaching aphorism	What it means/example
Mind: patterns of cognitive decline	The ability to have a pleasant conversation or remember old memories does not mean the patient does not have dementia: you must probe cognition with screening tools	Trainees may miss the diagnosis of early-stage dementia as social graces and crystalized memories remain intact in early stages of dementia. The use of validated screening tools to test cognition may be required to uncover the diagnosis
Mobility: homeostenosis and maintenance of functional status	It takes a lot of energy to tread water (…but you have to keep doing it or you sink!)	Maintenance of function can require significant effort in older patients without visible progress, but helps prevent decline, similar to a person treading water in the pool. This statement can be used to encourage patients who are frustrated that their exercise routine is not resulting in increased strength, as the prevention of decline is not visible
Mobility: importance of functional status and mobility assessment	Watch 'em walk!	Much can be gained from watching a patient walk, including gait speed, balance, frailty status, and cardiopulmonary function
Medications: vigilance about medication side effects/polypharmacy	You can cure many "diseases" by stopping medicines rather than starting them	Expect variability in response to medications. Any new symptoms in an older person should be considered a medication side effect until proven otherwise
Medications: medication dosing in older patients	Start low and go slow… (but get there!)	Age-related changes in drug metabolism can lead to altered or unexpected medication effects. Start with a low dose and observe for side effects as titrating to the desired dose but also don't underdose medications (such as anticoagulants) just because someone is older [19]

Table 4.1 (continued)

Geriatric principle/5M	Teaching aphorism	What it means/example
Multicomplexity: heterogeneity of aging	If you've seen one 80 year-old patient, you've seen one 80-year old patient!	A fit 80-year-old and a frail 80-year-old have very different risk profiles. Consider the 5Ms, assess frailty status, complete assessments such as gait speed, grip strength, and mobility assessments and use these to guide care
Multicomplexity: Limits of simple illness scripts	The "atypical" presentation of illness is typical in older patients	Age-related physiologic changes combined with underlying chronic illnesses may result in symptoms or presentations that are not "textbook" and may result in missed diagnosis. For example, missing a myocardial infarction in an older patient with dyspnea rather than chest pain as the presenting symptom
Multicomplexity: geriatric syndromes have multifactorial causes	A single presenting symptom may have many contributing etiologies	Geriatric syndromes rarely have just one cause, for example, falls, which typically are multifactorial
Multicomplexity: Geriatric syndromes often require multifactorial solutions	Multifactorial syndromes need multifactorial solutions	Prevention or treatment of geriatric syndromes such as falls or delirium which typically have multiple contributing causes will often require a multi-pronged approach to treat or reduce risk. For example, multifactorial interventions for fall prevention or delirium risk reduction for hospitalized patients
Multicomplexity: interprofessional care	It takes a village	Geriatric medicine emphasizes the importance of collaborative interdisciplinary teams to optimize health outcomes, such as a physician, physical therapist, optometrist, and social worker working together to help a patient who has vision impairment and severe arthritis who is falling to get the appropriate assessment, therapy, equipment, and glasses to reduce falls
Multicomplexity: hazards of hospitalization	You can win the battle but lose the war	Albeit necessary at times, hospitals can be dangerous places for the older adult. Iatrogenic events, adverse drug events, delirium, malnutrition, and functional decline are common outcomes for older adults in the hospital [20] You can fix the acute problem ("win the battle") but without attention to functional decline and rehabilitation both during and after the hospitalization, the overall "war" can be lost through complications and functional decline in spite of the acute issue being addressed
Matters most: goals of care	You are not treating a disease but a *person* with diseases. Find out what is important to the patient	Avoid the temptation to fixate on the problem list/medical conditions without considering the patient's preferences and goals

(continued)

Table 4.1 (continued)

Geriatric principle/5M	Teaching aphorism	What it means/example
Matters most: addressing loneliness, existential distress, and purpose	Having a reason to get up each morning is what keeps us going! Ask your patient about what gives them meaning and purpose in life and address spiritual needs	Purpose in life is associated with positive health outcomes. Part of good geriatrics care is helping patients or referring patients for help in maintaining or finding purpose to reduce loneliness, isolation, and loss of will to live [21]
Matters most: modification of preventative care with advanced age and frailty	Screen the strong and will the weak	Consider life expectancy, frailty status, goals of care and risks-vs-benefits of routine screening tests in a shared decision-making process with older patients. As life expectancy declines and frailty becomes more severe, a shift from screening for cancer to discussions about advance care planning/living wills and other interventions is more likely to help with shorter time frames [22]
Matters most: comfort with discussing advance care planning	"Death" and "dying" are not 4-letter words	It's okay to talk about death and assist with decision-making related to dying. Older patients appreciate the opportunity to make their wishes known

Teaching Explicitly About Multicomplexity

Another approach to teaching complexity is the four functional domain approach and the Geriatrics 5Ms can be applied in each of these domains. In this method, ask your learners to approach every geriatric patient from the perspective of four functional domains: physical functioning, social functioning, psychological functioning, and cognitive functioning (Fig. 4.1). Physical functioning includes questions such as "how many falls have you had in the last 12-months" and assessments of mobility, such as the "get-up and go" test. This can be followed by a question about the patient's current physical activity level and inquiry into the ability to perform activities of daily living (ADLs) and instrumental activities of daily living (IADLs). The geriatric medicine teacher should provide an example of questions that can assist the learner in collecting the most meaningful data. For instance, if the learner asks an older patient if they can cook, they may reply that they are an excellent cook. Whereas if the learner asks "who cooks your meals for you?" they may respond that a family member brings over meals for them to reheat during the week and this may be a clue that the family is intervening to ensure proper nutrition. Similarly, if a learner asks a patient if they manage their own finances, they may receive an affirmative response; however, if the question was changed to "who manages your finances?" additional insights may be gained if the patient responds that their son or daughter put all of their bills on auto payment so they didn't need to worry about that any longer. Impairment in these areas may correlate with the ability to live

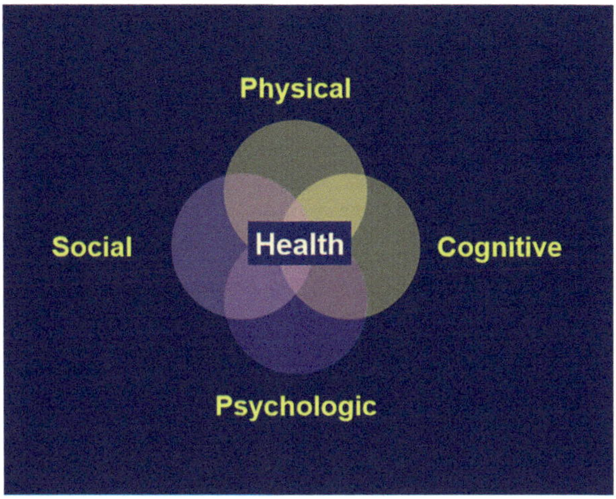

Fig. 4.1 Four-domain thinking approach (figure created by author (HL))

independently, risk of further functional loss, and increased mortality [23]. Assessment of social functioning can be obtained by asking the patient what they do for enjoyment and who they socialize with. Psychological functioning can be obtained by using standardized objective assessment forms, such as the PHQ-9, Geriatric Depression Scale (GDS), or GAD-7. Responses to these questions may reveal additional information about sources of psychological distress or worry and goals of care. Cognitive functioning should also be evaluated utilizing a standardized mental status assessment form (MMSE) which can be tracked over time and will further identify areas where additional resources may be needed. Examples of these would be the Folstein MMSE, Kokmen MMSE, MoCA Cognitive Assessment, or Mini-Cog. Once learners have assembled information in these four domains, it becomes less daunting to see the big picture and will assist them in assembling a goal-directed treatment plan. It can also be an ideal time to introduce students to interprofessional care teams, and all that other team members bring to help address the care of complex geriatric patients. The Geriatrics 5Ms can be applied to these four domains as we describe in an example patient in Table 4.2.

The 85-year-old patient has congestive heart failure and worsening cognitive impairment and mild to moderate dementia. She is being seen in the clinic for a complaint of weakness, frequent falls, and inability to drive any longer.

A final strategy a geriatric medicine teacher can use is to teach about clinical reasoning and how this differs with the complex older patient [25]. It can be instructive to explicitly explain to trainees through a clinical case as additional data is presented [26]. There are many models of clinical reasoning. One useful approach divides clinical reasoning into various aspects, broken down into those affecting diagnosis and those affecting treatment [27, 28]. These areas are listed in Table 4.3, along with some examples that the geriatric medicine teacher can use to teach how clinical reasoning is modified for older adults. These approaches can be incorporated into rounds and case presentations by the teacher, making clear to the learner how the faculty came to the diagnosis or treatment decision for the older patient.

Table 4.2 Example of the Geriatrics 5Ms applied to each of the 4 domains of health for an 85-year-old patient

	Physical functioning	Social functioning	Psychological functioning	Cognitive functioning
Mind	Inquire about the impact of cognition and memory on the patient's ability to remember self-care tasks, such as daily weights and remembering to take medications	Ask about the impact of cognitive changes on social networks and inquire if the patient is avoiding social situations due to cognitive changes	Use a standardized depression screening tool, such as the PHQ-9 Depression Scale Evaluate for mental distress impacting quality of life Refer or treat as appropriate	Use a standardized objective measurement tool of cognition Provide resources for patients with early dementia and caregiving resources
Mobility	Perform a mobility assessment and refer the patient to physical therapy Identify performance deficiencies in ADLs and IADLs and recommend solutions and resources to assist with ADL/IADL deficits that you find	Consider the impact of social isolation as the patient has stopped leaving home due to falls and the inability to drive	Consider the impact on mood on the ability of the patient to do the things she enjoyed	Consider the impact of mobility and driving limitations on the ability to attend things such as dementia support group meetings
Medications	Review medications for optimal care of the patient's congestive heart failure Review medications for side effects, such as orthostasis causing falls	Review timing and dosing of medications, such as diuretics, which may impact the patient's ability to attend social events due to frequent urination	Review medications for side effects on mood, cognition, and falls Treat mood symptoms with medications with favorable side effect profiles when indicated	Review medications for anticholinergic activity, sedation, or other adverse impacts on cognition

Table 4.2 (continued)

	Physical functioning	Social functioning	Psychological functioning	Cognitive functioning
Multicomplexity	Consider impact of aging-related physiological changes, the patient's multiple comorbidities, frailty status, and prognosis to make treatment changes and recommendations to optimize physical functioning, such as checking orthostatics, discovering she has orthostasis and prescribing compression stockings and adjusting her diuretic dose to reduce the frequency of falls	Address social determinants of health that impact the care plans for each of her conditions and individualize recommendations, such as working with a social worker to help with transportation needs to reduce social isolation	Recognize that depression may present atypically in this patient and use instruments with better sensitivity and specificity for older patients who have dementia, such as the Cornell Scale for Depression in Dementia [24]	Assess other factors that may be impacting cognition and assessment of cognition, such as hearing or vision impairment Recognize that the patient is at increased risk for delirium if hospitalized due to dementia diagnosis
Matters most	Address symptoms that are bothering the patient, such as lightheadedness or fatigue, instead of insisting patient take her beta-blocker for mortality reduction	Identify social isolation. Refer to community resources as indicated. Find out if patient has a healthcare proxy, has advance directives Screen for elder abuse or self-neglect	Address spiritual and psychological needs arising from patient's worsening health status Ask patient what matters most to her and work with care team to optimize these priorities	Account for her diagnosis of dementia when communicating with patient and patient's caregiver in ways that are respectful, culturally sensitive, and do not marginalize her or make assumptions that she cannot provide her preferences

Table 4.3 Aspects of clinical reasoning and application to Geriatrics

Concepts and aspects of clinical reasoning [27, 28]	Definition of concept	Application and modifications for Geriatrics clinical reasoning
Diagnosis		
Hypothesis generation	Clinicians make initial hypotheses based on the patient's demographic data, initial appearance, etc.	"Atypical" presentations of illness. e.g., fever may not be present in an older patient with an infection due to immunosenescence, and so infection should not be removed from the hypothesis
Context formulation	The initial hypothesis provides the constraints and framing for the next steps of hypothesis refinement	Importance of understanding the setting from which the patient came; e.g., calling the nursing home for a corollary informant to avoid being prematurely constrained in the hypothesis generation stage
Hypothesis refinement	Also known as "case building" when new data and information obtained is used to help rule in or rule out a diagnosis	A consideration that multiple issues may be going on simultaneously or the patient may have a geriatric syndrome as the presentation of illness which could lead to errors in hypothesis refinement
Test interpretation	Interpretation of data is used for hypothesis refinement	Test interpretation is more challenging with older patients, as there may be different "normal" ranges and findings, e.g., lower testosterone level, pyuria, or bacteriuria on urinalysis, a moderately elevated sedimentation rate, or lower titer positive ANA test all of which may be normal but lead to erroneous diagnoses
Bayesian reasoning	The application of probability theory to inductive reasoning, with updating the probability of a hypothesis as more data comes in	Thinking about how a low pretest probability affects the interpretation of test results, for example, a positive autoimmune test for lupus in an older patient without any symptoms of lupus
Probabilistic, physiologic, and causal reasoning	Causal reasoning is used to build a physiologic model and checks the patient's findings and results for coherence with this model	Consideration of precipitating and predisposing factors and comorbidities and the impact on the presentation of illness and diagnosis
Assessing for adequacy, coherence, and parsimony	Assessing the data gathered from the patient for when sufficient data is present to make a working diagnosis and stop gathering additional data or doing further testing	See "*Hickam's Dictum*" vs. "*Occam's Razor*" in the text above. Older patients have different illness scripts and may also have multiple diagnoses simultaneously, which must be considered when deciding no more data needs to be collected. For example, not stopping the assessment and examination of a nursing home patient who presents to the emergency room with delirium when the urinalysis comes back positive

(continued)

Table 4.3 (continued)

Concepts and aspects of clinical reasoning [27, 28]	Definition of concept	Application and modifications for Geriatrics clinical reasoning
Working (final) diagnosis	The diagnosis is decided upon once the assessment for adequacy, coherence, and parsimony is completed	In geriatric medicine, there must be consideration of multiple diagnoses, e.g. a hospitalized patient with pneumonia and whose worsening shortness of breath is attributed to pneumonia rather than an acute myocardial infarction occurring with concomitant pneumonia
Cognitive errors	Errors which occur due to subconscious biases, limitations of heuristics used in clinical reasoning, or other cognitive factors	Many different types apply to the older patient. A few examples: • Premature closure (e.g. stopping work-up for a delirious patient when the urinalysis is "positive") • Framing bias/diagnosis momentum (e.g. relying on the ER diagnosis for an admitted patient rather than taking a comprehensive H&P or using a patient's past medical history to attribute to an existing problem to rather than a new illness)
Treatment		
Treatment under conditions of uncertainty	What to do when there is not strong evidence of the next best step in the literature	In past years, older patients were often left out of clinical trials, especially those over age 85, therefore we often make decisions based on "expert opinion" or in the absence of a robust evidence-base in geriatric medicine
Tradeoffs between risks and benefits of tests and treatments	Clinical reasoning of treatment involves nuanced discussions of pros and cons	Prostate cancer screening in patients over age 70 results in overdiagnosis and overtreatment; consideration of life expectancy for screening tests such as colonoscopy and ability to communicate these to patients
Test-treatment thresholds	The point at which the decision to treat (or not treat) has been reached, resulting in no further testing or data is needed	Checking lipids on a patient over age 90 for primary prevention. Goals of care impact treatment thresholds and the necessity to test, for example, ordering a mammogram on a 90-year-old patient who does not want a breast biopsy or further investigation if positive
Decisional close-calls and "toss-ups"	Acknowledgment at times in clinical reasoning, multiple options may have equivalent risks and benefits	Whether or not to continue anticoagulation on a patient at high risk for stroke but also with multiple severe falls
Therapeutic trial as a diagnostic test	In the setting of uncertainty about the outcome, providing a time-limited trial to see if a particular treatment will be effective	Trialing an SSRI medication to help ease agitation in a patient with severe dementia who is unable to express their emotions

(continued)

Table 4.3 (continued)

Concepts and aspects of clinical reasoning [27, 28]	Definition of concept	Application and modifications for Geriatrics clinical reasoning
Watchful waiting versus immediate action	At times, the diagnosis and treatment plans can only be refined when time elapses	Not treating a biopsy-proven low-grade cancer in a patient with a limited life expectancy

Faculty may also use tests of clinical reasoning, such as the script concordance test, to test clinical reasoning [29, 30].

In conclusion, the complexities of caring for older adults may overwhelm some learners as each patient presents unique challenges and opportunities. However, it is critical that medical students have the tools to provide appropriate care to this segment of the population. We have outlined several approaches to assist educators in teaching learners how to think like a geriatrician. Broadening and adding nuance to typical illness scripts can assist learners in expanding their differential diagnosis. Helping trainees make clinical decisions in the setting of uncertainty avoids excess ordering of tests or therapeutic decision paralysis. Deconstructing multiple issues into smaller domains or components while incorporating goals of care aids in enhanced clinical reasoning. Modifying concepts of clinical reasoning pertinent to geriatric patients and presentations allows expansion of learning concepts and decreases cognitive errors. These approaches take time and deliberate practice and we should ensure learners have ample time to complete the process, interpret their findings, and analyze their recommendations. It is also important that we take the time and effort to verbalize our clinical reasoning process when working with learners. Indeed, this enhanced and nuanced approach to clinical reasoning may be the most important gift the Geriatric Medicine educator has to offer our trainees and impact of the care of the older patients they will care for and make them all masters of "subtlety and complexity" [1].

References

1. Hazzard WR. I am a geriatrician. J Am Geriatr Soc. 2004;52(1):161.
2. van Zuilen MH, Rubert MP, Silverman M, Lewis J. Medical students' positive and negative misconceptions about the elderly. Gerontol Geriatr Educ. 2001;21(3):31–40.
3. Meiboom AA, de Vries H, Hertogh CM, Scheele F. Why medical students do not choose a career in geriatrics: a systematic review. BMC Med Educ. 2015;15:101.
4. Gavinski K, Covin YN, Longo PJ. Learning how to build illness scripts. Acad Med. 2019;94(2):293.
5. Custers EJ. Thirty years of illness scripts: theoretical origins and practical applications. Med Teach. 2015;37(5):457–62.

6. Schmidt HG, Rikers RM. How expertise develops in medicine: knowledge encapsulation and illness script formation. Med Educ. 2007;41(12):1133–9.
7. Nguyen QD, Moodie EM, Forget MF, Desmarais P, Keezer MR, Wolfson C. Health heterogeneity in older adults: exploration in the canadian longitudinal study on aging. J Am Geriatr Soc. 2021;69(3):678–87.
8. Nicolle LE, Gupta K, Bradley SF, Colgan R, DeMuri GP, Drekonja D, et al. Clinical practice guideline for the management of asymptomatic bacteriuria: 2019 update by the Infectious Diseases Society of America. Clin Infect Dis. 2019;68(10):1611–5.
9. Gallegos-Orozco JF, Foxx-Orenstein AE, Sterler SM, Stoa JM. Chronic constipation in the elderly. Am J Gastroenterol. 2012;107(1):18–25; quiz 6.
10. Inouye SK, Studenski S, Tinetti ME, Kuchel GA. Geriatric syndromes: clinical, research, and policy implications of a core geriatric concept. J Am Geriatr Soc. 2007;55(5):780–91.
11. Hilliard AA, Weinberger SE, Tierney LM Jr, Midthun DE, Saint S. Clinical problem-solving. Occam's razor versus Saint's triad. N Engl J Med. 2004;350(6):599–603.
12. Mani N, Slevin N, Hudson A. What three wise men have to say about diagnosis. Br Med J. 2011;343:7769.
13. Lochner KA, Cox CS. Prevalence of multiple chronic conditions among Medicare beneficiaries, United States, 2010. Prev Chronic Dis. 2013;10:E61.
14. van Iersel MB, Brantjes E, de Visser M, Looman N, Bazelmans E, van Asselt D. Tolerance of clinical uncertainty by geriatric residents: a qualitative study. Eur Geriatr Med. 2019;10(3):517–22.
15. Gheihman G, Johnson M, Simpkin AL. Twelve tips for thriving in the face of clinical uncertainty. Med Teach. 2020;42(5):493–9.
16. Minimum Geriatric Competencies for Medical Students. Available https://adgap.americangeriatrics.org/education-training/competencies/geriatrics-competencies-medical-students.
17. Savitz HA. Geriatric axioms, aphorisms and proverbs. J Am Geriatr Soc. 1968;16(7):752–9.
18. Shah A. Identifying the unique needs of the aging population. In: Chun A, editor. Geriatric practice: a competency based approach to caring for older adults. Cham: Springer; 2020. p. 13–9.
19. American Geriatrics Society. American Geriatrics Society 2019 updated AGS Beers Criteria® for potentially inappropriate medication use in older adults. J Am Geriatr Soc. 2019;67(4):674–94.
20. Fernandez HM, Callahan KE, Likourezos A, Leipzig RM. House staff member awareness of older inpatients' risks for hazards of hospitalization. Arch Intern Med. 2008;168(4):390–6.
21. Musich S, Wang SS, Kraemer S, Hawkins K, Wicker E. Purpose in life and positive health outcomes among older adults. Popul Health Manag. 2018;21(2):139–47.
22. Tazkarji B, Lam R, Lee S, Meiyappan S. Approach to preventive care in the elderly. Can Fam Physician. 2016;62(9):717–21.
23. Covinsky KE, Palmer RM, Counsell SR, Pine ZM, Walter LC, Chren MM. Functional status before hospitalization in acutely ill older adults: validity and clinical importance of retrospective reports. J Am Geriatr Soc. 2000;48(2):164–9.
24. Brown EL, Raue P, Halpert KD, Adams S, Titler MG. Detection of depression in older adults with dementia. J Gerontol Nurs. 2009;35(2):11–5.
25. Shah A, Brown C, Javedan H. Teaching students to think geriatrically. 2011. Available https://pogoe.org/sites/default/files/Teaching%20Students%20to%20Think%20Geriatrically%20(handout%201).pdf.
26. Loewenthal J, Javedan H, Schwartz AW. Overcoming inertia: an exercise in clinical reasoning. J Gen Intern Med. 2020;35(9):2771–5.
27. Kassirer JP, Wong JB, Kopelman RI. Learning clinical reasoning. 2nd ed. Baltimore: Lippincott Williams & Wilkins Health; 2010. p. 329.
28. Kassirer JP. Teaching clinical reasoning: case-based and coached. Acad Med. 2010;85(7):1118–24.

29. Piovezan RD, Custódio O, Cendoroglo MS, Batista NA, Lubarsky S, Charlin B. Assessment of undergraduate clinical reasoning in geriatric medicine: application of a script concordance test. J Am Geriatr Soc. 2012;60(10):1946–50.
30. Ruiz JG, Tunuguntla R, Charlin B, Ouslander JG, Symes SN, Gagnon R, et al. The script concordance test as a measure of clinical reasoning skills in geriatric urinary incontinence. J Am Geriatr Soc. 2010;58(11):2178–84.

Chapter 5
Teaching Residents: Applying Clinical Frameworks to Older Adults

Steven R. Barczi and Elizabeth N. Chapman

Introduction

People aged 65 years old and older account for the largest proportion of acute and ambulatory medical care delivered in the USA of any age group, and this population continues to increase [1, 2]. Despite this growth, the number of residents who go on to pursue training in geriatric medicine has declined in recent decades [3]. Most older adults receive care from physicians who have not completed a geriatric medicine fellowship, making basic competence in caring for older adults critical, regardless of a resident physician's ultimate specialty or practice location.

Residency Education Requirements in Geriatrics

For many physicians, residency is the final opportunity for formal training in geriatric medicine before entering into independent practice. Recognizing this, the Accreditation Council for Graduate Medical Education (ACGME) has set requirements for exposure to geriatrics in the Common Program Requirements for Psychiatry, Physical Medicine and Rehabilitation, and Family Medicine, and Internal Medicine residency programs (Table 5.1). Internal Medicine programs must have a subspecialty education coordinator in geriatric medicine and provide

S. R. Barczi (✉) · E. N. Chapman
Madison VA Geriatric Research, Education, and Clinical Center, William S. Middleton Memorial Veterans Hospital, University of Wisconsin-Madison School of Medicine and Public Health, Madison, WI, USA
e-mail: Steven.barczi@va.gov; enchapman@medicine.wisc.edu

A. W. Schwartz (ed.), *Medical Education in Geriatrics*,
https://doi.org/10.1007/978-3-031-32499-4_5

Table 5.1 Summary of ACGME geriatrics requirements, published competencies, available toolkits, and fellowship training opportunities. [Compiled from Accreditation Council for Graduate Medical Education, Hogan et al. 2010; Association of Directors of Geriatrics Academic Programs, Lieff et al. 2005; American Geriatrics Society]

Discipline	Rotation requirements	Published competencies	Available toolkit [4–11]	Geriatrics fellowship
Anesthesiology	None	None	The Geriatrics for Specialty Residents Toolkit: Anesthesiology. https://geriatricscareonline.org	No
Emergency medicine	None	Hogan T et al. Academic Emergency Medicine 2010 [12]	The Geriatrics for Specialty Residents Toolkit: Emergency Medicine. https://geriatricscareonline.org	Yes
Family medicine	10% primary care site encounters with age 60+ and 125 visits with older adults or 100 h of Geriatrics [13]	*Minimum Geriatric Competencies for IM-FM Residents*. https://adgap.americangeriatrics.org [14]	None	Yes
General surgery	None	None	The Geriatrics for Specialty Residents Toolkit: General Surgery. https://geriatricscareonline.org	No
Gynecology-urology	None	None	The Geriatrics for Specialty Residents Toolkit: Gynecology-Urology. https://geriatricscareonline.org	No
Internal medicine	Clinical experiences in geriatric medicine required as part of foundational experiences in Internal Medicine [15]	*Minimum Geriatric Competencies for IM-FM Residents*. https://adgap.americangeriatrics.org [14]	American Geriatrics Society Resident Competencies for IM and FM residency- 2023.	Yes
Ophthalmology	None	None	The Geriatrics for Specialty Residents Toolkit: Ophthalmology. https://geriatricscareonline.org	No
Orthopedic surgery	None	None	The Geriatrics for Specialty Residents Toolkit: Orthopedic Surgery. https://geriatricscareonline.org	No

Discipline	Rotation requirements	Published competencies	Available toolkit [4–11]	Geriatrics fellowship
Otolaryngology	None	None	The Geriatrics for Specialty Residents Toolkit: Otolaryngology. https://geriatricscareonline.org	No
Physical medicine and rehabilitation	Competence in geriatric rehabilitation, including those with physical and/or cognitive impairments [16]	None	The Geriatrics for Specialty Residents Toolkit: Physical Medicine and Rehabilitation. https://geriatricscareonline.org	No
Psychiatry	One month of Geriatric Psychiatry [17]	Geriatric Core Competencies. https://www.aagponline.org [18]	None	Yes

clinical exposure to the specialty [15]. In family medicine, 10% of the required patient encounters in their primary care site must include adults aged 60 years and older. Additionally, residents must either participate in 125 patient encounters with older adults or spend 100 h devoted specifically to the care of the older adult during the program [13]. Psychiatry residency programs similarly must include a month of training in geriatric psychiatry. Within this month, training must include diagnosis and management of mental disorders in older adults with multiple comorbid conditions, diagnosis and management of neurodegenerative disorders, basic neuropsychological testing, and management of drug interactions [17]. Finally, residents in physical medicine and rehabilitation must demonstrate competence in geriatric rehabilitation, including the evaluation and management of patients with physical and/or cognitive impairments, disabilities, and functional limitations [16].

Tools for Teaching Geriatrics to Residents

Within these general mandates for geriatrics exposure, programs have significant latitude regarding how they provide this instruction (Table 5.1). To help standardize the expectations for resident trainees in Internal and Family Medicine and Psychiatry, the Association of Directors for Geriatrics Academic Programs (ADGAP) and the American Association for Geriatric Psychiatry (AAGP) have developed lists of key competencies in geriatrics [19, 20]. For internal medicine and family medicine trainees, critical competencies include evaluating and treating patients for common geriatric syndromes, avoidance of iatrogenic harms, working in an interprofessional team, facilitating safe hospital discharges, and assisting in advance care planning [19, 21]. Psychiatry resident competencies include development of communication skills to account for cognitive and sensory impairment, recognition and treatment of geriatric syndromes pertinent to psychiatry, appropriate prescribing in the context of medical complexity, and working with interdisciplinary teams [18].

Even with well-defined geriatrics competencies available to training programs, residents may struggle to incorporate these principles into daily patient care [21]. Leading educators from AGS and ADGAP have therefore developed a flexible curriculum for trainees in internal medicine and family medicine that can help programs to integrate geriatric medicine effectively into residency training [14]. This curriculum organizes its content using the Geriatrics 5Ms framework. It provides introductory materials to be used as part of immersive onboarding and two different models for covering critical topics in geriatrics—a longitudinal curriculum for use over the course of a three-year residency program and a focused curriculum for a traditional 2- or 4-week geriatrics rotation block. It also furnishes references and links to multiple teaching tools and other geriatrics education resources available for educators (Table 5.1).

Although the ACGME does not require specific exposure to geriatrics during most other residency training programs, leaders in these disciplines have recognized the importance of competence in the care of older adults and have created documents to guide residency programs in this regard (Table 5.1). Emergency medicine educators developed a set of core geriatrics competencies in response to the growing proportion of emergency department visits that involve older adults. The expert panel listed seven key areas for focus: atypical presentation of disease, geriatric trauma, including falls, cognitive and behavioral disorders, adaptation of usual emergency interventions to the older adult population, appropriate prescribing, safe transitions, and consideration of comorbid conditions [12]. Additionally, the American Geriatrics Society (AGS) has created toolkits for specialty residents in Orthopedic surgery, Anesthesiology, Emergency Medicine, General Surgery, Gynecology-Urology, Ophthalmology, Otolaryngology, and Physical Medicine and Rehabilitation. These toolkits include curricula, evaluation tools, and slide show presentations targeted to the specific needs of residents in the specialty caring for older adults [4–11].

Considerations for Teaching Residents About Geriatrics

Diagnosing the Learner The standardized curricula and core competencies provide useful general approaches to teaching geriatrics within a training program. Each trainee enters residency with different background and different career goals and therefore has unique learning needs. Approaching resident physicians as adult learners and applying andragogy theories can help create more meaningful and impactful experiences. As a first step, understanding previous exposures to geriatrics can assist an educator in more effectively engaging residents. To date, there are no requirements for dedicated exposure to geriatrics in undergraduate medical education, though there are recommended minimum competencies [22]. As such, medical school curricula vary widely with regard to the breadth and depth of experiences in geriatric medicine. While some programs have robust rotations that include dedicated time working with geriatricians across an array of settings, some may have no formal geriatrics exposures at all. When approaching a resident without previous geriatrics experiences versus a resident physician who has already spent considerable time in geriatrics during medical school, the educator may need to adjust content to ensure the learner is neither overwhelmed by new information nor bored by discussions that are too elementary.

Just as medical school experiences vary for resident physicians, so, too, will their personal and professional experiences prior to their undergraduate medical education years. Some trainees may have close, intergenerational family relationships that have afforded them perspectives on being a caregiver for an aging parent or grandparent. Some may have worked with older adult populations in other roles prior to medical school, perhaps as an emergency medical technician, a volunteer for a hospice agency, or a nursing assistant in a long-term care facility. These exposures in capacities outside their current medical training may influence their outlook on aging, older adults, and geriatric care, and may, in turn, provide a source for further engaging them as adult learners.

Finally, most resident physicians will not pursue geriatrics as a career but will still interact with older adults in whatever specialty they choose. Knowledge of a trainee's career plans provides opportunities to align geriatrics teaching and clinical encounters with the resident physician's career focus, which may improve engagement and deepen their interest. The future hospitalists will undoubtedly encounter delirium in their practice, budding primary care physicians will have complex older patients in their panels who require a team-based approach and knowledge of geriatric syndromes, and nascent proceduralists will need to obtain consent from adults with cognitive impairment and titrate sedation appropriately.

Mapping the Learning Environment Depending on the training program's setting, the resources for teaching geriatrics will vary regarding the time allocated within the curriculum that can be devoted to geriatrics education, the number of physicians with geriatrics expertise, the types of learning venues where instruction in geriatric medicine can occur, and the availability of interprofessional teams to provide instruction. To create an effective residency education experience in geriatrics, an educator must work within the constraints of the individual program landscape and the available learning venues to structure the exposure. While the ACGME Common Program Requirements for Internal Medicine, Family Medicine, Psychiatry, and Physical Medicine and Rehabilitation require geriatrics training, competing demands for resident time may limit the actual hours available for the experience [13, 15–17]. To that end, securing space within the curriculum is often the first challenge. Buy-in from residency program leadership is key to providing a high-quality geriatrics experience. In addition to helping the residency meet ACGME program requirements, there are other attributes that can make geriatric education attractive for program and associate program directors. Emphasizing team-based competencies, teaching effective communication skills, linking geriatric syndromes with patient safety issues, providing role models for healthy work–life balance, and providing thoughtful and useful trainee evaluations can help make the case for increasing the footprint of geriatrics in residency curricula.

Another limiting factor for geriatrics experiences within residency training is the small size of the geriatrics workforce. Outside of academic centers, there are fewer practicing geriatricians available to teach learners. Payment structures make practice of geriatrics in the community more challenging, and community-based residency programs can struggle to find geriatricians to precept trainees. Additionally, even within academic centers, substantial clinical, administrative, or research responsibilities may limit the ability of geriatricians to engage in teaching. The increasing urgency to educate trainees in the care of older adults as the population continues to grow also leads to multiple other learners from different disciplines and levels vying for time with geriatricians in shared clinical settings.

This mismatch between the number of geriatricians and the many health professional trainees who seek training in the care of older adults may require other physicians and members of the workforce to take on the role of teaching geriatrics. Fortunately, faculty development programs exist that can bring geriatrics teaching expertise to these clinicians, including the Curriculum for the Hospitalized Aging

Medical Patient (CHAMP) Program, which incorporates geriatrics content into a faculty development program for teaching in the acute care setting [23]. Similarly, the Reynolds Program for Advancing Geriatrics Education (PAGE) curriculum provides geriatrics teaching points to hospitalists during regularly scheduled staff meetings and enhances the provision of geriatrics teaching to resident physicians working with hospitalists [24]. Further, web-based and virtual modules can also be resources for effective geriatrics teaching when access to local geriatricians is limited. The Extension for Community Healthcare Outcomes (ECHO) program has successfully provided longitudinal geriatrics teaching to resident physicians in primary care settings through their Project ECHO-Geriatrics intervention, which uses videoconferencing to provide didactics and case-based discussions on geriatrics topics [25]. Other webinar-based geriatrics educational programs have also successfully improved resident physician knowledge while having a broad geographic reach due to their virtual nature [26].

Experiences in geriatrics are valuable, regardless of the site, but programs will vary in terms of the number of sites where geriatricians practice. In some areas, residents may have access to Acute Care for Elders (ACE) units, ambulatory primary and specialty care, home care, and long-term care settings. Other programs may have fewer or even one site where geriatricians practice. When settings are more limited, applying a standardized clinical framework can ensure adequate coverage of core geriatrics topics. It can allow trainees to develop a general approach to older adults, independent of the venue where their geriatrics exposure occurs, that they can replicate elsewhere.

In all venues, the practice of Geriatric Medicine relies heavily on collaboration with interprofessional teams. Not all training programs have embedded interprofessional teams that can provide resident education, however. Non-physicians who contribute to the care of older adults may have limited time or training to engage in teaching. While some centers may support robust interprofessional teams, other health systems could have fewer embedded team members who can participate in resident teaching. When direct interactions with interprofessional team members are in short supply, the educator may need to be deliberate about describing the ways in which they engage team members, their roles and how this enhances patient care. Asynchronous didactics created as enduring learning objects or teleconference teaching sessions by interprofessional team members can help provide insight into discipline-specific skillsets and team-based competencies, even if team members have limited bandwidth for daily teaching.

Clinical Frameworks for Teaching Geriatrics to Residents

Acknowledging these differences related to residents' backgrounds, program resources and settings, a standardized clinical framework to teach geriatrics can help ensure that residents receive consistent instruction on core geriatrics content using easily understood and remembered terms. In recent years, the geriatrics 5Ms have become a leading clinical framework that educators can adapt when teaching trainees of different experience levels and in different settings. This tool effectively conveys geriatric core competencies in a simple yet comprehensive method. Historically, some educators have used other strategies, like the Wisconsin Star Method, to ensure all components of Geriatrics care receive attention, or have instead focused on function as the central structure for teaching the care of older adults. Each of these approaches can be useful for helping resident physicians grow their geriatrics knowledge, skills, and attitudes. When discussing application of clinical frameworks, the geriatrics 5Ms will receive emphasis, but any of these options could be utilized to help provide structure to teaching residents.

The Geriatrics 5Ms Applied to Residency Education The AGS/ADGAP Geriatrics Curriculum for Residency Programs provides extensive guidance for incorporating the Geriatrics 5Ms into training for internal medicine and family medicine residents. The authors describe ways to introduce the 5Ms in an early introduction to geriatrics as part of an intern immersive training experience, followed by either a longitudinal geriatrics experience or a geriatrics block rotation where clinical and didactic sessions cover elements of each domain (mind, medications, multicomplexity, mobility, and matters most). The IM/FM Minimum Competencies for Geriatrics are cross-referenced with the Geriatrics 5Ms categories to help ensure that residents cover the key material [20]. Applying the 5Ms to resident training has been shown to improve both knowledge and self-efficacy regarding the care of older adults [27]. In most clinical settings, each of the geriatric 5Ms is likely covered, though some may be more highly emphasized than others. For example, a subspecialty Geriatrics Falls Clinic might put the greatest emphasis on mobility and medications while addressing to a lesser extent mind (e.g. whether cognitive impairment is a contributor to falls), multicomplexity (specifically the contribution of existing medical problems to fall risk), and what matters most (when weighing the risks versus benefits of a given drug that might increase fall risk or worsen sequelae of falls). In a primary care clinic where routine follow-up visits occupy much of the time, multicomplexity might be the main point of conversation, while the backdrop of mind, mobility, medications, and matters most might guide decision-making regarding treatments and preventive care. An inpatient geriatrics venue could underscore the importance of mind due to the high prevalence of delirium among hospitalized older adults. Specific medications contributing to delirium and the impact of hospitalization on mobility and functional decline may also take precedence, while consideration of multicomplexity and what matters most may receive less attention unless an older adult is nearing end of life or facing a major treatment decision.

The Wisconsin Star Method Developed initially for geriatric psychiatry, the Wisconsin Star Method helps frame the approach to complex older adults by considering the ways that five different factors contribute to a pressing clinical issue: medication factors, medical factors, behavioral factors, personal factors, and social factors [28]. By considering each of these, a resident can develop a more complete picture of the patient's situation that, in turn, can help uncover solutions that might not have been apparent from simply considering the medical problem at hand. The Wisconsin Star Method also provides opportunities for residents to understand team roles when utilized in a huddle or visit debriefing where each represented discipline provides input on a given point of the star. For example, a pharmacist could discuss medications, while the resident physician or other provider on the team could review the medical factors. A social worker may offer insight into social factors, and the patient themselves or a caregiver might provide the best insight into behavioral and personal factors. The team can then work together to develop solutions that address different contributors based on their area of expertise.

Functional History Framework Another approach to teaching residents about geriatrics is to make functional status the focus of the assessment. By having trainees inquire about functional history, specifically instrumental and basic activities of daily living, and explore reasons for functional decline, they can develop a differential diagnosis that includes common geriatric syndromes. For example, in an older adult with falls, exploring function might help identify triggers for falls (e.g. carrying laundry baskets down basement stairs). It may also provide clues about an underlying medical etiology (e.g. a person who has recently been less able to manage finances because of difficulty writing checks might be experiencing micrographia due to parkinsonism). Finally, it may help emphasize the impact of falls on quality of life (e.g. development of fear of falling causing an older adult to stop grocery shopping). The functional history focus also provides an opportunity to engage other disciplines, including physical and occupational therapists, speech language pathologists, social workers, neuropsychologists, and nursing professionals in diagnosis and management. For an older adult with memory impairment, for example, neuropsychologists could comment on how deficits in different cognitive domains might impact function, a social worker may be able to help connect with community resources to compensate for functional losses, and a pharmacist could offer solutions for simplifying medications in light of cognitive challenges. In the acute setting, recognizing how function changes in the context of illness and hospitalization can help inspire discussion about pertinent geriatrics syndromes and the hazards of hospitalization, particularly in the context of frailty.

Application of Clinical Frameworks

All learners can benefit from explicit discussion of the Geriatrics 5Ms at the start of a geriatrics experience. While residents may have previously participated in a geriatrics rotation, the 5Ms may not have been a part of the experience. Initial review of the meaning of each M and the key geriatrics concepts they represent will set the stage for subsequent discussions. For those who are familiar with them, brief review can help reacquaint the trainee and reinforce their existing knowledge. The RIME (Reporter, Interpreter, Manager, Educator) model can be helpful to keep in mind when targeting the 5Ms to an individual learner's needs [29] (Fig. 5.1). The following learner and learning environment vignettes demonstrate how to apply the 5Ms to trainees from a variety of backgrounds and in various settings in order to optimize learning (Tables 5.2 and 5.3). For a trainee like Dr. Brown in Vignette 2, selecting a single M—Mind, in this case, and asking him to obtain a focused cognitive history and apply the diagnostic criteria for dementia may be an appropriate starting point for teaching (Table 5.1). For Dr. Adams, in contrast, these reporting and interpretation tasks might not stimulate her interest (Table 5.1). She could leave with the impression that there is not much more to learn in geriatrics and have lower motivation to pursue fellowship training. To engage her effectively, a better fit may be emphasizing the manager role by talking through the merits of different cholinesterase inhibitor treatment options in a person with a new diagnosis of dementia. Alternatively, her preceptor could ask her to explain the diagnostic criteria of dementia to more junior trainees and offer feedback. This approach can solidify her knowledge and allow her to grow skills as an educator herself. While both trainees might be considering the same subject area and working in the same clinical setting, their learning experiences will be strategically different to account for their differing knowledge bases (Fig. 5.1).

Considering Previous Exposures to Older Adults in Personal or Professional Life Adult learners often benefit from connecting lessons to previous life experiences. Fortunately, exposures to older adults in another career often engender more positive feelings regarding geriatric populations [30]. For Dr. Clark, their experi-

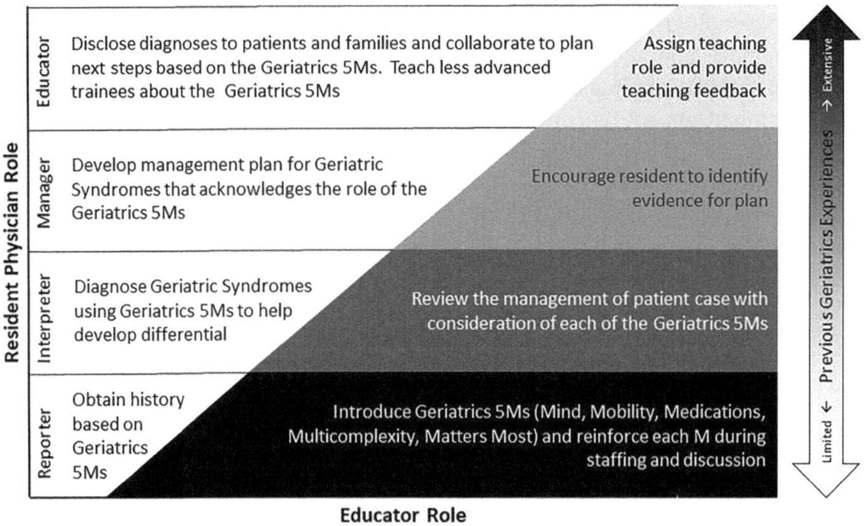

Fig. 5.1 Model for teaching geriatrics based on a resident physician's previous exposures to geriatrics using the 5Ms and RIME frameworks [Adapted from: Pangaro L. A new vocabulary and other innovations for improving descriptive in-training evaluations. *Academic Medicine* 1999; 74: 1203-7. doi: https://doi.org/10.1097/00001888-199911000-00012, Molnar F. The public launch of the Geriatric 5Ms (online). Available at http://canadiangeriatrics.ca/2017/04/update-the-public-launch-of-the-geriatric-5ms/. Accessed 2021 December 16]

Table 5.2 Learner vignettes with trainees highlighting the variety of geriatrics experiences and career goals that educators may encounter

Learner vignette 1: interested in geriatrics Dr. Adams (she/her/hers) is an intern in internal medicine on a geriatrics block rotation who is attending a memory evaluation clinic. She enjoyed her geriatrics rotation in medical school and has an interest in geriatric medicine as a career. She was exposed to ambulatory geriatrics care as a student, largely in a geriatrics primary care but also in some subspecialties, including falls and memory evaluation clinics
Learner vignette 2: little geriatrics experience Dr. Brown (he/him/his) is an intern in family medicine on a geriatrics block rotation who is attending a memory evaluation clinic. He is interested in primary care with an obstetrics practice. He did not have a specific geriatrics rotation during medical school but has worked with older adults during a hospice rotation and when on acute care clerkships. The bulk of his primary care exposures thus far have involved middle-aged and young adults, as well as children
Learner vignette 3: prior experience with geriatrics in another role Dr. Clark (they/them/theirs) is a Family Medicine resident on a Geriatrics block rotation who is working on an inpatient Geriatrics service, primarily seeing patients with delirium. Prior to starting medical school, they worked as a Certified Nursing Assistant in a nursing home. They spent time in both rehabilitation and long term care wings in the facility and encountered many people with cognitive impairment
Learner vignette 4: future subspecialist Dr. Dean (she/her/hers) is an internal medicine resident in a primary care clinic with a longitudinal geriatrics curriculum. She plans to become an oncologist. She had limited exposure to geriatrics in medical school but sees older adults regularly in her primary care continuity clinic experience

Table 5.3 Learning environment vignettes that demonstrate the variety of local resources in geriatrics a training program may provide

Learning environment 1: resource-rich geriatrics environment A university-based Family Medicine program includes a month-long geriatrics rotation with time spent in subspecialty geriatrics clinics like Memory and Falls, an inpatient geriatrics consultation service, a geriatric psychiatry clinic, and a teaching nursing home. Residents can see a driving safety assessment in an Occupational Therapy clinic if interested and can tour an adult day center. Preceptors include family medicine physicians with geriatrics fellowship training and internal medicine-trained geriatricians
Learning environment 2: limited geriatrics-specific teaching venues A community-based internal medicine program has a longitudinal geriatrics curriculum where trainees spend one half day per month in a nursing home setting with a board-certified geriatrician. There are no inpatient or subspecialty geriatrics practices in the area, but the residents work with a group of highly engaged hospitalists on the wards who manage many complex, elderly adults
Learning environment 3: no formal geriatrics exposure A university-based physical medicine and rehabilitation program offers rotations in acute rehabilitation at a freestanding rehabilitation hospital and consultations at the main hospital campus and a pediatrics hospital. Residents also rotate through ambulatory settings, including pediatrics, pain, spine, sports medicine, and electrodiagnostics clinics. There is no formal geriatrics rotation, but trainees have a flexible elective rotation and see many older adults in their non-pediatrics rotations

ences as a nursing assistant may have sparked an interest in older adults, and it is likely that they had to find ways to manage challenging behaviors related to cognitive impairment while working in that role (Table 5.1). When Dr. Clark sees a hospitalized older adult with delirium, they could be prompted to draw on previous experiences with nursing home residents to think about the geriatrics 5Ms. Their observations as a nursing assistant when caring for residents recently discharged from the hospital with delirium could help form the basis for discussions about the signs and symptoms that bedside nursing staff might observe (mind). They could also draw on their role as a caregiver to consider what non-pharmacologic interventions might help avoid potentially inappropriate medications to treat behaviors (medications). Reflecting on functional declines they may have observed in the post-acute setting could help them identify mitigation strategies (mobility), and having worked with residents at end of life might help frame conversations about goals with significantly ill delirious adults (matters most). While not every learner will have had these experiences, those who have can connect their current learning to previous events and can offer insight to other trainee colleagues from the perspective of another interprofessional team member.

Incorporating Career Goals Into Resident Teaching Most resident physicians will not pursue geriatric medicine, but almost all will encounter older adults in their practices. Drawing on this inevitability can help them appreciate the benefit of the instruction and find meaningful takeaways relevant to their interests. For Dr. Dean, the future oncologist, applying the 5Ms framework to the cancer patient can help her recognize the value of the approach (Table 5.2). Lessons about mobility and multicomplexity, for example, could touch on how comorbidity and frailty predict survival in some cancer types and how comprehensive geriatric assessment may improve the care of oncologic patients [31]. It may also help guide discussions about appropriateness of cancer screening in multimorbid, frail older adults. Discussion of mind could review the normal, gradual progression of dementia over many years and differentiate this from a more rapid presentation that could signify an alternative etiology for cognitive change such as a primary CNS lymphoma and paraneoplastic limbic encephalitis. When reviewing medications, older adults' increased sensitivity to side effects of drugs, including those used in chemotherapy, may offer useful insight. The emphasis on consideration of what Matters Most for older adults applies to the management of the geriatric oncology patient, as well. Using examples of geriatric patient cases or situations that align with trainee's interests may be an effective teaching strategy that can kindle excitement about caring for geriatric patients going forward [32].

Adapting Frameworks to the Learning Environment

High Resource Learning Environments In a resource-rich geriatrics environment, trainees may work in many different settings over the course of a rotation. These types of rotations offer significant breadth and allow residents opportunities to see the richness and diversity of geriatric practice. Learning Environment 1, for example, offers a myriad of exposures (Table 5.3). The variety of experiences can broaden the learner's perspective on geriatrics as a specialty and provide more opportunities to connect rotation activities with future career goals. With this variety, however, might come a lack of continuity with faculty mentors, decreased opportunities for meaningful evaluation and can leave trainees unsure of what to expect each day. To combat the limitations of consistency in such a rotation, robust orientation materials for each experience can be employed, and attention can be directed toward creating recurring experiences within these complex schedules. Faculty development that emphasizes setting expectations for trainees, promoting targeted learning objectives, and providing real time feedback can increase teaching efficacy. Additionally, the use of a single clinical framework across all sites can also help residents find a common thread among their experiences. Residents can begin the rotation with an introduction to the Geriatrics 5Ms. Faculty development trainings can similarly acquaint preceptors with the Geriatrics 5Ms so that they are prepared to provide the residents with opportunities to apply the concepts of the Geriatrics 5Ms and reinforce these themes across sites. With this repetition, they can better understand each M itself and appreciate how the Geriatrics 5Ms could relate to their own future practices.

Limited Geriatrics Teaching Settings A training program with fewer types of geriatrics experiences also has advantages for residents and likewise benefits from application of the Geriatrics 5Ms to teaching sessions. Education leaders in internal medicine and geriatric medicine have identified proficiency with collaboration in interprofessional teams as a priority for resident education, and geriatrics experiences that span several days or months can develop these skills effectively [33]. When residents have longitudinal or repeated exposures to the same setting, they can develop increased familiarity and self-efficacy with patient care in that environment. There may be more opportunities to understand the site's particular elements of systems-based practice, including how to facilitate efficient care and how to work with interdisciplinary teams on site. The supervising faculty member can develop more significant relationships with residents and observe trainees sequentially, thereby allowing potentially richer feedback sessions. Learning Environment 2, for example, could provide the residents with a solid understanding of nursing home care that is otherwise often lacking [34] (Table 5.3). Despite being a single site, there can be variety among patients; more robust seniors might be recovering from an elective joint replacement and transitioning home, while frailer long term care residents might be nearing end of life. In each case, the Geriatrics 5Ms can offer a standardized approach to help guide evaluation and management. If residents become adept at considering the Geriatrics 5Ms at this site, they will have developed a skill set that they can apply in others, as well. Further, in the presence of engaged teaching faculty outside of geriatrics, non-geriatrics rotations can be "geriatricized" through faculty development programs like CHAMP or PAGE [23, 24]. Within these programs, non-geriatrician clinicians can learn about the Geriatrics 5Ms and receive encouragement to apply the framework themselves. For a discussion of teaching in various clinical settings, see Chaps. 11–15.

Programs Without Geriatrics Rotation Requirements Residency programs outside of internal medicine, psychiatry, and family medicine are unlikely to have formal geriatrics rotations, but there still may be opportunities to reach the residents and share the concepts of the geriatrics 5Ms. In Learning Environment 3, a motivated teacher could incorporate geriatrics concepts into the curriculum through a series of lectures or clinical exposures (Table 5.3). Calling attention to ACGME requirements and board exam content areas may help bolster interest in specific geriatrics training experiences. Collaboration between residency programs (e.g. internal medicine and PM&R) can lead toward combined participation in lectures valuable for both learner groups such as sarcopenia or exercise in older adults. The American Geriatrics Society offers toolkits for teaching physical medicine and rehabilitation residents, including lecture slides, learning modules that can be preceptor-led or learner-led, and assessment tools, including quizzes and Objective Structured Clinical Examinations (OSCEs) [11]. Prefacing these materials with a discussion of the Geriatrics 5Ms or even introducing the Geriatrics 5Ms alone provides the residents an easy to remember approach to caring for their older adult patients. Distilling geriatrics down into a single clinical framework, whether it is the Geriatrics 5Ms or another approach, can make geriatrics more comprehensible to these trainees as a whole and could inspire greater interest in the population.

Conclusions and Future Directions for Teaching Geriatrics to Residents

Whether residents have a stated interest in geriatrics or not, the use of a standardized clinical framework for teaching about older adults creates opportunities to engage learners and adapt clinical experiences to ensure they achieve self-efficacy and competency. Residents enter their graduate medical education programs from a variety of backgrounds and with a variety of career goals that can be leveraged to increase interest and relevancy for core geriatrics topics. Training programs will have access to different settings and teachers, but with attentive instructional design and use of published curricula and resources, they can all provide meaningful and impactful educational experiences. Thoughtful application of a clinical framework can help standardize learning, increase awareness of "what geriatrics does," and develop confidence in caring for complex older adults no matter the learner or the environment.

References

1. Santo L, Okeyode T. National ambulatory medical care survey: 2018 national summary tables. https://www.cdc.gov/nchs/data/ahcd/namcs_summary/2018-namcs-web-tables-508.pdf. Accessed 1 September 2021.
2. Agency for Healthcare Research and Quality. HCUP fast stats. Healthcare cost and utilization project (HCUP). www.hcup-us.ahrq.gov/faststats/national/inpatienttrends.jsp?measure1=01

&characteristic1=02&time1=10&measure2=06&characteristic2=02&time2=10&expansionInfoState=hide&dataTablesState=hide&definitionsState=hide&exportState=hide. Accessed 1 September 2021.
3. Petriceks AH, Olivas JC, Srivstava S. Trends in geriatrics graduate medical education programs and positions, 2001 to 2018. Gerontol Geriatr Med. 2018;4:2333721418777659. https://doi.org/10.1177/2333721418777659.
4. American Geriatrics Society. The geriatrics for specialty residents toolkit: orthopedic surgery. https://geriatricscareonline.org/toc/the-geriatrics-for-specialty-residents-toolkit-orthopedic-surgery/TK006. Accessed 29 September 2021.
5. American Geriatrics Society. The geriatrics for specialty residents toolkit: anesthesiology. https://geriatricscareonline.org/toc/the-geriatrics-for-specialty-residents-toolkit-anesthesiology/TK002. Accessed 29 September 2021.
6. American Geriatrics Society. The geriatrics for specialty residents toolkit: emergency medicine. https://geriatricscareonline.org/toc/the-geriatrics-for-specialty-residents-toolkit-emergency-medicine/TK008. Accessed 29 September 2021.
7. American Geriatrics Society. The geriatrics for specialty residents toolkit: general surgery. https://geriatricscareonline.org/toc/the-geriatrics-for-specialty-residents-toolkit-general-surgery/TK003. Accessed 29 September 2021.
8. American Geriatrics Society. The geriatrics for specialty residents toolkit: gynecology-urology. https://geriatricscareonline.org/toc/the-geriatrics-for-specialty-residents-toolkit-gynecology-urology/TK009. Accessed 29 September 2021.
9. American Geriatrics Society. The geriatrics for specialty residents toolkit: ophthalmology. https://geriatricscareonline.org/toc/the-geriatrics-for-specialty-residents-toolkit-ophthalmology/TK005. Accessed 29 September 2021.
10. American Geriatrics Society. The geriatrics for specialty residents toolkit: otolaryngology. https://geriatricscareonline.org/toc/the-geriatrics-for-specialty-residents-toolkit-otolaryngology/TK007. Accessed 29 September 2021.
11. American Geriatrics Society. The geriatrics for specialty residents toolkit: physical medicine and rehabilitation. https://geriatricscareonline.org/toc/the-geriatrics-for-specialty-residents-toolkit-physical-medicine-rehabilitation/TK004. Accessed 29 September 2021.
12. Hogan T, Losman ED, Carpenter CR, et al. Development of geriatric competencies for emergency medicine residents using an expert consensus process. Acad Emerg Med. 2010;17(3):316–24. https://doi.org/10.1111/j.1553-2712.2010.00684.x.
13. Accreditation Council for Graduate Medical Education. ACGME program requirements for graduate medical education in family medicine. https://www.acgme.org/globalassets/PFAssets/ProgramRequirements/120_FamilyMedicine_2020.pdf. Accessed 29 September 2021.
14. Association of Directors of Geriatrics Academic Programs. Minimum geriatric competencies for IM-FM residents. Available https://adgap.americangeriatrics.org/education-training/competencies/minimum-geriatric-competencies-im-fm-residents. Accessed 1 September 2021.
15. Accreditation Council for Graduate Medical Education. ACGME program requirements for graduate medical education in internal medicine. https://www.acgme.org/globalassets/pfassets/programrequirements/140_internalmedicine_2022v3.pdf. Accessed 16 November 2022.
16. Accreditation Council for Graduate Medical Education. ACGME program requirements for graduate medical education in physical medicine and rehabilitation. Available https://www.acgme.org/Portals/0/PFAssets/ProgramRequirements/340_PhysicalMedicineRehabilitation_2020.pdf?ver=2020-06-29-163737-033. Accessed 1 September 2021.
17. Accreditation Council for Graduate Medical Education. ACGME program requirements for graduate medical education in psychiatry. https://www.acgme.org/globalassets/PFAssets/ProgramRequirements/400_Psychiatry_2020.pdf?ver=2020-06-19-123110-817&ver=2020-06-19-123110-817. Accessed 29 September 2021.
18. Lieff S, Kirwin P, Colenda CC. Proposed geriatric psychiatry core competencies for subspecialty training. Am J Geriatr Psychiatr. 2005;13(9):815–21. https://doi.org/10.1176/appi.ajgp.13.9.815.

19. Williams BC, Warshaw G, Fabiny AR, et al. Medicine in the 21st century: recommended competencies for internal medicine and family medicine residents. J Grad Med Educ. 2010;2(3):373–83. https://doi.org/10.4300/JGME-D-10-000651.
20. American Association for Geriatric Psychiatry. Geriatric core competencies. https://www.aagponline.org/index.php?src=gendocs&ref=GeriatricCoreCompetencies&category=Education. Accessed 1 September 2021.
21. Bynum D, Wilson LA, Ong T, et al. Meeting AGS competencies: are residents meeting expectations for quality care of older adults? J Am Geriatr Soc. 2015;63(9):1918–23. https://doi.org/10.1111/jgs.13598. Epub 2015 Aug 27.
22. Leipzig RM, Granville L, Simpson D, Anderson MB, Sauvigné K, Soriano RP. Keeping granny safe on July 1: a consensus on minimum geriatrics competencies for graduating medical students. Acad Med. 2009;84(5):604–10. https://doi.org/10.1097/ACM.0b013e31819fab70.
23. Podrazik PM, Levine S, Smith S, et al. The curriculum for the hospitalized aging medical patient program: a collaborative faculty development program for hospitalists, general internists, and geriatricians. J Hosp Med. 2008;3(5):384–93. https://doi.org/10.1002/jhm.348.
24. Mazotti L, Moylan A, Murphy E, et al. Advancing geriatrics education: an efficient faculty program for academic hospitalists increases Geriatrics teaching. J Hosp Med. 2010;5(9):541–6. https://doi.org/10.1002/jhm.791. Epub 2010 Aug 17.
25. Bennett KA, Ong T, Verrall A, et al. Project ECHO-geriatrics: training future primary care providers to meet the needs of older adults. J Grad Med Educ. 2018;10(3):311–5. https://doi.org/10.4300/JGME-D-17-01022.1.
26. Sedhom R, Barile D. Can webinar-based education improve geriatrics training in internal medicine residency programs? Am J Med Qual. 2016;31(6):606. https://doi.org/10.1177/1062860616653183. Epub 2016 Jun 2.
27. Phillips S, Hawley CE, Triantafylidis LK, et al. Geriatrics 5Ms for primary care workshop. J Teach Learn Resour. 2019;15:10814. https://doi.org/10.15766/mep_2374-8265.10814.
28. Howell T. The Wisconsin star method: understanding and addressing complexity in geriatrics. In: Malone ML, et al., editors. Geriatrics models of care: bringing 'best practice' to an aging America. Cham: Springer; 2015. p. 87–94.
29. Pangaro L. A new vocabulary and other innovations for improving descriptive in-training evaluations. Acad Med. 1999;74:1203–7. https://doi.org/10.1097/00001888-199911000-00012.
30. Fitzgerald JT, Wray LA, Halter JB, et al. Relating medical students' knowledge, attitudes, and experience to an interest in Geriatric Medicine. Gerontologist. 2003;43(6):849–55. https://doi.org/10.1093/geront/43.6.849.
31. Boakye D, Rillmann B, Walter V, et al. Impact of comorbidity and frailty on prognosis in colorectal cancer patients: a systematic review and meta-analysis. Cancer Treat Rev. 2018;64:30–9. https://doi.org/10.1016/j.ctrv.2018.02.003. Epub 2018 Feb 10.
32. Scheepers ERM, Vondeling AM, Thielen N, et al. Geriatric assessment in older patients with a hematologic malignancy: a systematic review. Haematologica. 2020;105(6):1484–93. https://doi.org/10.3324/haematol.2019.245803. Epub 2020 May 7.
33. Chang A, Fernandez H, Cayea D, et al. Complexity in graduate medical education: a collaborative education agenda for internal medicine and geriatric medicine. J Gen Intern Med. 2014;29(6):940–6. https://doi.org/10.1007/s11606-013-2752-2.
34. Ward KT, Eslami MS, Garcia MB, et al. Do internal medicine residents know enough about skilled nursing facilities to orchestrate a good care transition? J Am Med Dir Assoc. 2014;15(11):841–3. https://doi.org/10.1016/j.jamda.2014.08.004. Epub 2014 Oct 3. PMID: 25282630; PMCID: PMC4591026.

Chapter 6
Teaching Geriatric Fellows: Learning to Think Like a Geriatrician

Jeremy D. Whyman, Carolina Fonseca Valencia, and Helen Fernandez

Introduction

The world's population landscape is changing; however, an ever-present shortage of geriatricians and geriatrics trainees remains. In order to fulfill the needs of a growing number of older adults in the USA, an additional 30,000 geriatricians will need to be trained each year [1]. Several studies have highlighted that trainees who are more likely to choose a career in geriatric medicine tend to have had close relationships with older adults prior to medical school and have had early exposure to the field of geriatrics. Furthermore, the trainees who are more likely to pursue a career in geriatrics have often received early, strong guidance from a mentor and champion in the field; yet, these factors are not always easy to guarantee for all trainees [2].

These changes and challenges in the population landscape and workforce serve as a call to action for geriatrics' educators to adopt an innovative approach, ensuring that the next generation of geriatricians is equipped with the right tools to be "an elite workforce that discovers and tests geriatric principles through research; that teaches these geriatric principles to all health professionals and to the public; and that disseminates and implements these geriatric principles through health system and health policy leadership" [3]. Put simply, of course more board certified geriatricians ("Big G geriatricians" as defined by Dr. Tinetti [3]) are needed; however, the current "Big G geriatricians" must train thousands of non-geriatricians to empower them in becoming skilled and comfortable using geriatric principles in caring for older adults [4].

J. D. Whyman (✉) · C. Fonseca Valencia
Beth Israel Deaconess Medical Center, Harvard Medical School, Boston, MA, USA
e-mail: jwhyman@bidmc.harvard.edu; cfonseca@bidmc.harvard.edu

H. Fernandez
Mount Sinai Hospital, Icahn School of Medicine at Mount Sinai, New York, NY, USA

A. W. Schwartz (ed.), *Medical Education in Geriatrics*,
https://doi.org/10.1007/978-3-031-32499-4_6

In this chapter we present a road map for faculty working with geriatrics fellowship trainees, by describing some of the major challenges and opportunities encountered when training geriatrics fellows, as well as delineating the most important roles that define the work and identity of a geriatrician.

Becoming a Geriatrics Fellow

The Current Landscape

Despite that the first fellowship in geriatric medicine had already been established in 1966 at City Hospital Center (a Mount Sinai School of Medicine affiliate), in the years before 1978 Dr. William Hazzard remarked "there were no trained geriatricians; no geriatrics faculty to develop model geriatric care programs, train geriatricians, educate medical students, residents, or practicing physicians, or conduct aging-related research" [5]. While all medical schools and hospitals in the UK had departments of geriatrics in the 1970s, the US had no corresponding discipline.

It was not until the 1970s that this began to shift. In 1974 the National Institutes of Health established the National Institute on Aging and in 1975, the Veterans Health Administration (VA) established Geriatric Research Education and Clinical Care Centers (GRECCs) to improve the quality of care for older veterans. In 1978, Dr. Paul Beeson, a professor of Medicine at Oxford spearheaded the first of a series of Institute of Medicine (IOM) reports highlighting the challenges facing the medical profession as the population ages [5]. This work began to penetrate US fellowship training spurred on by a 2nd IOM study published in 1987 emphasizing the need to develop the capacity to train academic leaders in geriatrics and the recommendation to establish "Centers of Excellence" in geriatric medicine [6]. This effort was bolstered in 1988 when the American Boards of Family Practice and Internal Medicine chose to create a Certificate of Added Qualifications (CAQ) in Geriatric Medicine, which required 2 years of fellowship training [6]. This same year, 1988, the 2-year requirement for geriatrics fellowship training was reduced to 1 year. Subsequently 10,207 physicians (both from Internal Medicine and Family Medicine) would go on to receive geriatric medicine certification between 1988 and 2002 [6].

Between 1988 and the present the American College of Graduate Medical education (ACGME) has recognized that the traditional pathway to become a geriatrician includes completion of residency training in Internal Medicine (IM) or Family Medicine (FM) [7]. However, in most recent years several other pathways have emerged to advance geriatrics fellowship specialty training in other fields including Geriatric Psychiatry (ACGME accredited), Geriatric Emergency Medicine (non-ACGME accredited), Geriatric Oncology (non-ACGME accredited), and Geriatric Cardiology (non-ACGME accredited) among others. Although all geriatrics fellowships aim to educate the fellow in the principles of normal vs pathological aging, geriatric syndromes including frailty and cognitive impairment (amongst others),

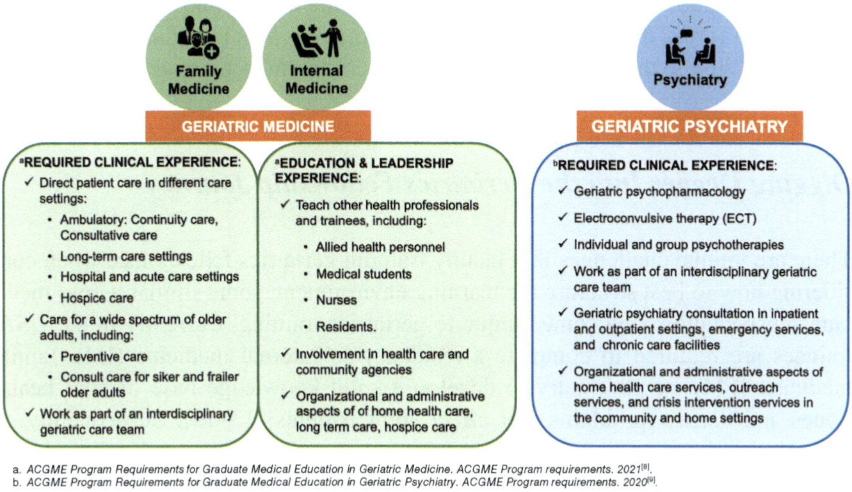

Fig. 6.1 ACGME curricular requirements for geriatrics training in different fields

and the complexities of how illness impairs independence, quality of life and patient goals and values [8, 9], the path of training may differ depending on the specialty. Figure 6.1 depicts common curricular requirements established by ACGME for Geriatric Medicine and Geriatric Psychiatry, illustrating some of the unique characteristics of each specialty when caring for older adults.

Mary Tinetti, a renowned Yale geriatrician, reflects, "Geriatrics is still a very new field and is still trying to compete for attention with more established disciplines like cardiology, nephrology, and others. We continue to need concerted efforts to enhance the visibility, credibility, and credentials of geriatrics to become embedded in academic medical centers in order to adequately research, teach, and care for older people" [10]. While efforts are ongoing to develop and implement many of the principles that Dr. Tinetti has laid out, the field has work to do to better understand how to increase the recruitment of future trainees.

Recent work done by Blachman and colleagues highlights that trainees pursuing geriatrics as a career path are a unique cohort [11]. They identified that geriatrics fellows tend to have a deep interest in working with complex patients, have often spent significant time with aging adults as a young person, and may have access to early intense geriatrics medical training, such as the Medical Student Training in Aging Research (MSTAR) program [12] or a geriatrics elective. Furthermore, many of these trainees are passionate about caring for underserved populations and have been noted to relish in the pursuit of following a path often less traveled [11]. However, Blachman and colleagues also identified that some of the trainees, when considering pursuing a geriatrics fellowship, vocalized concern about the lack of prestige associated with the field, and the persisting lower compensation geriatricians receive [11].

Given the above, more research needs to be done that will help to define further the positive forces that impact trainees taking them to pursue geriatrics as a career path in addition to the obstacles limiting the recruitment of more geriatricians.

Digging Deeper Into the Geriatrics Fellowship Journey

There are unique challenges that faculty training geriatrics fellows face when considering how to best structure the learning environment, some similar across medicine subspecialties, and some unique to geriatrics training. Currently in the USA, trainees are required to complete a residency in internal medicine (IM), family medicine (FM), or psychiatry to develop a solid knowledge base of core health issues and disease problems that affect adult patients [13–15]. Subsequently, to become a geriatrician the trainee is required to complete a 12-month fellowship in clinical geriatrics and demonstrate competency in understanding and differentiating normal aging from disease; diagnosing and managing a multitude of complex medical problems pertaining to the older adult known as the geriatrics syndromes; adapt to and understand different systems of care delivery; and begin to develop skills as educators and leaders in the field [16, 17].

The American Geriatric Society (AGS) and the Association of Directors of Geriatric Academic Programs (ADGAP) have defined Curricular Milestones (CM) which describe the learning trajectory within a sub-competency that takes a fellow from a novice in the subspecialty, to a proficient fellow or fellow expert [18]. The milestones are the "knowledge, skills, attitudes, and other attributes for each of the ACGME competences that describe the development of competence from an early subspecialty learner up to and beyond that expected for unsupervised practice" [19]. Figures 6.2 and 6.3 list the different CM expected to be attained by a geriatric medicine and a geriatric psychiatry fellow during their 1 year of training.

The AGS and ADGAP have also defined Entrustable Professional Activities (EPAs) for geriatric medicine which describe the core work that constitutes the discipline's specific expertise and provide the framework for faculty to perform meaningful assessment of geriatric fellows. These EPAs are critical, observable, measurable tasks, and responsibilities that practicing geriatricians can be trusted to perform proficiently, consistently, and unsupervised by the end of their training [20].

An example that helps illustrate the interplay between CM and the EPA framework can be reviewed in considering a fellow asked to evaluate a patient referred for geriatric consultation to evaluate cognitive impairment. During the first few months of fellowship, trainees learn to identify tools available for conducting a cognitive assessment. As the fellow reaches their fourth to fifth month of training, they are expected to demonstrate they can perform and interpret accurately these cognitive tests in an independent manner and use them as key aids in the diagnosis of cognitive impairment and/or dementia. Near completion of their training, fellows should be able to decipher normal and abnormal findings on these cognitive tests,

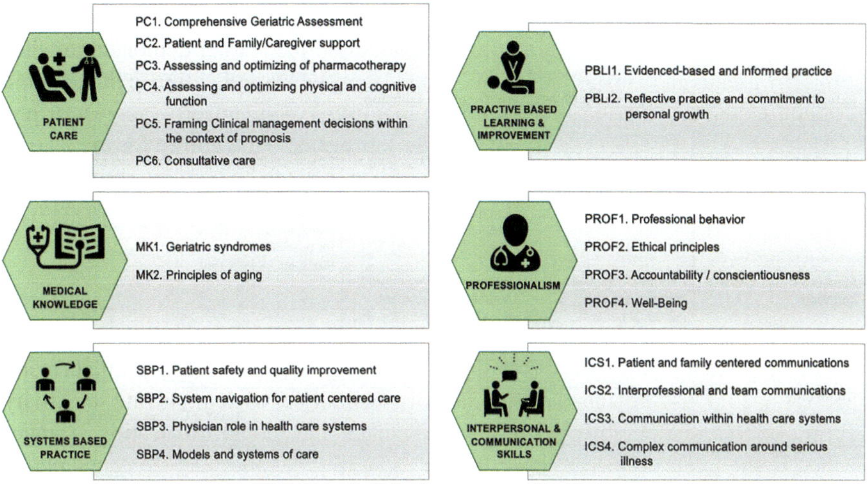

Fig. 6.2 ACGME geriatric medicine milestones [16]

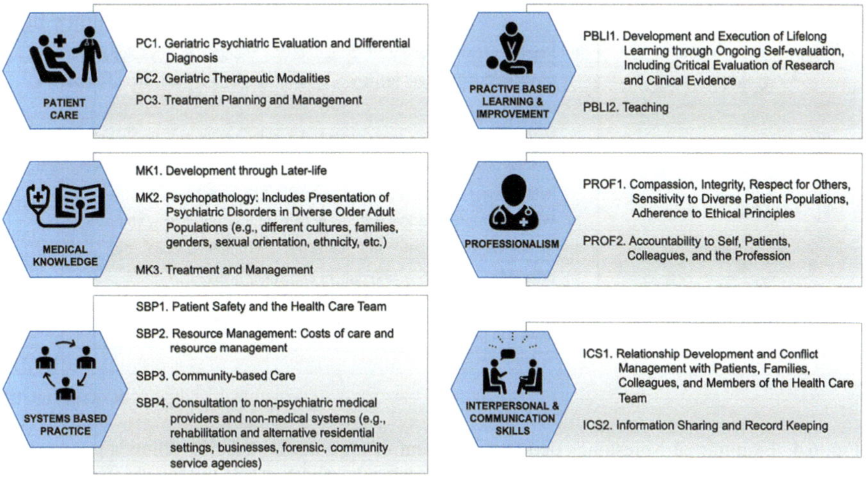

Fig. 6.3 ACGME geriatric psychiatry milestones [17]

incorporating performance of the functional assessment (Instrumental Activities of Daily Living (IADLS) and Activities of Daily Living (ADLS)) and integrating this assessment alongside the cognitive evaluation to properly diagnose dementia. Furthermore, by the time of graduation, fellows should be able to define an appropriate plan of care for the patient with cognitive impairment which will promote optimization of cognitive functioning across different care settings (Table 6.1) [8, 16].

The EPAs and their associated CMs provide the context for the IM subspecialty reporting milestones, allowing geriatrics fellowship directors to assess each fellow's

Table 6.1 ACGME milestone example of assessment and expected progression for geriatric fellows for 1 year fellowship [16]

Patient Care 4: Assessing and Optimizing Physical and Cognitive Function

Level 1	Level 2	Level 3	Level 4	Level 5
Identifies tools to assess physical function	Performs functional assessment of an individual patient	Interprets findings from a functional assessment, considering strengths and limitations of the assessment	Effectively integrates findings from functional and cognitive assessments into care plans, including referral for rehabilitative therapies as indicated	Promotes assessment and optimization of physical and cognitive functioning for patients across care systems
Identifies tools to assess cognition	Performs cognitive assessment of an individual patient	Interprets findings from a cognitive assessment, considering strengths and limitations of the assessment		

Comments:

Not Yet Completed Level 1 ☐
Not Yet Assessable ☐

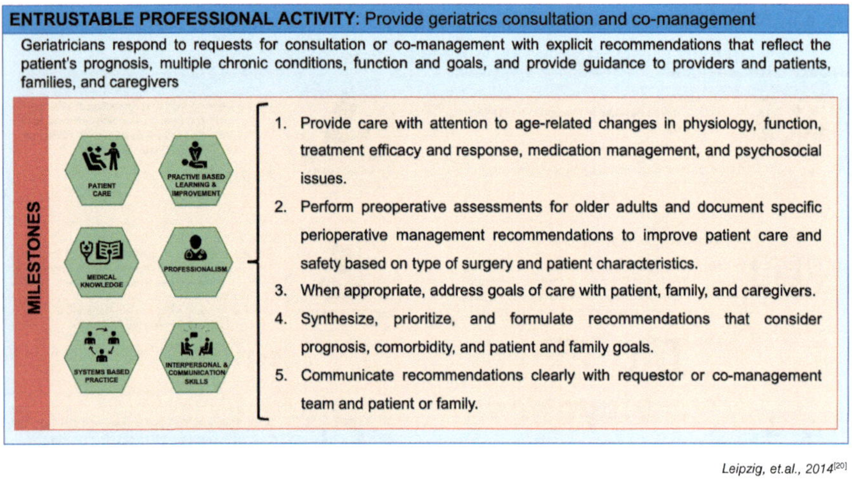

Fig. 6.4 Example of Milestones tied to assessment of a geriatric medicine fellow's progression toward attaining independence in entrustable professional activities (EPA) in the domain of geriatrics consultation and co-management

progress and to make an entrustment decision (whether the trainee can perform the activity without supervision) [20]. Furthermore, the geriatrics EPAs describe a geriatrician's expertise and help to frame how geriatricians differ from internists and family practitioners who care for older adults. The EPAs also emphasize the complexity of geriatric care and the greater likelihood of adverse events in those who are old, frail, or have multiple chronic conditions. Such complexity in turn requires prioritizing care with the individual and family and recognizing that definitive evidence can often be incomplete and that an individual's life expectancy can be uncertain [20]. Figure 6.4 illustrates this interplay.

Challenges and Opportunities

Teaching Geriatrics Fellows: Identity Formation

The term "geriatrician" was first coined by Dr. Ignatz Nascher, the father of geriatric medicine, in 1909 [21]. Over time the field of geriatric medicine has evolved, continuing its journey to define itself. Dr. Louise Aronson, a geriatrician and author explains in her book *Elderhood*, that Geriatricians use a blend of "scientific data, interpersonal skills, and pragmatic creativity" to care for older adults [22]. With these skills geriatricians are positioned as leaders who "take charge of caring for a rapidly evolving and diversifying aging population; educate the workforce to utilize the principles of geriatric care; and become agents of change by advocating and creating policies that will improve the care of this population" [4]. Dr. Mary Tinetti goes one step further in saying that geriatric medicine should be seen as "a 'meta-discipline'—perhaps the only one—that transcends and informs all other disciplines, and its knowledge base and principles should guide all care" [3].

Leaders like Dr. Aronson and Dr. Tinetti among others have pushed and challenged the discipline, a specialty still in its infancy, to continue to evolve, and we have seen this progression, as the field has embraced and incorporated complex concepts like frailty [23], geriatric syndromes [24], and by developing frameworks like the geriatrics 5M's [25, 26] and Patient Priorities Care [27] to help guide the care of complex older adults.

Against this evolving landscape, geriatric fellowships are charged with helping guide fellows as they craft new cognitive models to instill principles of aging and practice. This is done in part by building on their core medical knowledge, which was acquired during residency training (a foundation expected to be retained and built upon during the fellowship year). With this foundation as a starting point, geriatrics fellows are invited to reflect and consider early in their training what makes a geriatrician different from an internist/family physician or psychiatrist in order to help them develop their *geriatric identity*.

This evolution happens gradually during the 12-month fellowship year in a multistep process that requires the fellows to: (1) learn to identify normal physiological changes that occur with aging, to differentiate normal aging from pathology and disease; (2) incorporate into their reasoning the impact that a patient's environment and social determinants of health play on the aging process of the individual and the development of disease; (3) understand current medical guidelines (appreciating their limitations) and their implications for patient care, to provide evidence-based recommendations that will balance prevention and safety while incorporating concepts like "lag time to benefit" in their decision-making process [28]; (4) develop comfort and expertise in managing uncertainty as a foundational concept of geriatrics—the idea that in geriatrics many of the diseases and symptoms patients develop may be incurable, but that patients can still thrive despite living with illness [29, 30]; and (5) practice person-centered care by considering the patient's values, goals, and care preferences when making medical decisions [27].

The above concepts are illustrated with a case study (Case 6.1) of a patient with functional limitations and cognitive impairment who presents to a geriatrics clinic for preventive care and advice on cancer screening.

Case 6.1: What would you recommend for cancer screening in this patient?

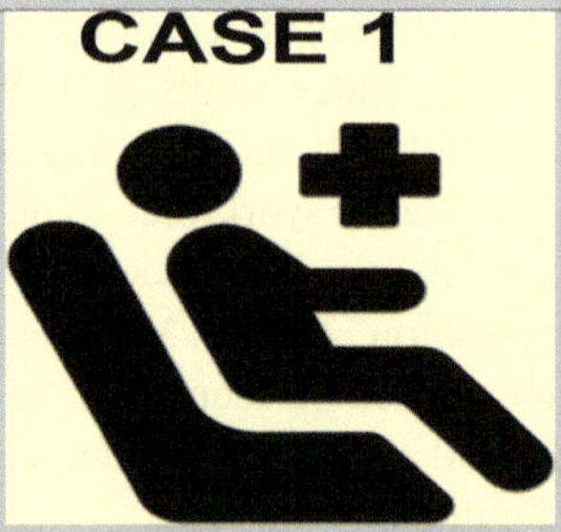

73-year-old community dwelling patient with a past medical history of coronary artery disease, heart failure, diabetes mellitus, cerebrovascular disease, falls, and depression, who is seen in the clinic for a regular follow-up.
They have been experiencing fatigue, as well as memory loss and weight loss. They live with their partner who is their primary caretaker and who reports assisting the patient with most of their activities of daily living (ADL's) including walking (uses a front wheel walker to ambulate), and some independent activities of daily living (IADL's) including medication and financial management as well as assisting with household chores.
On physical exam they are noted to have slow gait speed, and cognitive deficits.

In Table 6.2 we are able to appreciate a contrasting approach to the patient care when using a problem-centered approach, compared to a person-centered geriatric approach when guiding the decision of cancer screening.

Central to this framework is the fellow's understanding that in many ways age is an insufficient data point in considering the appropriateness of cancer screening, and that in geriatrics there are several additional crucial data points to consider, including but not limited to, functional performance by assessing gait speed [39] and frailty [35], as well as cognitive performance by assessing the level of cognitive impairment through tools like the MOCA® [33], and the impact that cognitive impairment has in the overall function of the patient [40].

The challenge that geriatrics educators face in this instance is in finding ways to guide the geriatric fellow into learning how to approach patient care through a more person-centered approach rather than a problem-centered approach. With a deliberate and targeted practice, the role of geriatrics educators is to coach fellows to transition the way they approach patient care from a primarily problem based structure where the focus is on finding solutions to fix specific problems, and instead using an approach that prioritizes geriatric syndromes and concepts like frailty and prognostication, integrating a patient's articulated priorities, goals, and values in the care plan, allowing for the fellow to build and develop an authentic geriatric identity. Table 6.3 highlights some of the tips we have found are helpful to assist fellows in this transition.

Table 6.2 Contrasting approach to the care of the patient in Case 6.1 when using the problem-centered approach vs the person-centered approach

PROBLEM-CENTERED APPROACH

REASONING

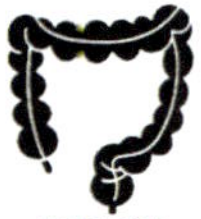

COLON CANCER

Population	Recommendation	Grade
Adults aged 50 to 75 years	The USPSTF recommends screening for colorectal cancer in all adults aged 50 to 75 years. See the "Practice Considerations" section and Table 1 for details about screening strategies.	A
Adults aged 45 to 49 years	The USPSTF recommends screening for colorectal cancer in adults aged 45 to 49 years. See the "Practice Considerations" section and Table 1 for details about screening strategies.	B
Adults aged 76 to 85 years	The USPSTF recommends that clinicians selectively offer screening for colorectal cancer in adults aged 76 to 85 years. Evidence indicates that the net benefit of screening all persons in this age group is small. In determining whether this service is appropriate in individual cases, patients and clinicians should consider the patient's overall health, prior screening history, and preferences.	C

Nee. Mayo Clinic Proceedings 2020[31]

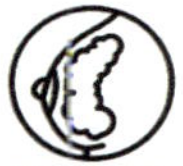

BREAST CANCER

Population	Recommendation	Grade
Women aged 50 to 74 years	The USPSTF recommends biennial screening mammography for women aged 50 to 74 years.	B
Women aged 40 to 49 years	The decision to start screening mammography in women prior to age 50 years should be an individual one. Women who place a higher value on the potential benefit than the potential harms may choose to begin biennial screening between the ages of 40 and 49 years.	C
Women aged 75 years or older	The USPSTF concludes that the current evidence is insufficient to assess the balance of benefits and harms of screening mammography in women aged 75 years or older.	I

Siu. Ann Intern Med. 2016[37]

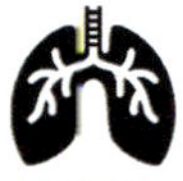

LUNG CANCER

Population	Recommendation	Grade
Adults aged 50 to 80 years who have a 20 pack-year smoking history and currently smoke or have quit within the past 15 years	The USPSTF recommends annual screening for lung cancer with low-dose computed tomography (LDCT) in adults aged 50 to 80 years who have a 20 pack-year smoking history and currently smoke or have quit within the past 15 years. Screening should be discontinued once a person has not smoked for 15 years or develops a health problem that substantially limits life expectancy or the ability or willingness to have curative lung surgery.	B

USPSTF. JAMA. 2021[38]

ADVISE

IN FAVOR of screening for the following cancers (as appropriate by gender and risk factors): Colorectal cancer, Breast cancer and/or Lung cancer

PERSON-CENTERED APPROACH

REASONING

This patient likely has a limited life expectancy of less than 10 years, which can be determined by assessing:

- **Functional status** (assessed by determining the presence or absence of impairment on *ADL's* and/or *IADL's*)
- **Cognitive status** (assessed with tools such as the *MiniCog®* [32] and/or *MOCA®* [33])
- The impact that **social determinants of health** have on the overall function and health trajectory of the patient
- **Values, goals, and care preferences**[27].

By using tools like the **Comprehensive Geriatric Assessment** (CGA)[34], **Frailty score calculator**[35] and/or **ePrognosis**[36] the fellow can estimate appropriately the likely life expectancy of the patient

In addition, the fellow would understand the concept of **"Lag time to benefit"** (LtB) defined as the time between the preventive intervention to the time when improved health outcomes are seen[28]; and know that most cancer screening tests have a LtB of less than 10 years

ADVISE

AGAINST any cancer screening given the patient's functional and cognitive limitations, as well as their health trajectory and life expectancy

Table 6.3 Proposed pearls to help geriatric fellows in developing their identity as geriatricians

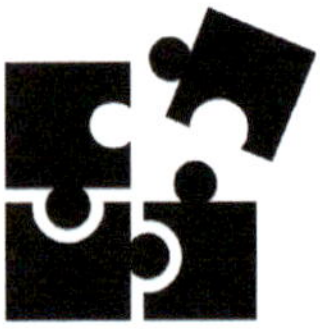

PEARLS FOR EDUCATORS:
Helping fellows develop their identity as Geriatricians

- ✓ Normalize for fellows that **developing the geriatrician's identity is an iterative process that takes time** and will depend on each fellow's individual journey.
- ✓ **Assist fellows in developing comfort managing uncertainty** by guiding and supporting them as they learn to manage patients with chronic and/or uncurable illness within the context of the patient's own goals and values[41].
- ✓ Model to fellows the **use of collaborative language with colleagues in other specialties and professions**, by recognizing that each one has a valuable set of skills that helps inform patient care[42].
- ✓ Coach fellows to **constantly seek improving the quality of care provided to the patients, and maximize patient safety** through system change, by encouraging involvement in scaled quality improvement initiatives during fellowship[43].
- ✓ Incorporate the ADGAP Fellowship Assessment Toolkit (developed by geriatrics fellowship directors across the US), as a tool that can help reduce variability of content emphasized across fellowships, standardizing the educational experiences and assist faculty in identifying the zone of proximal development[44] for individual learners in a more objective manner[19].
- ✓ Recognize fellows as **adult learners who are active participants in their own learning experience**, where faculty act as coaches in guiding them toward the required knowledge for the specialty as delineated by AGCME[8], and fostering a sense of "exploration and creativity" to allow them to continue advancing the specialty[45].

Teaching Geriatrics Fellows: Adapting Educational Strategies to Meet the Needs of a New Virtual Era

When the COVID pandemic began in March of 2020, the nature of work and medical training across the world changed for many. Applications to most medical subspecialties increased and geriatric medicine fellowship applications increased by 13% between 2020–2021 [46]. Geriatric fellowship recruitment transitioned to an entirely virtual platform. Through ADGAP, faculty developed and disseminated key strategies to improve the interview experience for geriatrics fellowship applicants with a focus on helping applicants understand institutional culture, community and geography, and at the same time helped support fellowship programs to optimize logistical and technology related challenges, enhance camera skill, navigation and comfort for faculty, and incorporating more intentional content to address issues around diversity, equity, and inclusion [47]. Geriatric fellowships training was impacted by the shift to virtual patient care, learning, and recruitment, a process that increased stress and burnout levels among trainees [48]. Geriatrics fellows were asked to use their broad and multidimensional, specialist training to participate in new programs and medical decision making related to COVID 19 in patient homes, long term care settings, hospice programs, via phone and virtually [49]. Fellows taught other physicians, nurses, and interdisciplinary faculty key skills [49]. Geriatrics fellowships across the country were assisted in their transition to incorporate telehealth training rapidly (this is addressed in more detail elsewhere within this book) [50].

Another important advance that added to geriatrics fellows' learning during the COVID-19 pandemic was the opportunity to learn virtually through live video-conferenced lectures, workshops, and seminars. Many fellowships had to migrate to fully virtual platforms for all their formal didactics and curriculum delivery (i.e., journal club, core lectures, morbidity, and mortality talks, etc.). *Geri-A-Float* has built on this platform by recruiting speakers from across the USA to deliver live and recorded sessions on diverse content not frequently covered in conventional fellowship curriculum and didactics [51]. This platform has also encouraged thoughtful reflection as to the reach that current educational platforms have. Traditionally each fellowship has been charged with building its own individual lectures, curriculum, and didactics, a paradigm that is now challenged by the connectivity social media has permitted in today's world. This paradigm shift should allow us to consider ways to foster better cross-institutional collaboration, particularly for smaller fellowship programs with limited faculty support. Future research on this area may allow new ways of streamlining cross-institutional curriculum and content delivery to reduce the time and resources each fellowship spends in building this material in siloed fashions. An example as to how this might look is to consider ADGAP hosting a monthly virtual national didactics morning where a speaker from an academic medical center gives a talk on incarceration in the elderly, a speaker from a community hospital might then lead a session on delirium assessment in the SNF, followed by a seminar on falls from a faculty member at a 3rd institution. New ways to better harness cross-institutional resources that all fellows could benefit from have the potential to strengthen geriatrics networks nationwide, deliver high quality educational content to all geriatrics fellows, and reduce inequities in specific geriatric curricula such as the gaps in educational content pertaining to social determinants of health (SDOH) [52].

Teaching Geriatrics Fellows: Teaching Geriatrics Fellows How to Teach

Simpson and colleagues wrote in *JAGS in 2017*, "over the last decade, the healthcare system and geriatricians' roles have been rapidly changing, but fellowship training has not" [53]. Simpson and colleagues defined the jobs of the geriatrician of the future (as seen in Fig. 6.5) highlighting the Geriatrician as a master educator for Big "G" and little "g" geriatricians [53]. However, helping geriatrics fellows develop skills as educators can present a real challenge given the multitude of clinical skills and knowledge base they are expected to master during a busy, and at times dizzying, 1 year training period.

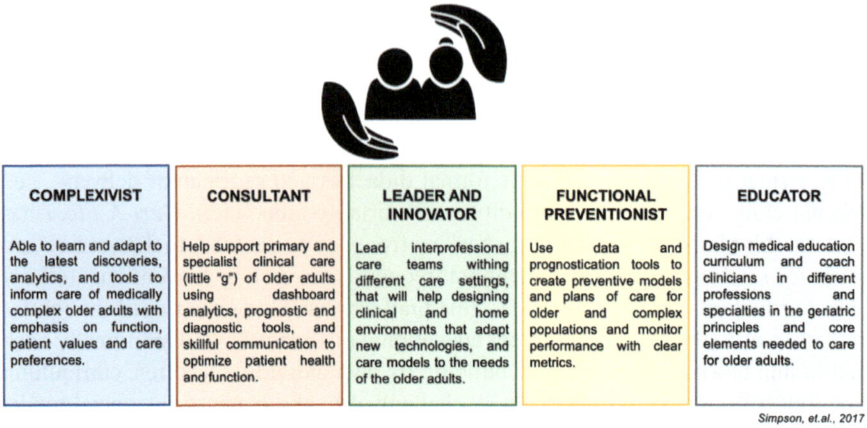

Fig. 6.5 Core roles of the geriatricians of 2025

Table 6.4 Proposed pearls to assist teaching geriatrics fellows how to teach

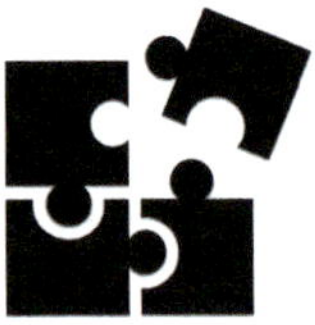 **PEARLS FOR EDUCATORS:** Teaching how to teach	✓ Educators must **advocate for and incorporate curriculum** covering topics such as **adult learning theory**[54], **setting goals and objectives**[55], **diagnosing the learner**[56], **receiving and giving feedback**[57], and **identifying the zone of proximal development**[44], which are key tools in helping fellows acquire skills to develop into "Big G" educators of the interdisciplinary teams they will be embedded in. ✓ Educators should **draw on tools that have already been created by other educators** fostering a sense of partnership and collaboration[58]. ✓ **Fellows should observe and be observed teaching in direct and indirect teaching activities across** different levels of learners (medical students, RNs, PAs, NPs, pharmacists, other physicians, patients, family members), over the course of their fellowship to help them foster diverse teaching experiences targeted to different audiences, which will allow fellows to build confidence and expertise in their roles as educators[59]. ✓ **Pair fellows with medical educators who have experience in mentoring and providing feedback**, encouraging these faculty to serve as coaches, frequently observing fellows teaching in real time and providing in-depth feedback to ensure growth occurs continuously across the fellowship year[60].

Major questions persist pertaining to the future of geriatrics fellowship training: *What would the ideal duration for geriatrics training be, knowing the inherited complexities that geriatrics medicine has accumulated over time? How should geriatricians define ourselves in the years ahead as medicine continues to change, adapt, and innovate at a rapid pace? What is the best way of teaching geriatrics fellows how to teach?*

Table 6.4 summarizes a few important themes and recommendations to help geriatric educators teach geriatrics fellows how to teach "Big G" and "little g" geriatricians, including but not limited to important concepts of aging in order to help develop other specialties and disciplines care for older adults.

Next Steps and Future Directions for Teaching Geriatrics Fellows

Geriatrics as a field has continued to grow, modernize, and adapt to a changing healthcare and societal landscape. With this progression the educational governing bodies that define how graduate medical education is delivered have established road maps that guide medical education in geriatric medicine through defining the Geriatric Medicine Milestones [16] and the Entrustable Professional Activities [20] which each fellow is expected to achieve by the completion of their training. At the same time, and perhaps in the hope of better defining geriatrics as a specialty, a core group of geriatric leaders and senior educators from across the USA came together in 2017 and defined the core roles of the geriatrician of 2025. These core features were enumerated to help ensure trainees will meet the needs of a growing and diversifying aging population (Fig. 6.5) [53].

As seen in Fig. 6.5, the jobs described by Simpson et al. define a geriatrician's role, not only as a physician caring for older adults, but as a "complexivist," "consultant," and "functional preventionist." Each of these roles is distinct and requires the development of specific knowledge and a skill set that will guide geriatricians through approaching the complexity that comes with aging, with the rigor of the scientific method, to deliver evidence based clinical care that is deeply person-centered [53].

Given the rapid evolution of geriatrics as a specialty, in depth and complexity, educators and leaders in geriatric medicine need to find new dynamic and creative avenues that allow geriatric fellows to develop the knowledge and skills required to become well-rounded geriatricians [61].

Training geriatrics fellows in leadership skill development is a priority that the field is beginning to tackle. Programs such as Tideswell Emerging Leaders in Aging (ELIA) [62] and the Health Policy in Aging Fellowship [63] have been crucial to bolstering leadership skills among faculty, the field has begun to provide leadership skill development earlier to fellows. Some notable initiatives include the *LEAP into Geriatrics Leadership Fellowship* developed by geriatricians at the Icahn School of Medicine at Mt. Sinai [64]. LEAP (Learn, Educate, Advocate, Promote) is a fellowship track, designed to give graduates core skill development to lead hospitals, health systems, quality improvement initiatives, and payer organizations. Fellows in this program pursue course development through the Institute for Health Care Improvement, patient safety and quality, and participate in committee leadership work across the health system, which helps them work on talent and leadership development initiatives alongside human resources (HR) [64]. Fellows also complete coursework on team building, emotional intelligence, and managing conflict. In addition to this, each fellow is also tasked with developing and piloting a project, alongside their mentor. It is hoped that this leadership track will serve as a model for other fellowships to build on across the country.

Another initiative includes the AGS/ADGAP Leadership and Life Skills Curriculum which was launched in 2021 through AGS and ADGAP, as an online course where all US geriatrics fellows have access to resources that will help cultivate and develop leadership skills [65].

Ensuring that the field of geriatrics remains committed to developing opportunities for advanced training for fellows beyond traditional internal medicine and family medicine residents remains crucial. In order to improve the training of Emergency Medicine physicians caring for aging adults, a small number of Geriatric Emergency Medicine (GEM) fellowship programs were developed [66] and although not ACGME accredited, they are regulated by academic bodies like the Society of Academic Emergency Medicine (SAEM) [67]. Likewise, Geriatric Oncology fellowship training opportunities have been developed and exist at a small number of large academic medical centers across the USA. Yet, while there is enthusiasm in other medicine sub-specialties, few of them have partnered with geriatrics to build combined fellowships in the ways that GEM and geriatric oncology have. Instead, fellows are left to pursue separate, distinct fellowships successively, like cardiology and then geriatrics [68]. In the years ahead, geriatric medicine fellowships and graduates must partner with training programs across the field of medicine to build collaboration and foster new opportunities for advanced training.

Leaders in medical education across the field of geriatrics have continued to innovate, create, and adapt new educational content and methods of delivery to meet the needs of present-day geriatrics fellows. Some examples of specific curricula that have been developed for this purpose can be found in Table 6.5.

The future of geriatric medicine is full of exciting opportunities for teaching geriatrics fellows. As geriatric educators continue to lead, evolve, and meet the next great challenges, it is important to recognize the enthusiasm and strengths that come from the diversity of training background and deep sense of teamwork and commitment advancing the field.

Table 6.5 Curricular innovations developed to deliver geriatrics content to different learners in diverse settings

Author/year	Title	Overview	Learners	Structure	Outcomes
Duggan M.C. et al. 2020 [51]	"Staying Afloat in the COVID-19 Storm: GERIAtrics Fellows Learning Online And Together (GERI-A-FLOAT)" https://doi.org/10.1111/jgs.16755	Educational series that uses virtual meetings to deepen knowledge of geriatric medicine and to convene fellows from across the country for networking and peer support	Geriatrics fellows in 1-year and advanced nonstandard programs from around the USA	• Weekly 1-h videoconferences • Instructional methods: flipped classroom, interactive lectures, workshops, and smaller breakout discussions	• Most benefit noted on sharing resources, clinical experiences, professional collaboration, and attention to mental health during a time of high stress • Most sessions were fellow led, allowing participants to learn from each other in diverse geographic regions and hospital systems
Robertson ML et al. 2022 [52]	"Inequities in the care of older adults: identifying education gaps in geriatric medicine fellowship" https://doi.org/10.1080/02701960.2022.2047037	Virtual learning collaborative GERIAtrics Fellows Learning Online And Together (GERI-A-FLOAT) developed to connect trainees nationwide A needs assessment was conducted to address gaps in education around social determinants of health (SDOH) and inform a curricular thread	Geriatrics fellows	• Voluntary, anonymous survey distributed to fellows through a broad network • The survey sought to understand prior curricula trainees had that were specifically focused on SDOH and older adults • Respondents prioritized topic areas for the curriculum	• This needs assessment is guiding a curricular thread for GERI-A-FLOAT and ideally larger milestones for fellowships • The most commonly taught concepts were ableism, ageism, and poverty • Respondents prioritized the topic of racism, ageism, and ableism • The survey identified a lack of consistent SDOH curricula pertaining to older adults across all levels of training
Danto-Nocton E.S. et al. 2018 [69]	"Strength in Numbers: A National Monthly Case Conference Series for Fellows" https://doi.org/10.1111/jgs.15448	The "Fellows Most Difficult Case Conference" is designed to broaden geriatric medicine fellows' exposure to cases and to faculty and fellows from around the country through a monthly telephone conference	Geriatrics fellow	• Monthly 60-min conference call • Fellow led, case-based presentation once a month • Teaching points provided by 2 faculty members	• Highly valued strategy for connecting fellows and faculty beyond their own programs to the wider community of geriatric medicine specialists • Allowed to broaden fellows' understanding of different approaches, perspectives, and frameworks that may be used to address the needs of complex older adults

(continued)

Table 6.5 (continued)

Author/year	Title	Overview	Learners	Structure	Outcomes
Ramaswamy R. et al. 2020 [70]	"Implementation of an evidence-based medicine curriculum in a fellowship program: Can it influence clinical practice?" https://doi.org/10.1080/02701960.2020.1777409	Implementation, and evaluation of a multi-pronged Evidence-Based Medicine (EBM) curriculum in a Geriatrics and Palliative Medicine fellowship program that included deliberate practice and feedback, and an emphasis on application to geriatric patient care	Geriatrics, Hospice, and Palliative Medicine fellows	• Two workshop-style sessions, each lasting 1–1.5 h, at the beginning of the academic year introduced fellows to the importance of EBM, clinical question formulation, relevant literature search strategies, and literature appraisal techniques • A longitudinal component included weekly JC discussions, monthly oral presentations at an EBM Case Conference, and quarterly EBM worksheet completion over the course of the academic year	• Pretest and posttest questionnaires revealed an increase in confidence in fellows' ability to teach not only specific EBM concepts but also the steps of EBM cycle question formulation, literature search, critical appraisal, and application to patient care
Denson K et al. 2014 [71]	"Geriatric Oncology OSCE: Using Geriatric Assessment Tools to Guide Patient Treatment Decisions" https://doi.org/10.15766/mep_2374-8265.9860	Development and implementation of a geriatric oncology educational OSCE for oncology fellows at the Medical College of Wisconsin (MCW)	Oncology fellows	• Initial 1-h didactic presentation/demonstration session introducing geriatric assessment tools • Second session, 1 week later, with a two-case OSCE session followed by a debrief session, designed to give learners practice using the tools with standardized patients as both an educational/assessment method	• This curriculum was successfully implemented in the oncology fellowship core curriculum • The OSCEs were an effective method for increasing fellows' confidence and skills in caring for elderly patients • The OSCE cases were believable and applicable to clinical practice

Sehgal M et al. 2019 [72]	"Introducing Aquifer Geriatrics, the American Geriatrics Society National Online Curriculum" https://doi.org/10.1111/jgs.15813	This curriculum aims to help address the national shortage of geriatrics educators, complement current teaching, bridge content gaps in geriatrics education, and standardize geriatrics-focused educational content	Learners in different professions and levels of training	• Evidence-based, peer-reviewed, online case-based modules based on the Association of American Medical Colleges/John A. Hartford Foundation Minimum Geriatrics Competencies for Medical Students	• Innovative online teaching resource for teaching geriatrics-focused content • Provides an efficient and engaging way to teach increasing numbers of healthcare trainees and professionals geriatric principles and evidence-based management of geriatric syndromes
Gardhouse AI et al. 2017 [73]	"#GeriMedJC: The Twitter Complement to the Traditional-Format Geriatric Medicine Journal Club" https://doi.org/10.1111/jgs.14920	A Twitter hashtag, #GeriMedJC, established in August 2014 to complement the traditional-format geriatric medicine journal club	Open to the public through the Twitter platform	• Monthly 1-h live, 23-h asynchronous Twitter-based complement to the traditional-format geriatric medicine journal club • The Twitter moderator tweets from the handle @ GeriMedJC; encourages use of #GeriMedJC; and invites content experts, study authors, and followers to participate in critical appraisal of medical literature	• Developing a Twitter complement to a live traditional geriatric medicine journal club is feasible • #GeriMedJC has demonstrated steady growth and global participation and that an online journal club can broaden the community of participants beyond what is typical of a traditional, isolated academic silo consisting of mainly geriatrician and trainee participants
Saraiva MD et al. 2016 [74]	"Evaluating Communication Skills of Geriatrics Fellows: Interrater Agreement of an Objective Structured Clinical Examination" https://doi.org/10.1111/jgs.13918	Evaluation of the interrater reliability of a communication assessment scale of the Objective Structured Clinical Examination (OSCE)	Geriatrics fellows in their first and second year of training	• A communication station, from a 10 station OSCE, was video recorded to analyze its reliability • Six examiners (five geriatricians, one psychologist) who had no previous contact with the fellows evaluated the video-recorded station • Examiners received written instructions on how to rate the fellow's performance according to a 16-item, 5-point Likert scale (1 = very poor, 2 = poor, 3 = fair, 4 = good, 5 = perfect)	• This study revealed that evaluating communication skills based on a single examiner results in considerably lower reliability levels than generally considered adequate • Grading systems need to be based on three or more examiners to achieve acceptable interrater agreement

(continued)

Table 6.5 (continued)

Author/year	Title	Overview	Learners	Structure	Outcomes
O'Sullivan P et al. 2008 [75]	"Development and Implementation of an Objective Structured Clinical Examination to Provide Formative Feedback on Communication and Interpersonal Skills in Geriatric Training" https://doi.org/10.1111/j.1532--5415.2008.01860.x	Pilot study in which clinician-educators affiliated with the geriatrics training programs at Beth Israel Deaconess Medical Center and Boston University Medical Center designed and piloted a novel Objective Structured Clinical Examination (OSCE) to assess the communication and interpersonal skills of medical, dental, and geriatric psychiatry fellows	Medical, dental, and geriatric psychiatry fellows	• The OSCE consisted of three stations where geriatricians and standardized patients evaluated candidates using specifically designed checklists and an abbreviated version of the Master Interview Rating Scale • Communication skills were assessed through performance of specific "real life" clinical tasks, such as obtaining a medical history, explaining a diagnosis and prognosis, giving therapeutic instructions, and counseling • Interpersonal skills were assessed through the effect of the communication between doctor and standardized patient on fostering trust, relieving anxiety, and establishing a therapeutic relationship	• This pilot study demonstrated that the OSCE format of assessment provides a valid means of evaluating the communication and interpersonal skills of interdisciplinary geriatric trainees and provides a valuable forum for formative assessment and feedback

Gelfman LP et al. 2014 [76]	"The Effectiveness of the Geritalk Communication Skills Course: A Real-Time Assessment of Skill Acquisition and Deliberate Practice" https://doi.org/10.1016/j.jpainsymman.2013.12.231	Evaluation of the effectiveness of the Geritalk communication skills course and impact on skill acquisition by directly observing participants leading family meetings before and after the course and the sustained deliberate practice of the participants two months after the course	First-year Geriatrics or Palliative Medicine fellows	• Two-day Geritalk program • Curriculum of didactic presentations and demonstrations, small-group communication skills practice, and future skills practice commitment • The didactic sessions addressed basic communication skills, giving bad news, negotiating goals of care, and forgoing life-sustaining treatment, including do-not-resuscitate orders	• The Geritalk communication skills course is effective at teaching both the fundamental communication skills necessary to lead a family meeting and advanced communication skills • The course was effective particularly with participant acquisition of "empathic continuers" skill • The study demonstrates that the participants reported continued deliberate practice of these skills two months after the course
Callahan KE et al. 2013 [43]	"A Longitudinal, Experiential Quality Improvement Curriculum Meeting ACGME Competencies for Geriatrics Fellows: Lessons Learned" https://doi.org/10.1080/02701960.2013.815179	Development, implementation, and evaluation of an evidence-based Quality Improvement (QI) curriculum for geriatrics fellows	Geriatrics fellows	• The evidence-based curriculum included didactics and a fellow-led QI intervention based on audit and feedback through the Practice Improvement Module in Care of the Vulnerable Elderly • QI knowledge, attitudes, and behaviors were assessed before and after the improvement project	• Fellows' knowledge of QI improved ($p = 0.0156$), but behavior did not change significantly across a short-term improvement project • A structured focus group with fellows revealed themes of accountability and the importance of interprofessional teamwork in QI • QI education for geriatrics fellows can be feasible, well received, and prepare future physician leaders for patient-centered care, performance measurement, and effecting systems change

(continued)

Table 6.5 (continued)

Author/year	Title	Overview	Learners	Structure	Outcomes
Higuchi M et al. 2013 [77]	"Developing Future Nursing Home Medical Directors: A Curriculum for Geriatric Medicine Fellows" https://doi.org/10.1016/j.jamda.2012.10.008	Novel medical director's curriculum for first-year geriatric medicine fellows to prepare them for the role of nursing home medical director	Geriatrics fellows	• The curriculum consists of seven seminars that have been integrated into the didactic sessions during the first year of fellowship • Core content areas include: (1) roles and responsibilities of the medical director, (2) infection control, (3) physician documentation, (4) federal regulations and state surveys, (5) quality improvement, (6) culture change in nursing homes, and (7) transitions in care • All topics were discussed using the framework described by the American Medical Directors Association's position statement on the roles and responsibilities of the nursing home medical director	• First curriculum described in the literature designed to prepare geriatric medicine fellows for the role of medical director in nursing homes • The curriculum format was redesigned to mirror AMDA's position statement regarding the roles and responsibilities of the medical director in LTC facilities • Content covered in the curriculum includes common issues that often need to be addressed by the medical director. It also addresses the need for fellows to understand the "big picture" context, as well as learn about the "basics" of nursing home operations • The instructional methods used in this curriculum provide more case-based, interactive learning and application, and the opportunity to share experiences. Ample time is provided for questions, answers, and discussion to review board examination type questions

Acknowledgements *Ryan Zitnay Chippendale, MD.* Assistant professor of medicine at Boston University School of Medicine. Geriatric Medicine Fellowship Program Director at BMC/BUSM and co-director for the Geriatric-Oncology combined Fellowship at BMC

Eric Widera, MD. Professor of Medicine, Director, Hospice & Palliative Care Service (SFVAMC), Associate Program Director, Geriatric Medicine Fellowship Program (UCSF).

Nina Blachman, MD. Assistant Professor, Department of Medicine at NYU Grossman School of Medicine. Director, Geriatrics Fellowship Program. Merrin Master Clinician Fellow

References

1. Fried LP, Hall WJ. Editorial: leading on behalf of an aging society: leading on behalf of an aging society. J Am Geriatr Soc. 2008;56(10):1791–5. https://doi.org/10.1111/j.1532-5415.2008.01939.x.
2. Petriceks AH, Olivas JC, Srivastava S. Trends in geriatrics graduate medical education programs and positions, 2001 to 2018. Gerontol Geriatr Med. 2018;4:2333721418777659. https://doi.org/10.1177/2333721418777659.
3. Tinetti M. Mainstream or extinction: can defining who we are save geriatrics? J Am Geriatr Soc. 2016;64(7):1400–4. https://doi.org/10.1111/jgs.14181.
4. Callahan KE, Tumosa N, Leipzig RM. Big 'G' and Little 'g' geriatrics education for physicians. J Am Geriatr Soc. 2017;65(10):2313–7. https://doi.org/10.1111/jgs.14996.
5. Morley JE. A brief history of geriatrics. J Gerontol Ser A Biol Med Sci. 2004;59(11):1132–52. https://doi.org/10.1093/gerona/59.11.1132.
6. Bragg EJ, Warshaw GA. Evolution of geriatric medicine fellowship training in the United States. Am J Geriatr Psychiatry. 2003;11(3):280–90. https://doi.org/10.1097/00019442-200305000-00005.
7. ACGME Home. 2022. https://www.acgme.org/.
8. ACGME. ACGME program requirements for graduate medical education in geriatric medicine. ACGME Program requirements. 2021, p. 52.
9. ACGME. ACGME program requirements for graduate medical education in geriatric psychiatry. ACGME program requirements. 2020, p. 50.
10. J. Hartford Foundation. A brief history of geriatrics. https://www.johnahartford.org/ar2005/2_a_brief_history.html. Accessed 29 September 2021.
11. Blachman NL, Blaum CS, Zabar S. Reasons geriatrics fellows choose geriatrics as a career, and implications for workforce recruitment. Gerontol Geriatr Educ. 2021;42(1):38–45. https://doi.org/10.1080/02701960.2019.1604341.
12. Medical Student Training in Aging Research (MSTAR) Program. American federation for aging research. https://www.afar.org/grants/mstar. Accessed 25 July 2022.
13. ACGME Internal Medicine Milestones.pdf. https://www.acgme.org/portals/0/pdfs/milestones/internalmedicinemilestones.pdf. Accessed 27 September 2021.
14. ACGME Family Medicine Milestones.pdf. https://www.acgme.org/portals/0/pdfs/milestones/familymedicinemilestones.pdf. Accessed September 27, 2021.
15. ACGME Psychiatry Medicine Milestones. https://www.acgme.org/globalassets/pdfs/milestones/psychiatrymilestones.pdf. Accessed 12 May 2022.
16. ACGME Geriatric Medicine Milestones.pdf. https://www.acgme.org/Portals/0/PDFs/Milestones/GeriatricMedicineMilestones.pdf. Accessed 4 August 2021.
17. ACGME Geriatric Psychiatry Milestones.pdf. https://www.acgme.org/globalassets/pdfs/milestones/geriatricpsychiatrymilestones.pdf. Accessed 3 May 2022.
18. Holmboe E. Competency-based training. The milestone guidebook. Chicago: ACGME; 2020. p. 41.
19. AGS. ADGAP fellowship assessment toolkit. https://geriatricscareonline.org/toc/fellowship_assessment/TK010#.
20. Leipzig RM, Sauvigné K, Granville LJ, et al. What is a geriatrician? American Geriatrics Society and Association of Directors of Geriatric Academic Programs End-of-Training Entrustable

Professional Activities for Geriatric Medicine. J Am Geriatr Soc. 2014;62(5):924–9. https://doi.org/10.1111/jgs.12825.
21. Clarfield AM. Dr. Ignatz Nascher and the birth of geriatrics. CMAJ. 1990;143(9):944–8.
22. Aronson L. Elderhood: redefining aging, transforming medicine, reimagining life. London: Bloomsbury Publishing; 2019.
23. Fried LP, Tangen CM, Walston J, et al. Frailty in older adults: evidence for a phenotype. J Gerontol Ser A Biol Med Sci. 2001;56(3):M146–57. https://doi.org/10.1093/gerona/56.3.M146.
24. Inouye SK, Studenski S, Tinetti ME, Kuchel GA. Geriatric syndromes: clinical, research and policy implications of a core geriatric concept. J Am Geriatr Soc. 2007;55(5):780–91. https://doi.org/10.1111/j.1532-5415.2007.01156.x.
25. Tinetti M, Huang A, Molnar F. The geriatrics 5M's: a new way of communicating what we do. J Am Geriatr Soc. 2017;65(9):2115. https://doi.org/10.1111/jgs.14979.
26. Schwartz AW, Hawley CE, Strong JV, et al. A workshop for interprofessional trainees using the geriatrics 5Ms framework. J Am Geriatr Soc. 2020;68(8):1857–63. https://doi.org/10.1111/jgs.16574.
27. Tinetti ME. Association of patient priorities–aligned decision-making with patient outcomes and ambulatory health care burden among older adults with multiple chronic conditions a non-randomized clinical trial. JAMA Intern Med. 2019;179(12):1688–97. https://doi.org/10.1001/jamainternmed.2019.4235.
28. Lee SJ, Leipzig RM, Walter LC. Incorporating lag time to benefit into prevention decisions for older adults. JAMA. 2013;310(24):2609. https://doi.org/10.1001/jama.2013.282612.
29. Ellis-Smith C, Tunnard I, Dawkins M, et al. Managing clinical uncertainty in older people towards the end of life: a systematic review of person-centred tools. BMC Palliat Care. 2021;20(1):168. https://doi.org/10.1186/s12904-021-00845-9.
30. Ghosh AK, Joshi S. Tools to manage medical uncertainty. Diabetes Metab Syndr Clin Res Rev. 2020;14(5):1529–33. https://doi.org/10.1016/j.dsx.2020.07.055.
31. Nee J, Chippendale RZ, Feuerstein JD. Screening for colon cancer in older adults: risks, benefits, and when to stop. Mayo Clin Proc. 2020;95(1):184–96. https://doi.org/10.1016/j.mayocp.2019.02.021.
32. Mini-Cog©. Quick screening for early dementia detection. https://mini-cog.com/. Accessed 25 July 2022.
33. MoCA. Cognitive assessment. https://www.mocatest.org/. Accessed 25 July 2022.
34. Parker SG, McCue P, Phelps K, et al. What is comprehensive geriatric assessment (CGA)? An umbrella review. Age Ageing. 2018;47(1):149–55. https://doi.org/10.1093/ageing/afx166.
35. Clegg A, Bates C, Young J, et al. Development and validation of an electronic frailty index using routine primary care electronic health record data. Age Ageing. 2016;45(3):353–60. https://doi.org/10.1093/ageing/afw039.
36. ePrognosis. https://eprognosis.ucsf.edu/. Accessed 25 July 2022.
37. Siu AL, U.S. Preventive Services Task Force. Screening for breast cancer: U.S. Preventive Services Task Force recommendation statement. Ann Intern Med. 2016;164(4):279. https://doi.org/10.7326/M15-2886.
38. Krist AH, Davidson KW, et al. Screening for lung cancer: US preventive services task force recommendation statement. JAMA. 2021;325(10):962. https://doi.org/10.1001/jama.2021.1117.
39. Studenski S. Gait speed and survival in older adults. JAMA. 2011;305(1):50. https://doi.org/10.1001/jama.2010.1923.
40. Mitchell SL. Advanced dementia. N Engl J Med. 2015;372(26):2533–40. https://doi.org/10.1056/NEJMcp1412652.
41. Gheihman G, Johnson M, Simpkin AL. Twelve tips for thriving in the face of clinical uncertainty. Med Teach. 2020;42(5):493–9. https://doi.org/10.1080/0142159X.2019.1579308.
42. Chang A, Fernandez H, Cayea D, et al. Complexity in graduate medical education: a collaborative education agenda for internal medicine and geriatric medicine. J Gen Intern Med. 2014;29(6):940–6. https://doi.org/10.1007/s11606-013-2752-2.
43. Callahan KE, Rogers MT, Lovato JF, Fernandez HM. A longitudinal, experiential quality improvement curriculum meeting ACGME competencies for geriatrics fellows: lessons learned. Gerontol Geriatr Educ. 2013;34(4):372–92. https://doi.org/10.1080/02701960.2013.815179.

44. Dunphy BC, Dunphy SL. Assisted performance and the zone of proximal development (ZPD); a potential framework for providing surgical education. Austr J Educ Dev Psychol. 2003;3:48–58.
45. Palamara K, Kauffman C, Chang Y, et al. Professional development coaching for residents: results of a 3-year positive psychology coaching intervention. J Gen Intern Med. 2018;33(11):1842–4. https://doi.org/10.1007/s11606-018-4589-1.
46. Huppert LA, Santhosh L, Babik JM. Trends in US internal medicine residency and fellowship applications during the COVID-19 pandemic vs previous years. JAMA Netw Open. 2021;4(4):e218199. https://doi.org/10.1001/jamanetworkopen.2021.8199.
47. ADGAP_Tip_Sheet_on_Virtual_Interviewing.pdf.
48. Mezera V, Ekdahl AW, Bertschi D, et al. The experiences of early career geriatricians throughout Europe during the COVID-19 pandemic. Eur Geriatr Med. 2022;13(3):719–24. https://doi.org/10.1007/s41999-021-00605-1.
49. Chopra S, Solomon P, Goldhirsch SL, Fernandez H, Cummings K. Geriatrics fellowship during COVID-19: expanding impact, using innovation and maintaining balance. Gerontol Geriatr Educ. 2022;43(1):55–63. https://doi.org/10.1080/02701960.2021.1968855.
50. Nearing KA, Lum HD, Dang S, et al. National geriatric network rapidly addresses trainee telehealth needs in response to COVID-19. J Am Geriatr Soc. 2020;68(9):1907–12. https://doi.org/10.1111/jgs.16704.
51. Duggan MC, Goroncy A, Christmas C, Chippendale R. Staying afloat in the COVID-19 storm: GERIAtrics fellows learning online and together (GERI-A-FLOAT). J Am Geriatr Soc. 2020;68(10):E54–6. https://doi.org/10.1111/jgs.16755.
52. Robertson ML, Mushero N, Demers L, Goroncy A, Chippendale R. Inequities in the care of older adults: identifying education gaps in geriatric medicine fellowship. Gerontol Geriatr Educ. 2022;2022:1–7. https://doi.org/10.1080/02701960.2022.2047037.
53. Simpson D, Leipzig RM, Sauvigné K. The 2025 big "G" geriatrician: defining job roles to guide fellowship training. J Am Geriatr Soc. 2017;65(10):2308–12. https://doi.org/10.1111/jgs.14995.
54. Taylor DCM, Hamdy H. Adult learning theories: implications for learning and teaching in medical education: AMEE Guide No. 83. Med Teach. 2013;35(11):e1561–72. https://doi.org/10.3109/0142159X.2013.828153.
55. Mullan PB, Lypson ML. Communicating your program's goals and objectives. J Grad Med Educ. 2011;3(4):574–6. https://doi.org/10.4300/JGME-03-04-31.
56. Knowles MS, Holton EF, Swanson RA. The adult learner: the definitive classic in adult education and human resource development. 6th ed. Amsterdam: Elsevier; 2005.
57. Thach S. Managing the difficult learning situation. Fam Med. 2000;32(5):307–9.
58. Miloslavsky EM, Degnan K, McNeill J, McSparron JI. Use of fellow as clinical teacher (FACT) curriculum for teaching during consultation: effect on subspecialty fellow teaching skills. J Grad Med Educ. 2017;9(3):345–50. https://doi.org/10.4300/JGME-D-16-00464.1.
59. Streiter S, Loewenthal J, Berry S, Schwartz AW. Better together: promoting geriatrics education across residency specialties with a pilot peer teaching exchange. J Am Geriatr Soc. 2019;67(10):E1–3. https://doi.org/10.1111/jgs.16170.
60. Parks K, Miller J, Westcott A. Chapter 8: coaching in graduate medical education, 2017, p. 5.
61. Pelleg AR, Schiller G, Goldhirsch SL, Fernandez HM, Lindenberger EC. Geriatrics and palliative medicine leadership is needed now more than ever: what are the training gaps? J Am Geriatr Soc. 2021;69(4):1063–70. https://doi.org/10.1111/jgs.17050.
62. Foley KT, Farrell TW, Salzman B, et al. Learning to lead: reflections from the Tideswell-AGS-ADGAP emerging leaders in aging program scholars. J Am Geriatr Soc. 2019;67(3):434–6. https://doi.org/10.1111/jgs.15701.
63. Medina-Walpole A, Fonzi J, Katz PR. Academic career development in geriatric fellowship training. J Am Geriatr Soc. 2007;55(12):2061–7. https://doi.org/10.1111/j.1532-5415.2007.01425.x.
64. Icahn School of Medicine at Mount Sinai. LEAP into geriatrics leadership fellowship. Icahn School of Medicine. https://icahn.mssm.edu/education/residencies-fellowships/list/leap-geriatrics-leadership. Accessed 22 July 2022.

65. AGS/ADGAP leadership and life skills curriculum community. https://myagsonline.americangeriatrics.org/llsc/home. Accessed 22 July 2022.
66. Rosen T, Liu SW, Cameron-Comasco L, et al. Geriatric emergency medicine fellowships: current state of specialized training for emergency physicians in optimizing care for older adults. AEM Educ Train. 2020;4(1):S122–9. https://doi.org/10.1002/aet2.10428.
67. Society for academic emergency medicine (SAEM). https://www.saem.org/. Accessed 22 July 2022.
68. Hummel SL, Alpert CM, Galatas C, Afilalo J. Training geriatric cardiologists for an aging population: time to get going. Am J Med. 2017;130(4):385–6. https://doi.org/10.1016/j.amjmed.2016.10.031.
69. Danto-Nocton ES, Simpson D, Rasansky M, Pascarella LC, Malone ML. Strength in numbers: a national monthly case conference series for fellows. J Am Geriatr Soc. 2018;66(7):1404–8. https://doi.org/10.1111/jgs.15448.
70. Ramaswamy R, Leipzig RM, Hung WW. Implementation of an evidence-based medicine curriculum in a fellowship program: can it influence clinical practice? Gerontol Geriatr Educ. 2020;2020:1–10. https://doi.org/10.1080/02701960.2020.1777409.
71. Denson K, Manzi G, Foy P, Giever T, Rehm J. Geriatric Oncology OSCE: using geriatric assessment tools to guide patient treatment decisions. MedEdPORTAL. 2014;10:9860. https://doi.org/10.15766/mep_2374-8265.9860.
72. Sehgal M, Syed Q, Callahan KE, et al. Introducing aquifer geriatrics, the American Geriatrics Society National Online Curriculum. J Am Geriatr Soc. 2019;67(4):811–7. https://doi.org/10.1111/jgs.15813.
73. Gardhouse AI, Budd L, Yang SYC, Wong CL. #GeriMedJC: The Twitter complement to the traditional-format geriatric medicine journal club. J Am Geriatr Soc. 2017;65(6):1347–51. https://doi.org/10.1111/jgs.14920.
74. Saraiva MD, de Paulo ML, Avelino-Silva TJ, et al. Evaluating communication skills of geriatrics fellows: interrater agreement of an objective structured clinical examination. J Am Geriatr Soc. 2016;64(1):206–7. https://doi.org/10.1111/jgs.13918.
75. O'Sullivan P, Chao S, Russell M, Levine S, Fabiny A. Development and implementation of an objective structured clinical examination to provide formative feedback on communication and interpersonal skills in geriatric training. J Am Geriatr Soc. 2008;56(9):1730–5. https://doi.org/10.1111/j.1532-5415.2008.01860.x.
76. Gelfman LP, Lindenberger E, Fernandez H, et al. The effectiveness of the geritalk communication skills course: a real-time assessment of skill acquisition and deliberate practice. J Pain Symptom Manag. 2014;48(4):738–44. https://doi.org/10.1016/j.jpainsymman.2013.12.231.
77. Higuchi M, Wen A, Masaki K. Developing future nursing home medical directors: a curriculum for geriatric medicine fellows. J Am Med Dir Assoc. 2013;14(3):157–60. https://doi.org/10.1016/j.jamda.2012.10.008.

Chapter 7
Continuing Medical Education in Geriatric Medicine

Rachel Stark and Reena Karani

An urgent need exists to develop and implement high quality continuing medical education (CME) in geriatrics. The growth of the older adult population in the USA, evidence that a large majority of this group has at least one chronic disease requiring consistent care and management [1], and the ongoing shortage of specialty trained geriatricians have important implications for CME of providers. In order to meet the medical and psychosocial needs of this growing population, in an environment of constantly evolving scientific evidence, providers must be offered CME opportunities that are relevant, evidence-based, practical, and ultimately improve patient experiences and outcomes.

We observe that this need is not new [2], nor has it evolved suddenly. Rather, core education in the care of the aging adult has persistently comprised a narrow sliver of curricular time in formal undergraduate and graduate medical education for decades, often leaving practicing medical providers without the basic skills and knowledge they need to provide high quality, evidence-based, patient-centered care to an aging population. Indeed, this observation does not even account for the dynamic nature of the evolving knowledge base in geriatrics, on which the principle of continuing medical education should be overlaid. If our observation is not new, and this need has existed and has been recognized for decades, why do we find ourselves without adequate CME to address knowledge gaps in providers caring for older adults? Likely part of the reason rests in our inadequate understanding of optimal ways to deliver CME, in general, and lack of optimal models to address geriatrics CME

R. Stark (✉)
Veterans Affairs Boston Healthcare System, Boston, MA, USA
e-mail: rachel.stark@va.gov

R. Karani
Icahn School of Medicine at Mount Sinai, New York, NY, USA
e-mail: reena.karani@mssm.edu

A. W. Schwartz (ed.), *Medical Education in Geriatrics*,
https://doi.org/10.1007/978-3-031-32499-4_7

specifically. In this chapter we aim to provide an overview of CME best practices, the state of CME in geriatrics to date, and recommendations for the optimal practical design and implementation of CME in geriatrics going forward.

Principles of an Optimal Continuing Medical Education Program

An optimal CME program should be designed with the goal of meeting learning objectives for participants and, ultimately, that participants implement what was learned to improve health outcomes for patients. A review of the CME literature identifies few studies that have carefully examined the impact of CME programs on learners, and even fewer that have identified patient-related outcomes. Yet higher quality studies indicate that CME can positively impact physician performance. CME programs are more likely to impact patient-related outcomes if designed to be interactive, to utilize multiple methods, to include multiple exposures, are of longer duration, and focus on content that has been identified to be important to physicians [3]. Spaced learning, which involves [specified] educational encounters that are devoted to the same [specified] material, and distributed over a [specified] number of periods separated by a [specified] interstudy interval, with a [specified] learning outcome after a [specified] retention interval, has also been utilized in CME [4]. Spaced learning, using online platforms has been a successful tool to improve clinical knowledge and foster changes in clinical practice [5].

It has been difficult to study the impact of CME programs, as there are many outcome variables to consider, and these can be difficult to measure because of confounders. Allen et al. [6] conducted a review of the CME literature identifying twelve categories of impact that emerged: knowledge, practice change, skill, confidence, attitudes, career development, networking, user outcomes, intention to change, organizational change, personal change, and scholarly accomplishments. Unsurprisingly, knowledge was the most commonly measured outcome in CME studies, and scholarly accomplishments were the least common. This same group developed the Continuing Professional Development Impacts Survey (CPDIS) [7], a tool to measure the impact of CME on participants, beyond knowledge, skills, and attitudes. The CPDIS measures domains of learning and self-efficacy, networking and building community, and achievement and validation, providing a practical resource for researchers and educators to measure the impact of their programs using more relevant outcome measures.

Continuing Medical Education Programs in Geriatrics

While CME is most often targeted toward members of one specialty, CME in the area of geriatrics presents some particular challenges. Given that older adults receive care from physicians across the breadth of medical specialties and that comprehensive geriatric care requires high levels of interprofessional collaboration, CME efforts must be developed for geriatricians, other specialties that have significant numbers of older adult patients (such as general internal medicine, family medicine, surgery, etc.) and interprofessional healthcare team members. Moreover, the content and focus of geriatrics CME must be tailored to the particular roles and responsibilities of the practitioner as well as be calibrated to previous training received by them. As a result, teachers of geriatrics CME need to have a broad understanding of scope of practice in various clinical contexts, as well as expertise in medical education to facilitate participants' achieving their learning goals.

Thomas and colleagues reviewed papers published on CME in geriatrics and interviewed authors to gain insights about effective CME programs in the field [8]. The authors noted that despite many existing opportunities for CME programs in geriatrics, there is a dearth of publications related to these programs, confirming that while there may be adequate access to CME in geriatrics, very little is known about best practices and outcomes of these programs. Their review of published papers, and complementary structured interviews with CME leaders, identified important areas of consideration when developing CME in geriatrics, including elements of successful program implementation and participant recruitment, as well as considerations for optimal train the trainer courses in geriatrics (Table 7.1). Additionally, they identified many barriers to developing successful CME programs, not unique to geriatrics, including the time and expense to develop programs, lack of standard on best practices for effective CME, and physical space constraints. Barriers also exist at the level of the learner, including time, geographic and financial limitations, as well as perception of utility of the program. The pivot to more online learning during the COVID-19 pandemic may demonstrate opportunities for the development and growth of future online CME programs in geriatrics that are accessible to more learners and would address the barriers of geography, space constraints, and travel limitations.

Our review of the literature identifies several themes that emerge in the approach to CME programs in geriatrics, many of which reflect best practices from the limited CME literature. Several approaches to CME have been utilized, including a train the trainer model, immersive learning (i.e. workshops), and longitudinal learning, with ongoing education over time (Table 7.2). CME courses in geriatrics with an emphasis on interprofessional training have also had important impacts. Additionally, some teaching tools have been utilized with particular success, including the use of toolkits, or online resources, that can be utilized by learners indefinitely after course completion.

Train the Trainer

One frequently utilized approach for CME is the "train the trainer" model (TTT), in which a group of learners are trained in content mastery such that they can then, in turn, disseminate knowledge and skills as teachers of larger groups of learners themselves. This model has been successfully utilized in many geriatrics CME

Table 7.1 Areas of consideration for developing and implementing geriatrics CME (this is Table 3 from Thomas et al. [8])

Program development	• Allow ample time for development of training • Address known or commonly experienced barriers • Use high quality existing products to avoid "reinventing the wheel" • Involve trainers in development from the start to increase investment • Use templates in developing electronic products to increase efficiency • Use highly interactive multimedia simulations to save time • Design quick interventions for clinical practice • Connect interventions to activities physicians are already doing in practice • Use case-based training to make content come alive • Use different strategies for training precontemplative and contemplative learners • Create public awareness of health issues to motivate physician change
Participant recruitment	• Provide CME credit • Identify thought leaders or "stars" in community and get them on board • Incorporate a "carrot" into training, such as recertification, performance improvement, generation of more revenue
Implementation	• Hold trainings in a nice setting with good food • Use technology to reach physicians who have access to equipment • Offer participants templates for obtaining CME credit
Train the trainer programs	• Focus on teaching skills in model development so that trainers will have the skills to teach others effectively • Assure peer educators that is okay to teach colleagues about geriatrics even though they themselves are not geriatric specialists • Engage in regular one-on-one communication to keep trainers actively enthusiastic about the program • Network with opinion leaders at training sessions

programs. TTT is an attractive approach to CME because it is cost efficient and has the potential to impact a large number of learners. TTT models also have the flexibility to be structured as a longitudinal curriculum or as immersive workshops and can be successfully implemented at a single institution or include learners from across large regions.

Mazotti et al. [9] describe a TTT model of geriatrics faculty development in which hospitalists at a single academic medical center participated in a curriculum in the care of older adults, embedded within the structure of already existing faculty meetings. In turn, these hospitalists then taught the same curriculum to residents they supervised on the inpatient wards. Program participants reported greater confidence in their care of older adults, as did the residents who learned from these hospitalists. Similarly, a single day immersive TTT workshop of faculty at 2 Oregon hospitals [10] utilized multiple educational modalities (i.e. didactic teaching methods, small group sessions with scripted cases and standardized learners, and pocket teaching guides) and demonstrated increased knowledge and self-reported confidence in caring for geriatric populations, as well as in teaching geriatric-specific content to residents.

Table 7.2 Summary of selected geriatric CME programs

Authors	Program description	TTT (Yes/No)	Outcomes measured (Yes/No)
Mazotti et al.	TTT model of geriatrics curriculum for hospitalist faculty	Yes	Yes
Eckstrom et al.	Single day TTT geriatrics workshop using multiple educational modalities	Yes	Yes
Levine et al.	Geriatricians trained 60 non-expert peers, who then trained over 1000 learners; sessions centered around 3 core concepts using toolkits	Yes	Yes
Christmas et al.	Three day geriatrics mini with optional one year longitudinal mentorship by geriatrician faculty	No	Yes
Willett et al.	Three year community based CME program for generalists	No	Yes
Kramer et al.	Longitudinal geriatrics CME for physicians and other members of the interprofessional team who care for the elderly in rural areas; involves didactic components as well as QI project, and face-to-face and distance learning components	No	Yes
Ford et al.	Yearlong curriculum for physicians and interprofessional team members	No	No
Podrazik et al.	CME program for physicians providing care to hospitalized older adults; involves use of portable teaching modules	Yes	No
Toner et al.	CME program aimed at the team of caregivers for the elderly in rural and underserved areas	No	No

TTT models can also be utilized to train a core faculty, who will then reach a large audience of learners beyond a single institution or region. Levine et al. [11] developed a geriatrics CME program centered around three core topic areas including memory loss, incontinence, and depression, wherein expert geriatrics faculty trained 60 non-expert peers to facilitate small group teaching on the same topics using evidence-based toolkits. This relatively small group of trainers were then able to reach an audience of over 1000 learners, and measured positive outcomes from them having participated in the program including improved self-reported knowledge, attitudes, and office practices measured at the time of training and six months later. In this study, the use of toolkits that were used in the session, and then referred to later, was felt to be integral to the success of the CME program. Further discussion of faculty development training appears in Chap. 22.

Longitudinal Impacts Following an Intensive Course

Because less is known about optimal CME teaching approaches that result in sustained meaningful impact, it is imperative for CME developers to evaluate relevant educational and clinical outcomes at the end of an experience and, whenever possible, at more distant time points following program completion. Christmas et al. [12] reported on their implementation of a geriatrics "mini-fellowship" CME program for non-geriatric clinician educators, delivered as a 3 days intensive curriculum followed by the option of up to a year of mentorship by a geriatrics faculty upon completion of the course. The program was evaluated at the time of course completion, and again six months later. Importantly, the authors designed their intervention to assess sustainability of the lessons and skills learned in the curriculum and noted a small proportion of participants were meeting their teaching goals six months after the course completion.

CME programs are particularly important for community-based providers, who frequently serve as preceptors and teachers for students' and residents' clinical training. Targeting CME to this population of providers has implications for training future providers, as well as clinical outcomes for the aging population. Willett et al. [13] developed a 3 year community based CME program for generalist physicians after which learners reported improved efficacy at caring for elderly patients, improved ability to teach geriatrics concepts to clinical learners, and improved clinical care in specific realms of geriatrics. Like most other CME programs, there was no comparison group for measurement of educational and clinical outcomes, nor was there long term follow-up of learners following the completion of the CME program.

Longitudinal CME

Traditional CME programs are structured as immersive programs or workshops, but there is also evidence of successful implementation of geriatrics CME delivered longitudinally. The Veteran's Affairs Geriatric Scholars Program (GSP) is an example of a successful longitudinal CME program for primary care providers and other members of the health care team who care for older adults [14]. The GSP was developed to improve the skills of clinicians caring for older adults and also to meet the need for high quality care for elderly populations in rural areas, noting particular inequities in the care of older adults in rural settings. The GSP involved both face-to-face education and distance learning, had mandatory and elective components, and involved didactic teaching as well as experiential learning through the implementation of a quality improvement (QI) project over a six month time period. Didactic components of the GSP were taught as immersive courses, and the QI project was implemented over six months. As part of longitudinal professional accountability, participants were surveyed monthly about their clinical progress, as well as the status of the QI project. Using a retrospective pre/post design, the authors reported improvement in participants' use of evidence-based brief standardized assessments, clinical decision-making, and standards of care.

Ford and colleagues [15] described a robust year-long longitudinal curriculum in geriatrics designed to improve participants' knowledge, skills, and abilities related to geriatric health care while also highlighting work with an interprofessional team. Course leaders used feedback from participants to revise the curriculum yearly. While the curriculum was not intended to be a TTT model, the authors note that many of the scholars who completed the course went on to participate in scholarly work, leadership, and teaching in geriatrics as a result of the course, impacting a broad number of learners beyond the CME course.

Provision of Educational and/or Clinical Resources for Future Reference

Another practical and meaningful approach from the CME literature includes the provision of resources or toolkits that can be accessed by participants following formal program completion. The Curriculum for the Hospitalized Aging Medical Patient (CHAMP) faculty development course [16] was a model of faculty development implemented at the University of Chicago, designed for hospitalists, internists, and geriatricians who care for older adults in the hospital setting. The model integrated clinical content and teaching techniques, so that participants could improve clinical skills and also be prepared to teach other learners. Moreover, the CHAMP program involved the development of portable and highly accessible teaching modules in the care of geriatric hospitalized patients that are easily accessed and used by clinicians and clinical educators [17].

Interprofessional Training

Comprehensive clinical care in geriatrics relies heavily on high functioning interprofessional teams, thus geriatric CME programs need to consider the needs of learners from across disciplines. The Program for Outreach to Interprofessional Services and Education (POISE) in medically underserved areas [18] is a model of interprofessional development in geriatrics with a wide scope, intended to improve the care of the elderly populations in rural and largely underserved areas in New York state. POISE emphasized teamwork, roles of team members, communication skills, leadership, and problem solving skills. We highlight the POISE project in our review of geriatrics CME because of its innovative structure and successful inclusion of interprofessional team members as learners, though the authors did not measure the impact of this curriculum on clinical outcomes. Further discussion of interprofessional training appears in Chap. 8.

Next Steps, Call to Action and Recommendations for Geriatrics CME

The population of older adults continues to grow in the USA, and providing evidence-based, patient-centered care to all is critical for the health of our nation. These older adults will receive their care across a variety of clinical settings and from interprofessional health practitioners across specialties. As a result, we have a critical imperative to develop and evaluate continuing medical education in geriatric medicine for all those who care for this vulnerable population across specialties and settings.

CME in geriatrics need not be delivered in typical conference format in order to be of high quality. Indeed, born out of the COVID-19 pandemic has been the development and delivery of online CME content for providers, who have had the opportunity to access learning without the need to travel to a conference or CME event. Such courses have the possibility of reaching many more learners and removing geography and travel expense as an impediment to access for a large group of learners. Accredited CME courses may now be used by physicians for credit in maintenance of certification (MOC) in internal medicine and geriatrics, allowing clinicians to participate in self-directed and spaced learning opportunities that will augment their clinical practice. Thus, the timing is optimal for the development of high quality geriatrics CME, and for its use by a large number of learners.

This chapter reviewed approaches and strategies derived from the literature to guide educators seeking to develop or enhance CME experiences for practitioners. We believe that the optimal construct for CME in geriatrics will be designed by leaders with content expertise in geriatrics, in partnership with expert educators. CME programs should be relevant to adult, interprofessional learners, should offer opportunities for learning in virtual and in-person environments, should harness opportunities for spaced learning when possible, and should be linked to practice. Importantly, the optimal geriatrics CME program will have measurable outcomes that highlight knowledge, skills, and attitudes of learners, but will go beyond these measures to include clinical outcomes and variables that can be captured using tools like CPDIS. It is our hope that these principles can be used to develop high quality, rigorously designed evidenced-based CME that is easily accessible to clinicians, thereby improving the quality of care delivered to our older adult patient population.

Acknowledgment The authors thank Carrie Levinson, Manager of Reference and Instruction Services at the Icahn School of Medicine at Mount Sinai, for her expertise and support of the in-depth reference search related to this chapter.

References

1. Institute of Medicine (US) Committee on the Future Health Care Workforce for Older Americans. Retooling for an aging America: building the health care workforce. Washington: National Academies Press; 2008. Available https://www.ncbi.nlm.nih.gov/books/NBK215400/.
2. Wessler S. Continuing medical education and geriatrics. Bull N Y Acad Med. 1985;61(6):558–64.
3. Cervero RM, Gaines JK. The impact of CME on physician performance and patient health outcomes: an updated synthesis of systematic reviews. J Contin Educ Heal Prof. 2015;35(2):131–8. https://doi.org/10.1002/chp.21290.
4. Versteeg M, Hendriks RA, Thomas A, Ommering BWC, Steendijk P. Conceptualising spaced learning in health professions education: a scoping review. Med Educ. 2020;54:205–16. https://doi.org/10.1111/medu.14025.

5. Phillips JL, Heneka N, Bhattarai P, Fraser C, Shaw T. Effectiveness of the spaced education pedagogy for clinicians' continuing professional development: a systematic review. Med Educ. 2019;53:886–90.
6. Allen LM, Palermo C, Armstrong E, Hay M. Categorising the broad impacts of continuing professional development: a scoping review. Med Educ. 2019;53(11):1087–99. https://doi.org/10.1111/medu.13922.
7. Allen LM, Palermo C, Armstrong E, Hay M. Measuring impacts of continuing professional development (CPD): the development of the CPD impacts survey (CPDIS). Med Teach. 2021;43(6):677–85. https://doi.org/10.1080/0142159X.2021.1887834.
8. Thomas DC, Johnston B, Dunn K, Sullivan GM, Brett B, Matzko M, Levine SA. Continuing medical education, continuing professional development, and knowledge translation: improving care of older patients by practicing physicians. J Am Geriatr Soc. 2006;54:1610–8.
9. Mazotti L, Moylan A, Murphy E, Harper GM, Johnston CB, Hauer KE. Advancing geriatrics education: an efficient faculty development program for academic hospitalists increases geriatric teaching. J Hosp Med. 2010;5(9):541–6. https://doi.org/10.1002/jhm.791.
10. Eckstrom E, Desai SS, Hunter AJ, Allen E, Tanner CE, Lucas LM, Joseph CL, Ririe MR, Doak MN, Humphrey LL, Bowen JL. Aiming to improve care of older adults: an innovative faculty development workshop. J Gen Intern Med. 2008;23(7):1053–6. https://doi.org/10.1007/s11606-008-0593-1.
11. Levine SA, Brett B, Robinson BE, Stratos GA, Lascher SM, Granville L, Goodwin C, Dunn K, Barry PP. Practicing physician education in geriatrics: lessons learned from a train-the-trainer model. J Am Geriatr Soc. 2007;55(8):1281–6. https://doi.org/10.1111/j.1532-5415.2007.01205.x.
12. Christmas C, Park E, Schmaltz H, Gozu A, Durso SC. A model intensive course in geriatric teaching for non-geriatrician educators. J Gen Intern Med. 2008;23(7):1048–52. https://doi.org/10.1007/s11606-008-0585-1.
13. Willett RM, Boling PA, Meyers ME, Hoban JD, Lawson SR, Schlesinger JB. Professional development in geriatrics for community-based generalist faculty. J Am Geriatr Soc. 2007;55(2):300–4. https://doi.org/10.1111/j.1532-5415.2007.01050.x.
14. Kramer BJ, Creekmur B, Howe JL, Trudeau S, Douglas JR, Garner K, Bales C, Callaway-Lane C, Barczi S. Veterans affairs geriatric scholars program: enhancing existing primary care clinician skills in caring for older veterans. J Am Geriatr Soc. 2016;64(11):2343–8. https://doi.org/10.1111/jgs.14382.
15. Ford CR, Brown CJ, Sawyer P, Rothrock AG, Ritchie CS. Advancing geriatric education: development of an interprofessional program for health care faculty. Gerontol Geriatr Educ. 2015;36(4):365–83. https://doi.org/10.1080/02701960.2014.925889.
16. Podrazik PM, Levine S, Smith S, Scott D, DuBeau CE, Baron A, Whelan C, Johnson J, Cook S, Arora V, Meltzer D, Sachs G. The curriculum for the hospitalized aging medical patient program: a collaborative faculty development program for hospitalists, general internists, and geriatricians. J Hosp Med. 2008;3(5):384–93. https://doi.org/10.1002/jhm.348.
17. Curriculum for the hospitalized aging medical patient (CHAMP). n.d. http://champ.bsd.uchicago.edu/index.html. Retrieved 22 January 2022.
18. Toner JA, Ferguson KD, Sokal RD. Continuing interprofessional education in geriatrics and gerontology in medically underserved areas. J Contin Educ Heal Prof. 2009;29(3):157–60. https://doi.org/10.1002/chp.20029.

Chapter 8
Teaching Geriatrics to Interprofessional Teams

Andrea Justine Landi and Lauren Jan Gleason

Interprofessional Education and Collaboration

The complexity of care for older adults requires the interprofessional collaboration to provide goal-concordant, holistic care. The first step to achieving this level of collaboration is with interprofessional education, the work of multiple professions "learning about, from and with each other" in interprofessional education (IPE) [1]. In this chapter we will first discuss general principles of IPE, followed by characteristics of geriatrics IPE, a review of the landscape of geriatric IPE, and examples of successful models of IPE.

In 2009, a group of six professional organizations—dentistry, nursing, allopathic and osteopathic medicine, pharmacy, and public health—recognized the need for collaboration and formed the Interprofessional Education Collaborative (IPEC). This group developed the core competencies for interprofessional collaborative education and practice. In 2016, an additional nine professional organizations joined IPEC—podiatry, physical therapy, occupational therapy, psychology, veterinary, optometry, allied health professions,[1] social work, and physician assistants [2].

[1] Not defined specifically by IPEC but the Association of Schools Advancing Health Professions defines it as: the segment of the workforce that delivers services involving the identification, evaluation and prevention of diseases and disorders; dietary and nutrition services; and rehabilitation and health systems management.

A. J. Landi · L. J. Gleason (✉)
University of Chicago School of Medicine, Chicago, IL, USA
e-mail: alandi@bsd.uchicago.edu; lgleason@bsd.uchicago.edu

A. W. Schwartz (ed.), *Medical Education in Geriatrics*,
https://doi.org/10.1007/978-3-031-32499-4_8

Table 8.1 IPEC Interprofessional Education Collaborative (IPEC) competencies

Competency 1—values/ethics for interprofessional practice
• Develop a trusting relationship with patients, families, other team members by respecting dignity and privacy, embracing individual differences and cultural diversity, and acting with honesty and integrity
• Work with individuals of other professions to maintain a climate of mutual respect, shared values, and high standards of ethical conduct
Competency 2—roles and responsibilities for collaborative practice
• Clear communication about one's roles and responsibilities, as well as limitations in skills, knowledge, and abilities, and then engage diverse populations who complement one's own professional expertise to develop strategies to meet the needs of patients and populations
• Use the knowledge of one's own role and those of other professions to appropriately assess and address the health care needs of patients and to promote and advance the health of populations
Competency 3—interprofessional communication practices
• Communicate with patients, families, communities, and professionals in health and other fields in a responsive, responsible, and understandable manner that supports a team approach to the promotion and maintenance of health and the prevention and treatment of disease
• Encourage the ideas and opinions of other team members and recognize how one's uniqueness contributes value to interprofessional working relationships
Competency 4—interprofessional teamwork and team-based practices
• Apply relationship-building values and the principles of team dynamics to perform effectively in different team roles to plan, deliver, and evaluate patient/population centered care and population health programs and policies that are safe, timely, efficient, effective, and equitable
• Reflect on individual and team performance and use processes for improvement to increase effectiveness of interprofessional teamwork and team-based care

In 2016, the IPEC board released an update to the core competencies by incorporating population health outcomes alongside individual care competencies for the goal of improving health and health equity across the lifespan. The four core competencies and the related sub-competencies all fall under one domain—Interprofessional Collaboration (Table 8.1).

The first step toward breaking down the silos of health care is to start at the individual accreditation board level where educational goals and core competencies necessary to becoming an independent practitioner are determined. With each school and program having its own accreditation process and curriculum, it was important to create a space where accreditors could collaborate and so in 2014 the Health Professions Accreditors Collaborative (HPAC) was created. By 2019, twenty-five health professions accreditors harmonized their accreditation standards related to interprofessional practice and education [3]. The harmonization and integration of interprofessional education competencies into any healthcare professional curriculum allows for learners from different professions to learn about, from and with one another.

The aspect that has been missing is the incorporation of accreditation standards for Geriatrics, Age-Friendly Concepts [4] (IPEC).

Interprofessional Geriatric Education

The comprehensive care of older adults with complex needs requires an approach where providers from multiple different professions with different sets of knowledge and skills collaborate to provide patient-centered, evidence-based care in a coordinated fashion. Therefore, programs should include interprofessional education (IPE) as a part of geriatric education in the curriculum. *Interprofessional Geriatrics Education*, the teaching of interprofessional collaboration, is defined as when students from different professional training programs learn about, from and with each other, for the care of older adults [5].

Landscape of Interprofessional Geriatrics Education (Summarized in Fig. 8.1)

The early 1900s marked the development of medical specialties and the need for clear communication between medical specialties and general practitioners. In the 1930s, nurses were advocating for team-based approaches to care in the hospital setting, and by the 1950s this team-based approach spanned across settings to the care of chronically ill patients in the outpatient, mental health, and rehabilitation settings. Federal funding for training students in the interdisciplinary team (IDT) approach to health care delivery came in the 1970s when the healthcare field was experiencing a shortage of health professionals [6].

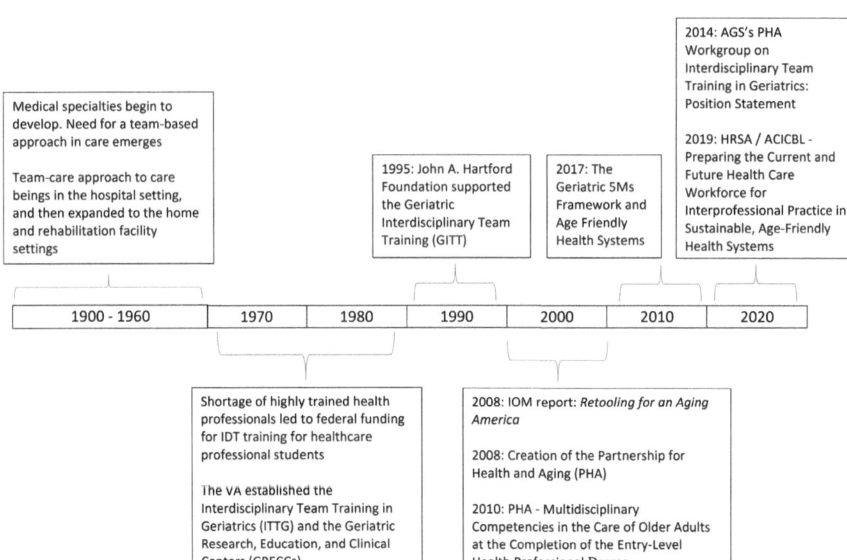

Fig. 8.1 Timeline of interprofessional work in geriatrics. *IOM* Institute for medicine, *AGS* American Geriatrics Society, *HRSA* Health Resources and Services Administration, *ACICBL* Advisory Committee on Interdisciplinary, community-based linkages

In light of the rapid growth in the aging population, particularly in the number of veterans 75 years and older, the Department of Veterans Affairs (VA) took action in the 1970s by implementing the clinical-based education program for staff and students called the Interdisciplinary Team Training in Geriatrics (ITTG) [6]. In 1973, the VA also established the Geriatric Research, Education, and Clinical Centers (GRECCs) by designating 8 medical centers as "geriatric centers of excellence" in geriatric clinical care, research, and education, which has now grown to 20 GRECC sites across the country. By designating centers that would excel in all three tenets of geriatrics, it avoided the fragmentation of efforts and facilitated quality research, enhanced education, and improvement in clinical care of older veterans. All GRECCs are required to be affiliated with medical schools and major health professional schools; therefore, they are not only associated with the improved care of older veterans but also all older Americans [7].

In 1995, the John A. Hartford Foundation (JAHF) supported the Geriatric Interdisciplinary Team Training (GITT) initiative that provided grants to eight institutions to develop GITT training models for three core disciplines: nursing, social work, and medicine [8]. The goal was to determine the effect of the GITT experience on: trainee's attitudes toward health care teams, self-perceived team skills, interest in geriatrics and teams, trainee's knowledge of geriatric IDT care planning, and knowledge of team dynamics. Post-program analysis showed a significant improvement in the attitudes toward teams and team skills across all disciplines, although less so among physicians. These findings highlight the history of disciplinary hierarchy within medicine, the years physicians spend training with and working on teams made up of other physicians, and the need for interdisciplinary team training to be integrated into medical school and residency curricula [6].

In 2008, The Institute of Medicine issued a report titled *Retooling for an Aging America: Building the Health Care Workforce*, calling for bold initiatives starting immediately to train the principles of geriatric medicine to all healthcare professionals [9]. Later that year, the American Society of Geriatrics (AGS) assembled 21 health care professional organizations to create a plan of action in response to the IOM recommendations. This led to the creation of the Partnership for Health in Aging (PHA) [4].

A PHA working group made up of representatives from 10 health care disciplines—dentistry, medicine, nursing, nutrition, occupational therapy, pharmacy, physical therapy, physician assistants, psychology, and social work—collaborated to develop multidisciplinary core competencies for the care of older adults. After reviewing the feedback of more than 25 professional organizations, the group finalized the set of competencies referred to as the "Multidisciplinary Competencies in the Care of Older Adults at the Completion of the Entry-Level Health Professional Degree" [10]. The competencies include:

- Domain #1: Health Promotion and Safety
- Domain #2: Evaluation and Assessment
- Domain #3: Care Planning and Coordination Across the Care Spectrum (Including End-of-Life Care)

- Domain #4: Interdisciplinary and Team Care
- Domain #5: Caregiver Support
- Domain #6: Healthcare System and Benefits

The PHA Workgroup on Interdisciplinary Team Training in Geriatrics met to review the literature on the use of a geriatric IDT. The group found that geriatric IDT is an accepted, well-developed care model that is versatile across a variety of care settings and has been shown to improve healthcare outcomes. The PHA endorsed all efforts to support and implement IDT in geriatrics, recommended any groups well positioned to support its advocacy to do so, and emphasized the urgent need to incorporate Interprofessional Geriatric Education [5].

Most recently, the Health Resources and Services Administration (HRSA) and the Advisory Committee on Interdisciplinary, Community-Based Linkages (ACICBL) reviewed the issues related to interprofessional education, interprofessional practice, and building an Age-Friendly Health System, and provided recommendations for preparing the healthcare workforce for interprofessional and age-friendly practice in their 2019 annual report. Two notable recommendations being that health professions programs integrate age-friendly, interprofessional principles into their curricula, and that HRSA collaborates with health professional organizations, academia, and other agencies to develop age-friendly, interprofessional practice competencies.

We summarize the landscape of interprofessional geriatrics education in Fig. 8.1.

Age-Friendly Health Systems

The health care system and the community at large has been unprepared for the aging population and the complexity of caring for older adults. Older adults often have multiple functional, medical, cognitive, and social factors that influence care, in addition to the fact that they are also interacting with a built environment that inadequately meets their needs. All of these layers of complexity have ultimately led to disproportionate amount of harm that older adults face in the health care system [11].

In 2017, the Geriatrics 5Ms Framework: What Matters, Medications, Mind, Mobility, and Multi-Complexity was introduced as a tool that helps make the complexity of caring for older adults more manageable, as well as help organize and focus attention to the older adult's wellness and strengths and away from only thinking about their disease [11].

As mentioned earlier, current accreditation standards of health professions schools and programs do reflect the harmonization of IPEC in most curricula, but the same cannot be said for the integration of the 5Ms. The ACICBL review identified that most curricula have their own set of geriatric core competencies or required proficiencies in the care of *older patients, elderly patients, patients with a mix of ages, patients of all ages, diverse age populations, and/or patients across the lifespan*. The Commission on Accreditation in Physical Therapy Education is the only professional program to mention two of the 5Ms—mentation and mobility—in the context of caring for older adults [4]. The American Geriatrics Society updated the geriatric core competencies for medical students in 2021 to now have the competencies categorized by the 5Ms instead of the previous 8 domains [12].

The practice of age-friendly care for older adults starts with education. Geriatric medicine through the framework of both the 5Ms and interprofessional education and collaboration are the key elements to providing age-friendly care and developing an Age-Friendly Health System [13].

Teaching Geriatrics to Interprofessional Teams

When teaching interprofessional geriatrics education it is important for all learners to understand each other's roles and how providers can work together to provide the highest quality of care. There are various ways to do this ranging from in-person sessions, virtual meetings, videos, observations all reported in the medical education literature.

The first educational program for interprofessional trainees using the geriatric 5Ms entailed a half-day workshop of trainees from 10 different professions—Pharmacy, Rehabilitation Sciences, Physician Assistant Studies, Nursing, Medicine, Optometry, Psychology, Audiology, Social Work, and Speech-Language Pathology [13]. This workshop model provided interprofessional trainees the opportunity to understand one another's professions and then immediately apply that knowledge by working on a case together while also strengthening their interest in caring for older adults and was able to also be adopted to a virtual platform [13, 14]. We summarize some examples of models of interprofessional geriatrics education in Table 8.2.

The Future of Interprofessional Geriatric Education

The future of Interprofessional Geriatric Education requires using the geriatric 5Ms as the framework to grow the interprofessional team-based and an age-friendly workforce where a common language is spoken among all professions that interact with older adults.

To accomplish this goal there needs to be additional outreach to and training for all medical specialties and other patient facing professionals that have not yet participated in age-friendly, IPE efforts so far, including, but not limited to, certified nursing assistants, medical assistants, radiology technicians, patient transporters, phlebotomy technicians, healthcare administrators, and language interpreters. The health and well-being of older adults are also influenced by their built environment outside of the healthcare system; therefore, it is important to consider effective methods in engaging emergency medical service professionals, the police and fire

Table 8.2 Examples to engage interprofessional learners in geriatric education

Teaching strategy	Title/author/year	Participants students/trainees	Teaching content	Results
Interactive Workshop	A workshop for interprofessional trainees using the geriatrics 5Ms framework [13]; implementing an interprofessional workshop based on the 4Ms for an age-friendly health system [14]	Professional school trainees: nursing, medicine, physician assistant, pharmacy, speech-language pathology, social work, audiology, psychology, rehabilitation sciences	Case-based learning with interprofessional groups using the geriatrics 5Ms framework with a modified jigsaw format and virtually	Improved understanding of training and background of other healthcare professionals, improved familiarity, and applicability of 5Ms framework in older adults
Participation in an interprofessional team-based geriatric home training program. Led by IP faculty teams	Interprofessional, older adult, team-based home visits: a 6-year prospective analysis [15]; assessment of student interprofessional education (IPE) training for team-based geriatric home care: does IPE training change students' knowledge and attitudes? [15]	Dental, medical, occupational therapy, pharmacy, physical therapy, and physician assistant students	5-four-hour sessions over one academic year. Teams met with a community-dwelling older adult three times	Higher likelihood of understanding their roles in an interprofessional health team Improvement in attitudes toward older adults
Video-based workshop	Interprofessional education without limits: a video-based workshop [16]	Medical students[a]	Video-based workshop introducing professional providers and roles to medical students	Improved students' self-related understanding of IP team members' roles and increased confidence in interaction within IP health care team; beneficial in schools without other health care professions for interactive learning
Interprofessional geriatric case competition	Interprofessional competencies of students in a geriatric case competition [17]	Professional graduate health care studies representing 13 disciplines	Interprofessional care plan of a simulated complex geriatric patient	Evaluations based on IPEC competencies: (1) values/ethics for IP Practice; (2) roles/ responsibilities; (3) IP communication; (4) teams and teamwork

(continued)

Table 8.2 (continued)

Teaching strategy	Title/author/year	Participants students/trainees	Teaching content	Results
Simulation training with role playing	Evaluation of a simulation training program for geriatric medicine [18]	Trainees in geriatric medicine, trainees in medicine, nurses in geriatric medicine	Different scenarios: acute illness, continence care, dementia care, complex discharge planning, delirium, end-of-life care	Improved self-confidence across all scenarios
Interactive, case-based workshop	Innovative interprofessional geriatric education for medical and nursing students: focus on transitions in care [19]	Medical and nursing students	Transitions of care	90% of students were better able to describe the necessary IP communication; 80% of students reported an enhanced appreciation of IP teamwork
Interprofessional medication management module	Improving medical and pharmacy student confidence in medication management and attitudes about interprofessional collaboration by utilizing an interprofessional module [20]; First do no "pharm": Educating medical and pharmacy students on the essentials of medication management [21]	Medical students and pharmacy students	IP group didactic, IP group case-based breakout sessions	Improvement in student's attitudes about IP collaboration with regard to understanding roles and teamwork; improvement in medication management competencies
Conduct comprehensive geriatric assessment in patients followed by a clinic-based consultation session	Impact of a collaborative interprofessional learning experience upon medical and social work students in geriatric health care [22]	Medical students, residents, social workers	Interprofessional team	Participants' perception of interprofessional collaboration increased

Table 8.2 (continued)

Teaching strategy	Title/author/year	Participants students/trainees	Teaching content	Results
Peer teaching exchange	Promoting geriatrics education across residency specialties with a pilot peer teaching Exchange [23]	Geriatric fellows, dermatology, anesthesia, and interventional radiology, physical medicine and rehabilitation	Geriatric fellows led didactics to the specialty residents and vice versa to promote knowledge and collaboration	Improved communication and knowledge shared among professional specialties
Professional development				
Boot camp: combination of traditional didactic and experiential, discussion-based learning	Geriatric care boot cAMP: an interprofessional education program for healthcare professionals [24]; Geriatric care boot camp series: Interprofessional education for a new training paradigm [25]	Nursing, research coordination, pharmacy, medicine, psychology, physical therapy, dentistry, faculty	Half-day course covering topics core concepts in geriatric care, including characteristics of older adults, delirium and dementia, medication management, palliative care, and ethical questions; 30- to 45-min session, for a total of five sessions	Improved knowledge in caring for older adults; attendees found the interprofessional nature of the program beneficial
Lectures, workshops, conference presentations, e-learning	Advancing geriatric education: development of an interprofessional program for health care faculty [26]	Dentistry, family medicine, internal medicine, nursing, occupational therapy, physical therapy, psychology, social work, cell biology, communication studies, emergency medicine, nutrition, pharmacy GPs, and practice nurses	Advanced illness including multiple chronic conditions, frailty, symptom management, and medication management. The importance of health care teams and care coordination	Positive faculty reports of the program, information gained and expressed intent by each scholar to apply learned content to teaching and/or clinical practice

(continued)

Table 8.2 (continued)

Teaching strategy	Title/author/year	Participants students/trainees	Teaching content	Results
Faculty development program (FDP)	Infusing geriatrics expertise in health professions education through interprofessional faculty development [27]	Academic or clinical faculty from nursing (including nurse practitioners), medicine, pharmacy, social work, dentistry, gerontology, health administration, nursing home administration, occupational therapy, physician assistant, speech/ language pathology, public administration	10-month FDP, 7 face-to-face seminars (5 h each), three weekend retreats (12–13 h each)	Increased knowledge with significant gains in self-efficacy in Partnership for health in aging domains (PHA)
Virtual telementoring series	An innovative model using telementoring to provide geriatrics education for nurses and social workers at skilled nursing facilities [28]	Nursing professionals, social workers, physicians	One-hour ECHO [b] sessions on geriatric topics weekly for 10–12 weeks	Improvement in self-efficacy to treat patients with dementia, educate about hospice and palliative medicine options, and assess and manage infections in older adults

IP interprofessional, *5Ms* - Geriatrics 5Ms
[a] Not technically IPE as single group
[b] Extension for Community Healthcare Outcomes

departments, public health professionals, local government officials, policymakers, town planners, and architects.

Success in geriatrics depends on teamwork. It is essential that all healthcare professionals are knowledgeable in geriatrics regardless of specialty and learn to work as members of a healthcare team. IPE expands learner's knowledge and attitudes about working in teams and should be an essential part of any curriculum. It will take continued healthcare reform and legislative initiatives and the full support of professional associations, credentialing and licensing groups, accreditation bodies, healthcare institutions, and all healthcare providers to create a culture where interprofessional geriatric education and practice is embraced by all members of the team and integrated into the curriculum and culture [5].

References

1. Framework for action on interprofessional education and collaborative practice. http://apps.who.int/iris/bitstream/handle/10665/70185/WHO_HRH_HPN_10.3_eng.pdf.
2. Collaborative IE. Core competencies for interprofessional collaborative practice: 2016 update. Washington: Interprofessional Education Collaborative; 2016.
3. Collaborative HPA. Guidance on developing quality interprofessional education for the health profession, 2019. https://healthprofessionsaccreditors.org/wp-content/uploads/2019/02/HPACGuidance02-01-19.pdf.
4. Preparing the current and future health care workforce for interprofessional practice in sustainable, age-friendly health systems. 2019. https://www.hrsa.gov/sites/default/files/hrsa/advisory-committees/community-based-linkages/reports/seventeenth-2019.pdf.
5. Partnership for Health in Aging Workgroup on Interdisciplinary Team Training in Geriatrics. Position statement on interdisciplinary team training in geriatrics: an essential component of quality health care for older adults. J Am Geriatr Soc. 2014;62(5):961–5.
6. Reuben DB, Levy-Storms L, Yee MN, Lee M, Cole K, Waite M, et al. Disciplinary split: a threat to geriatrics interdisciplinary team training. J Am Geriatr Soc. 2004;52(6):1000–6.
7. Goodwin M, Morley JE. Geriatric research, education and clinical centers: their impact in the development of American geriatrics. J Am Geriatr Soc. 1994;42(9):1012–9.
8. Fulmer T, Flaherty E, Hyer K. The geriatric interdisciplinary team training (GITT) program. Gerontol Geriatr Educ. 2004;24(2):3–12.
9. Institute of Medicine (US) Committee on the Future Health Care Workforce for Older Americans. Retooling for an aging America: building the health care workforce. Washington: National Academies Press; 2008.
10. Partnership for health in aging. https://aptageriatrics.org/pdfs/PHA-Multidisc-Competencies.pdf.
11. Age-friendly health systems: guide to using the 4Ms in the care of older adults. 2020. http://www.ihi.org/Engage/Initiatives/Age-Friendly-Health-Systems/Documents/IHIAgeFriendlyHealthSystems_GuidetoUsing4MsCare.pdf.
12. Competencies and milestones. https://adgap.americangeriatrics.org/education-training/competencies-and-milestones.
13. Schwartz AW, Hawley CE, Strong JV, Phillips SC, Amir O, Ludwin BM, et al. A workshop for interprofessional trainees using the geriatrics 5Ms framework. J Am Geriatr Soc. 2020;68(8):1857–63.
14. Hawley CE, Doherty K, Moye J, Phillips SC, Ngoc Phung ET, Dawson CMP, et al. Implementing an interprofessional workshop based on the 4Ms for an age-friendly health system. J Am Geriatr Soc. 2021;69(12):E27–30.
15. Reilly JM, Aranda MP, Segal-Gidan F, Halle A, Han PP, Harris P, et al. Assessment of student interprofessional education (IPE) training for team-based geriatric home care: does IPE training change students' knowledge and attitudes? Home Health Care Serv Q. 2014;33(4):177–93.
16. Szafran JCH, Thompson K, Pincavage AT, Saathoff M, Kostas T. Interprofessional education without limits: a video-based workshop. MedEdPORTAL. 2021;17:11125.
17. Lach HW, Little MO, Zubatsky M, Kuljeerung O, Berg-Weger M. Interprofessional competencies of students in a geriatric case competition. Gerontol Geriatr Educ. 2021;42(2):243–51.
18. Braude P, Reedy G, Dasgupta D, Dimmock V, Jaye P, Birns J. Evaluation of a simulation training programme for geriatric medicine. Age Ageing. 2015;44(4):677–82.
19. Balogun SA, Rose K, Thomas S, Owen J, Brashers V. Innovative interprofessional geriatric education for medical and nursing students: focus on transitions in care. QJM. 2015;108(6):465–71.
20. Kostas T, Thomas J, Thompson K, Poston J, Levine S. Improving medical and pharmacy student confidence in medication management and attitudes about interprofessional collaboration by utilizing an interprofessional module. J Interprof Care. 2018;32(6):790–3.

21. Sehgal M, Nassetta KR, Bamdas JAM, Sourial M. First do no 'pharm': educating medical and pharmacy students on the essentials of medication management. Curr Pharm Teach Learn. 2019;11(9):920–7.
22. Gould PR, Lee Y, Berkowitz S, Bronstein L. Impact of a collaborative interprofessional learning experience upon medical and social work students in geriatric health care. J Interprof Care. 2015;29(4):372–3.
23. Streiter S, Loewenthal J, Berry S, Schwartz AW. Better together: promoting geriatrics education across residency specialties with a pilot peer teaching exchange. J Am Geriatr Soc. 2019;67(10):E1–3.
24. Solberg LB, Solberg LM, Carter CS. Geriatric care boot cAMP: an interprofessional education program for healthcare professionals. J Am Geriatr Soc. 2015;63(5):997–1001.
25. Solberg LB, Carter CS, Solberg LM. Geriatric Care Boot Camp Series: interprofessional education for a new training paradigm. Geriatr Nurs. 2019;40(6):579–83.
26. Ford CR, Brown CJ, Sawyer P, Rothrock AG, Ritchie CS. Advancing geriatric education: development of an interprofessional program for health care faculty. Gerontol Geriatr Educ. 2015;36(4):365–83.
27. Marrs SA, Ansello EF, Slattum PW, Davis K, Parsons PL, Zimmerman K, et al. Infusing geriatrics expertise in health professions education through interprofessional faculty development. Gerontol Geriatr Educ. 2021:1–13.
28. Gleason LJ, Martinchek M, Long M, Rapier N, Hamlish T, Johnson D, et al. An innovative model using telementoring to provide geriatrics education for nurses and social workers at skilled nursing facilities. Geriatr Nurs. 2019;40(5):517–21.

Part III
Teaching Geriatrics in Different Medical Education Settings

Chapter 9
Making Large Group Teaching Memorable

Colleen Christmas and Simone Lescott

Importance of and Challenges with Teaching Geriatrics in Large Groups

Healthcare professionals with knowledge, expertise, and compassion for caring for our aging populations are in demand worldwide. By extension, teachers of geriatric medicine are in very high demand and often are asked to deliver teaching to large groups and diverse learners. Teaching in the large group setting can be challenging to address the range of learners needs and interests simultaneously and traditionally has been a more passive, and less effective, means of teaching. Compounding these challenges, some learners may not highly value learning about geriatrics [1–3] presenting additional barriers to learner engagement and effectiveness in teaching sessions.

Meiboom and colleagues utilized a concept mapping approach to suggest the key areas geriatrics lectures could target to try to overcome the low levels of interest in the field and most important areas where education is lacking currently [4]. They describe 5 broad principles to incorporate in teaching about geriatrics to address these needs: keeping the teaching patient-centered and representative of the patient population served, emphasizing the intellectually and emotionally stimulating nature of the work, including exposure to role models in geriatrics, and emphasizing the incredible skill involved in caring for older adults. For example, for a group of primary care physicians most familiar with patients from their community seen in the office setting teaching could involve working through a patient scenario in this

C. Christmas (✉)
The Johns Hopkins University School of Medicine, Baltimore, MD, USA
e-mail: cchristm@jhmi.edu

S. Lescott
Yale School of Medicine, New Haven, CT, USA

A. W. Schwartz (ed.), *Medical Education in Geriatrics*,
https://doi.org/10.1007/978-3-031-32499-4_9

setting, including anecdotes from a local prominent role model in primary care and emphasizing aspects of care that are challenging but highly rewarding. In contrast, in teaching pre-clinical nursing students, a patient-centered discussion may center on an older family member, such as a parent or grandparent. As we consider pedagogy further in the next section, some of these themes will be revisited.

While there are many pedagogical approaches to teaching geriatrics in large groups, traditional lecture formats are the most commonly employed large group teaching method. Unfortunately, typical retention of information presented in a traditional large group lecture format is estimated at approximately 5% of the information presented, arguing for innovations in this approach [5]. Multiple scholars in medical education convincingly argue that the traditional lecture should be replaced by shorter and far more active modalities of learning [6–8] based on what is best known about how adult learners engage with new information and create long-term memories from research in the cognitive sciences. A few key principles of adult learning theory are important to keep in mind when teaching in large groups to engage learners and to ensure what they learn about geriatrics is effectively retained.

Applying Adult Learning Theories to the Pedagogy of Teaching Geriatrics

Build on Baseline Geriatrics Knowledge

Many of the principles related to what is known about adult learning can be extraordinarily helpful as one prepares lectures in geriatric medicine. First, consider how the previous level of knowledge of a learner enhances their ability to acquire new information. When we explore the learner's existing knowledge of a subject, we can intentionally access that information to help build a scaffolding on which new information can be added. When the level of baseline knowledge of the audience is unknown, one risks providing information that is already known and thus the learner disengages, or providing information that is far too advanced and appropriate for the level of learner and the intervention is frustrating to the learners and ineffective. This area of the knowledge gap that builds on what is already known but feels withing the learner's abilities to learn is referred to as the "zone of proximal development" [9]. One way this principle of building on existing knowledge can be put into action in geriatrics teaching sessions is when planning to speak, for example, about delirium, first check and make sure that the learners you are engaging know the basic definition of delirium before going on to discuss signs, symptoms, and management. The teacher could ask for a volunteer to define delirium, then provide a definition that either affirms the responses or fills in the gaps before proceeding [10]. The approach to assessing the level of learner may depend on how confident one is already the audience has this information (in which case it would be a quick check-in) and how important having a particular piece of knowledge is to assimilate the rest of the lecture (arguing for more time-consuming assessments). This assessment not only tells the presenter what the level of understanding is already and helps the teacher adjust the content of information to be delivered accordingly, but also serves a second important function: to activate prior knowledge of the subject for the learner, readying their brains to more easily assimilate additional new information. Many options exist for assessing baseline knowledge and activating prior knowledge. For example, instead of asking for a volunteer to vocalize their baseline knowledge on behalf of a group, one could consider ensuring all participants activate their baseline knowledge by starting a session asking each person to write down what they know already and the questions they have on the subject, using an electronic polling device or show of hands to answer brief questions or engage participants in small or large group discussions about their knowledge. Active means of engaging groups to share prior knowledge could include inviting them to brainstorm about the topic utilizing sticky notes placed on a board to create a "graffiti wall" either physically or on a shared electronic document, co-creating an electronic word cloud, or sharing verbally with a partner or small group briefly at the start of a session before the lecturer provides new information [10].

Promote Self-Motivated Learning

A second principle of adult learning theory is that of self-determination, which posits that learning that is intrinsically motivated by a curiosity or perceived need to learn has a multitude of benefits. This learning that is intrinsically motivated is more readily retained, results in improved wellbeing, and is associated with deeper learning than that which is extrinsically motivated, such as learning done to please a teacher or to pass a test [11]. Self-determination theory further states that the needs for autonomy, competence, and connection underpin these intrinsic drivers; thus, teachers can intentionally try to promote teaching that facilitates autonomy, competence, and relatedness through their words and actions. The educator must help create a "need to know" of the information in the learner by helping them find for themselves the gap between what they already know and what they need to learn that will inform something of value to that learner. For example, orthopedic residents may become more interested in learning about postoperative delirium when the teacher helps guide the residents to make the connection between delirium and something they value, length of stay. Other devices here might include the use of dramatic statistics to demonstrate the importance of a certain topic or asking the audience to reflect for a moment on the last time they saw a person with whatever the topic of discussion is, and how they felt their ability to care for that person might be improved or where they struggled, perhaps even briefly sharing these "real world" stories.

Further, information presented in a lecture format that is more immediately used can increase the learner's sense of orientation to learning and thus is more readily retained [7] to make sure that the topic is relevant to whatever task is at hand for learners. For example, in teaching about conducting goals of care discussions the lecturer may solicit from the audience an example of a patient currently on the service who might benefit from this sort of discussion and weave information about that patient throughout their presentation of how to conduct goals of care discussion, challenging the learners to try to utilize the information later that day. Similarly, one might consider creating a mock assignment to utilize the information presented later in the day to practice its principles. In the goals of care discussion example, the lecturer can encourage each audience member to find one person—a patient, or friend, or family member—and discuss goals of care before the day ends and to reflect on the principles they utilized from the lecture, and which ones they would need to further learn about. Finally, people more readily recall stories than facts [10], so consider who is the sort of person that is impacted by your topic and tell a story about this person that invokes emotion and a sense of need to act as a means of "hooking" the learners into the topic at hand.

Provide Structure to Organize Information

The third principle to keep in mind is that information that is presented in an organized form is more readily retained by learners [10]. Invest time planning how the information to be delivered can best be organized and include introductory comments that reveal the organizational plan you will utilize in the lecture. This may involve the use of metaphors or mnemonics or careful use of diagrams and visuals to help focus on concepts and principles. A very effective and widely used format for presenting information related to geriatrics topics is to link to the Geriatric 5Ms, 5 key organizing concepts in communicating about geriatrics [12]. Not only does having 5 principles all starting with the letter M make retention and organization of information simpler, the wide-spread use of this framework means that learners take advantage of the principle of repetition. Studies from the cognitive sciences involving adult learners demonstrate clearly that repetition, particularly spaced in time, increases retention [13]. Often in planning lectures teachers feel that they need to put in so much information that they intentionally delete anything that seems redundant, however including a degree of repetition gives the learners the opportunity to practice and to repeat the principles and skills, modified for new scenarios. For example, after teaching a concept related to frailty early in the lecture perhaps later in the lecture one might include a question that prompts the learner to recall that same information and emphasize a principle that can be applied in other scenarios.

Promote Active Learning

Finally, the principle best demonstrated to impact long-term retention of information in educational sessions is that active learning far outpaces passive learning [7, 8, 10, 13]. This charge can often feel daunting in a lecture venue, particularly a large one with mixed levels of learners, more formal settings, and virtual lectures where the audience may not be fully visible. Like other pedagogical principles discussed above, careful planning and borrowing tips from other successful approaches in medical education can help ensure your teaching involves opportunities for active learning. Approaches to promoting active learning include addressing the culture of the learning environment, fostering a growth mindset, and using highly engaging techniques; each of these is described in more detail here.

Some learners are more extroverted and readily engaged in more public active approaches to learning than others for a variety of reasons. The teacher helps set the culture and tone of the learning environment. In some settings the teacher may already know the learners well and have already established a culture of inclusion, support, and learning; in other settings the teacher may have to overcome significant barriers to doing so. When one is unfamiliar with the learners and the typical culture at a place it can help to ask beforehand what the usual teaching structures are like, what the students may be expecting, and whether they are used to active approaches or more passive teaching.

In planning your geriatrics large group teaching session, the educator should consider how to foster an environment that is inclusive of all voices, safe to make mistakes, and supportive but challenging. What the teacher chooses to acknowledge, comment, or provide feedback on sends a message about the learning environment [10] indicating whether all voices are invited and received without judgment or criticism. Questions such as "Do the images and examples utilized center on the often-used white person experience or are they representative of diverse patients?" are often helpful. It may also be beneficial for the teacher to invite a colleague to examine the teaching materials, specifically assessing the materials through the lens of maximizing inclusion. In general, in building learning environments where risk taking and getting things wrong is valued, the ratio of positive reinforcement should outpace those of corrective feedback significantly [14]. In a lecture setting this might occur by posing questions periodically and when students answer, reinforcing what they got right in addition to what they further need to understand. While building this sense of community and promoting inclusiveness and support, the teacher can create a learning environment that also fosters a growth mindset [14] in learners by being both supportive yet challenging and by praising growth and effort, not only correct answers. An excellent way for the teacher to promote a growth mindset is to share their own failures and growth as an example of the growth mindset [10].

Studies of adult learners demonstrate that challenging information can still be learned when approached with a growth mindset within a supportive environment. To avoid frustrating learners in these situations, however, it can be very helpful if the teacher first explains the intention to purposely create a challenging environment for the purposes of maximal growth and engagement [10]. Consider posing questions that the learners likely do not immediately know the answer to, explicitly stating that they have not been given this information yet but that you are challenging them to find it and report back because that work will help them learn the material well. For example, in a lecture on the management of diabetes in older adults living in a skilled nursing facility could begin by asking the learners to predict what the most appropriate level of glycemic control is and challenging the learners to spend 5 min during class trying to identify clinical trials that included nursing home residents and then report back. The first person to find a good study is awarded some nominal prize or recognition, and in support of fostering growth mindsets, all are praised for the effort.

Once the principles of growth mindset and a challenging yet supportive environment are established, there are a variety of approaches [15] that can be used to maintain this learning culture during the teaching session. In the simplest approach, the lecturer may pause and ask questions of the audience periodically, using traditional (raise hands and answer, written quizzes) or more modern (audience response systems) approaches, or by encouraging students to interact by discussion questions in small groups for a limited time then reporting back. Other approaches to encourage active learning involve breaking into small groups to discuss clinical scenarios and problem solve as a team, periodically breaking into pairs to share personal stories with each other about a topic then sharing themes from those stories as a group, building in time for reflection and writing or drawing for participants (with or without sharing), and utilizing the arts in creative ways, such as encouraging participants to contribute to a playlist of songs or visual images related to the topic of the lecture. In the right setting, the majority of the teaching could be accomplished by nearly entirely active learning approaches interspersed with breaks to allow the learner to process the information [7, 15], such as by practicing role play scenarios and discussing what went well and what could be done differently, watching and discussing books or films, or utilizing games. Gamification of learning, while more challenging to create, has the added benefit that most learners are intrinsically motivated to win games, games are highly engaging, and they often provide a safe means for taking risks. There are commercial products available to simplify the creation of games, and multiple games for teaching geriatric principles have been studied and shown to be effective in motivating learners and establishing non-threating environments for active learning [16].

A summary of these 4 key principles is outlined in Fig. 9.1.

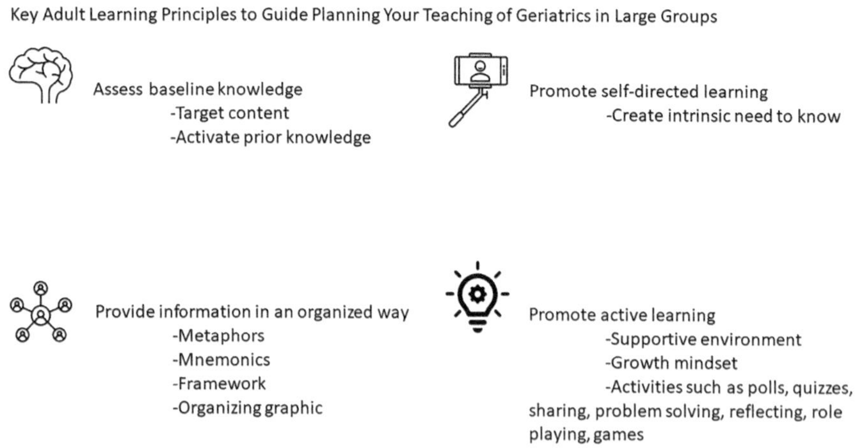

Fig. 9.1 Utilizing the cognitive sciences in the delivery of geriatrics lectures

Utilizing the Cognitive Sciences in the Delivery of Geriatrics Lectures

Understanding how memories are created, stored, and retrieved brings to bear principles to keep in mind in your delivery of information when teaching geriatrics in large group settings. The principles of sensory memory, working memory, and cognitive load (see Fig. 9.2) are important principles to consider when teaching geriatrics in large group settings given that the typical attention span of learners is only 15–20 min [17–19].

To retain information, a learner must first processes what is seen, heard, and felt through a system called sensory memory. Information delivered that utilizes all of these modalities synergistically will require less effort to process and store, thus the presentation can be designed to stimulate all modalities. While emotion is often undervalued in learning pedagogy, there is strong evidence to support its potent effect on linking to and storing knowledge [10]. After processing through sensory memory, information is then transferred to working memory where it is manipulated, often linked to prior knowledge, before transfer in the brain to areas of storage that represent long-term knowledge. Working memory is often the rate limiting step in formulating long-term memories and is impacted by cognitive load [18]. Cognitive load is the amount of effort it takes for the working memory to manipulate this information and is thus related both to the learners pre-existing familiarity with the information and the volume of information and the format in which it is delivered [18].Thus when planning large group teaching sessions in geriatric medicine, educators should consider both the abilities of the learner and the volume and structure of the information being delivered. There are ways to minimize the cognitive load in the delivery of information by including not only

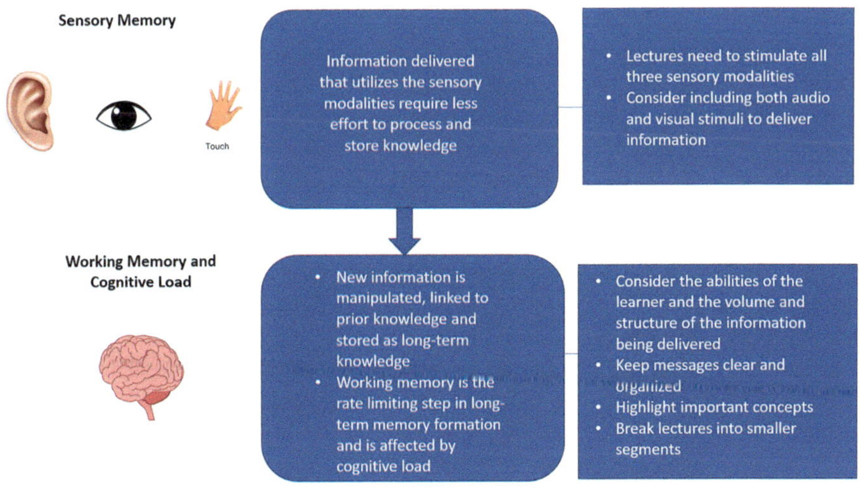

Fig. 9.2 The interactions between sensory memory, working memory, and cognitive load to create lasting storage of information

audio but also visual stimulus, ensuring that what is spoken and what is viewed on any slides are congruent and devoid of extraneous or distracting information, keeping messages simple, and highlighting when the most important concepts are shared to help the student focus. A 1 hour teaching session should contain no more than 20 minutes of lecture (ideally, broken into smaller segments divided between brief active learning activities) and the rest should be directed toward active learning, so lectures should convey no more than 2–3 key points [7]. These 2–3 key messages serve as guideposts for reviewing the content of the teaching session, and any information that is extraneous or does not help support making these 2–3 points should be eliminated. Text that is read is processed in the same area of the brain as verbal information, thus audiences cannot fully listen and fully read simultaneously. Combine verbal information with a simple, clear, congruent visual image utilizing "Dual Coding Theory" [19]. When used verbal and visual information are used synergistically, studies demonstrate that recall is increased significantly [19]. A great example of this could be utilizing a simplified graphic of an older adult's body with highlighted areas noting changes with aging and pointing at and talking through each of those changes, during a lecture on aging physiology. A good rule for large groups teaching sessions is the 10–20–30 rule promoted by innovator, businessman, and entrepreneur, Guy Kawasaki: most effective talks should include no more than 10 slides, last no longer than 20 minutes, and use no smaller than 30-point font [20]. In other words, simple is better. A very common mistake in large group teaching involves attempting to deliver all the information relevant to a topic in a short amount of time, but given the limits on working memory and attention, simple, clear messages are most effective in teaching. While traditionally, slides have been used to demonstrate information visually in large group teaching settings, but newer modalities such as concept maps on wipeboards may be just as or more effective, particularly when the subject matter is highly conceptual [21].

In teaching geriatrics in large group settings, it is also important for teachers to remember that they communicate not only verbally, but nonverbally through their facial expressions and body language. A good lecture is at least in part good theater; utilizing intentional body language can convey enthusiasm and generate interest in the subject from learners. During the session, teachers should actively monitor reactions of their learners and adjust their presentations accordingly. If the audience appears disinterested, the teacher should check in to understand that disinterest. This might mean asking a question of the audience to understand if the level of information delivery is appropriate and clearly conveyed or recreating a "need to know" to re-engage learners. During the teaching session, teachers should work continuously to build rapport by making eye contact, smiling, and perhaps even periodically referencing participants by name (facilitated by utilizing name tents or tags). Teachers should also signal key concepts by saying so, using highlighted visuals, pausing, repeating, or gesturing. End with a summary, or better yet, invite students to help generate a summary or key points they have learned.

Future Directions in Teaching Geriatrics

While examples of excellent educational programs (e.g., the Facilitated Learning to Advance Geriatrics (FLAG) [22] and the Reynolds Mini-fellowships in Geriatrics [23]) that seek to increase knowledge and teaching effectiveness about aging and the care of older adults exist, most lecturers in geriatrics utilize a passive, traditional format and fail to utilize new research in the cognitive sciences and new teaching pedagogies to engage learners and more effectively teach. More instruction for teachers in geriatrics is needed to most effectively spread geriatrics principles to meet the care needs of the aging population. Further, more evidence is needed to understand approaches to teaching geriatrics in large groups that maximally engage a variety of health professional learners and result in attitudes and behaviors that best serve our patients and society.

References

1. Samra R, Griffiths A, Cox T, Conroy S, Gordon A, Gladman JR. Medical students' and doctors' attitudes towards older patients and their care in hospital settings: a conceptualisation. Age Ageing. 2015;44(5):776–83. https://doi.org/10.1093/ageing/afv082.
2. Kishimoto M, Nagoshi M, Williams S, Masaki KH, Blanchette PL. Knowledge and attitudes about geriatrics of medical students, internal medicine residents, and geriatric medicine fellows. J Am Geriatr Soc. 2005;53(1):99–102. https://doi.org/10.1111/j.1532-5415.2005.53018.x.
3. Reuben DB, Fullerton JT, Tschann JM, Croughan-Minihane M. Attitudes of beginning medical students toward older persons: a five-campus study. The University of California Academic Geriatric Resource Program Student Survey Research Group. J Am Geriatr Soc. 1995;43(12):1430–6. https://doi.org/10.1111/j.1532-5415.1995.tb06626.x.
4. Meiboom AA, de Vries H, Scheele F, Hertogh CMPM. Raising enthusiasm for the medical care of elderly patients: a concept mapping study to find elements for an elderly friendly medical curriculum. BMC Med Educ. 2018;18(1):238. https://doi.org/10.1186/s12909-018-1344-6.
5. Masters K. Edgar Dale's pyramid of learning in medical education: a literature review. Med Teach. 2013;35(11):e1584–93. https://doi.org/10.3109/0142159X.2013.800636.
6. Sawatsky AP, Zickmund SL, Berlacher K, Lesky D, Granieri R. Understanding resident learning preferences within an internal medicine noon conference lecture series: a qualitative study. J Grad Med Educ. 2014;6(1):32–8. https://doi.org/10.4300/JGME-06-01-37.1.
7. Cooper AZ, Richards JB. Lectures for adult learners: breaking old habits in graduate medical education. Am J Med. 2017;130(3):376–81. https://doi.org/10.1016/j.amjmed.2016.11.009.
8. Freeman S, Eddy SL, McDonough M, Smith MK, Okoroafor N, Jordt H, Wenderoth MP. Active learning increases student performance in science, engineering, and mathematics. Proc Natl Acad Sci U S A. 2014;111(23):8410–5. https://doi.org/10.1073/pnas.1319030111.
9. Gauvain M. In: Benson JB, editor. Vygotsky's sociocultural theory in encyclopedia of infant and early childhood development. 2nd ed. Amsterdam: Elsevier; 2020.
10. Lang JM. Small teaching: everyday lessons from the science of learning. San Francisco, CA: Jossey-Bass; 2016.
11. Kusurkar RA, Croiset G, Ten Cate TJ. Twelve tips to stimulate intrinsic motivation in students through autonomy-supportive classroom teaching derived from self-determination theory. Med Teach. 2011;33(12):978–82. https://doi.org/10.3109/0142159X.2011.599896.

12. Tinetti M, Huang A, Molnar F. The geriatrics 5M's: a new way of communicating what we do. J Am Geriatr Soc. 2017;65(9):2115. https://doi.org/10.1111/jgs.14979.
13. Brown PC. Make it stick: the science of successful learning. Cambridge, MA: The Kelknap Press of Harvard University Press; 2014.
14. Dweck CS. Mindset: the new psychology of success. New York: Random House; 2006.
15. "Basic Active Learning Strategies". Center for Teaching and Learning, University of Minnesota. https://cei.umn.edu/teaching-resources/active-learning. Accessed 25 Jun 2022.
16. Schmall V, Grabinski CJ, Bowman S. Use of games as a learner-centered strategy in gerontology, geriatrics, and aging-related courses. Gerontol Geriatr Educ. 2008;29(3):225–33. https://doi.org/10.1080/07399330802359443.
17. Jeffries W. Teaching large groups. In: Jeffries W, Huggett K, editors. An introduction to medical teaching. Dordrecht: Springer; 2014. p. 11–26.
18. Young JQ, Van Merrienboer J, Durning S, Ten Cate O. Cognitive load theory: implications for medical education: AMEE guide no. 86. Med Teach. 2014;36(5):371–84. https://doi.org/10.3109/0142159X.2014.889290.
19. Clark J, Paivio A. A dual coding perspective on encoding processes. In: McDaniel M, Pressley M, editors. Imagery and related mnemonic processes: theories, individual differences, and applications. Berlin: Springer-Verlag; 1987. p. 5–33.
20. Kawasaki G. https://guykawasaki.com/the_102030_rule/. Accessed 10 Dec 2021.
21. Fischer K, Sullivan AM, Krupat E, Schwartzstein RM. Assessing the effectiveness of using mechanistic concept maps in case-based collaborative learning. Acad Med. 2019;94(2):208–12.
22. Krichbaum K, Kaas MJ, Wyman JF, Van Son CR. Facilitated learning to advance geriatrics: increasing the capacity of nurse faculty to teach students about caring for older adults. Gerontologist. 2015;55(Suppl 1):S154–64. https://doi.org/10.1093/geront/gnu165.
23. Heflin MT, Bragg EJ, Fernandez H, Christmas C, et al. The Donald W. Reynolds consortium for faculty development to advance geriatrics education (FD~AGE): a model for dissemination of subspecialty educational expertise. Acad Med. 2012;87(5):618–26. https://doi.org/10.1097/ACM.0b013e31824d5251.

Chapter 10
Teaching Geriatrics in the Classroom: Small Groups

Alyson Michener and Rachel Miller

Vignette: Small Group Teaching in Geriatrics
You have been asked to take over teaching an hour-long didactic session on mobility assessment and falls for the internal medicine residency program. The session is for second- and third-year internal medicine residents on their ambulatory rotations. There are 4 ambulatory sections, each with twenty residents. In past years, the resident feedback has been that the session could be more engaging, and thus the chief residents have asked you to make this teaching more interactive. Consider how you could apply principles of small group teaching to this assignment.

Introduction

Small group teaching is a collaborative learning endeavor [1] where students actively learn together via interaction between members of the group. The instructor deliberately employs teaching strategies that promote communication and participation among participants to facilitate learning [2]. Learning activities typically require application of knowledge through group discussion, deliberation, and reflection [1].

A. Michener (✉)
Perelman School of Medicine, University of Pennsylvania, Philadelphia, PA, USA
e-mail: alyson.michener@pennmedicine.upenn.edu

R. Miller
Corporal Michael J. Crescenz Veterans Philadephia Healthcare System, Perelman School of Medicine, University of Pennsylvania, Philadelphia, PA, USA
e-mail: rachel.miller@pennmedicine.upenn.edu

A. W. Schwartz (ed.), *Medical Education in Geriatrics*,
https://doi.org/10.1007/978-3-031-32499-4_10

A small group ideally consists of no more than 20 learners [2]. However, small group teaching is more defined by the process of instruction rather than by the group size [3]. In fact, small group teaching techniques can even be applied to larger groups in order to gain some of the benefits of these teaching methods. Small group teaching strategies are well suited to educating learners on geriatrics topics and can be applied when educating learners of all levels and health disciplines about geriatric principles.

Advantages of Small Group Teaching

Small group teaching methods are designed to engage adult learners who want to help set objectives, apply knowledge in real time, practice problem solving, and receive feedback [4]. In studies, they have been shown to be more effective than didactic lectures at increasing student engagement, improving retention of knowledge, self-directed learning, communication skills, teamwork, and peer discussion [1]. Students work collaboratively with peers and compare knowledge and build on their understanding of concepts [3]. This encourages higher order thinking, promotes lifelong learning skills, and allows students to practice communication skills [5]. Additionally, students may receive feedback in real time [1]. Further, students have the opportunity to establish closer contact with academic faculty [6].

For these reasons, small group teaching strategies fit well with medical training and are frequently applied to preclinical and clinical medical school curricula. These strategies allow for application of basic science knowledge to clinical case scenarios. Further, learners have the opportunity to practice working in teams and develop communication skills, all of which are essential to the practice of medicine [3]. Additionally, small group teaching techniques may be useful when teaching interprofessional learners to simulate team dynamics.

Small Group Teaching for Geriatrics

Small group teaching strategies are an effective method to teach geriatric principles. Small group activities allow students to enrich their preclinical content knowledge by enhancing the learning with discussion [7]. Many geriatric topics, including multimorbidity, polypharmacy, and goals of care are best taught through interactive methods. Students sometimes perceive geriatrics topics as complex [8], so small group activities may allow students to work through nuanced clinical challenges. A full discussion of addressing complexity in geriatrics can be found in Chap. 4. Geriatrics educators may wish to consider including learners from multiple disciplines in order to encourage collaboration and simulate real world interprofessional clinical scenarios, as discussed in Chap. 8.

Despite a need for education in geriatrics, due to curricular and faculty constraints, many medical schools lack the faculty and clinical opportunities to provide clinical exposure to geriatrics to all students. In some cases, small group teaching may even substitute for dedicated clinical exposure to geriatrics [9, 10]. Students can then apply knowledge obtained from small group teaching to real world patient scenarios involving older adults.

Small group teaching strategies can also be applied to teach geriatrics principles to learners of other levels of training. At the graduate medical education level, small group teaching strategies can be applied to teach geriatrics principles in the form of resident reports and didactics and fellow conferences. They can also be applied to faculty development, institutional grand rounds, and even on a broader scale at national meetings and conferences.

Best Practices for Small Group Teaching in Geriatrics

Designing a Geriatrics Teaching Session

Planning an effective small group teaching session requires deliberate planning and careful consideration of several factors (Table 10.1).

Target Audience Identify the number and level of learners who will be included in the activity. Consider the educational need of the learners and whether they have had any prior exposure to geriatrics education or the specific topics that will be taught. If the activity will include interprofessional learners, account for various levels of background knowledge and skillsets.

Faculty Availability The number of available faculty may determine the size of the small groups or type of teaching strategies that can be used. Several faculties may be required to host multiple small groups synchronously. As the average number of geriatrics faculty at US allopathic and osteopathic medical schools is only around ten to eleven [11], accommodating synchronous small groups for an entire medical school class may be difficult. For institutions with limited geriatrics faculty, sessions may be run asynchronously, meaning that small groups meet at separate times to allow each faculty to facilitate two or more small groups. Another strategy that has been used is a "train the trainer" method where other non-geriatric faculty are taught to teach selected geriatric medicine topics [12]. Moreover, some small group teaching strategies can be implemented in the context of a larger group or lecture format.

Allotted Time Consider the time allotted for the small group meeting and whether didactic content will be delivered during the session or if students will be expected to prepare outside of the small group session. Some small group teaching strategies

Table 10.1 Geriatrics small group teaching preparation worksheet

Component	Example from vignette
Background/Current Condition (Why) – *What is the geriatrics gap in knowledge, skills, attitudes that you plan to teach?*	*Mobility assessment and fall prevention and management*
Who are your intended learners? – *What is their geriatric education/knowledge background (can also review geriatrics-related competencies)*	*Second- and third-year internal medicine residents. No prior formal geriatrics education during residency, variable during medical school*
Resources – *Faculty availability* – *Setting/equipment*	*One faculty to teach all sections* *Conference room with a long rectangular table, seats set up around it. AV equipment available*
When/Where can this occur? – *Allotted time in schedule*	*1 h during ambulatory rotation* *Repeated 4 times to separate groups of learners*
Goals and Objectives (What) – *What geriatrics knowledge, skills, attitude do you plan to address?* – *Incorporate Geriatric 5Ms*	***Geriatrics** 5M domain: Mobility* *Objectives:* *1. Assess mobility in older adults* *2. Identify risk factors for falls in older adults* *3. Review evidence-based fall prevention strategies*
Instructional Strategies (How) – *What active small group learning techniques can be utilized?*	*Think-pair-share to have learners discuss recent fall-related hospital admission or ambulatory case* *Role play timed up-and-go* *Go round where learners share something they will implement in practice*
Evaluation – *How will you measure your baseline?* – *How will you know that your intervention made a difference?*	*Based on the responses to the go around at the end of the session*

Adapted from [13]

rely on a "flipped classroom" method where learners are required to work independently or in groups prior to or after small group sessions to review course materials or complete an assignment [14]. Other strategies minimize the amount of work required outside of the small group meeting, though may rely on a higher level of prior learner knowledge. If this is the case, the small group teacher may wish to check background knowledge by issuing a readiness assessment [15, 16]. The amount of learner preparation required is important to consider in the context of other educational demands and where this small group teaching will fit within the overall curriculum.

Learning Goals and Objectives Identify learning goals and objectives for the teaching session. The learning goals are the higher-level themes, whereas the learning objectives should describe specific knowledge, skills, and attitudes that should be achieved in the context of the teaching session.

Teaching Activities Plan purposeful learning activities to engage the learners. This is often centered around a clinical case with learners given questions or problems to solve. Specific small group teaching strategies are discussed below.

Evaluation The predetermined goals and objectives form the basis of evaluation. Learners should receive feedback on their performance relative to the identified learning goals and outcomes. This may be done in the context of a learning activity where learners can gauge their understanding of content relative to peers and fill in gaps with the facilitator providing feedback [1].

The Role of the Facilitator During the Session

Create and Manage the Learning Environment The facilitator needs to ensure a comfortable learning environment that promotes participation and engagement [17]. This starts with selecting an appropriate physical space and room layout which will promote discussion and participation in group activities. Seating may need to be arranged to accommodate smaller teams or breakout groups. A circular or ovular seating arrangement can help promote discussion. If technology will be used for the session, the facilitator should consider the availability of internet access and equipment availability such as computers, projectors, and sound.

At the start of the session, it is important for the facilitator to establish goals and expectations for the group dynamics. The facilitator should promote a learning environment that is relaxed and comfortable so that all learners feel that they are able to contribute.

Facilitate the Learning Learning objectives should be outlined at the start of the session and the facilitator should work to keep discussion flowing toward the established learning goals. The facilitator should vary teaching styles to reach different learning styles [1]. At times, this may even mean that the facilitation is done by the learners. Open-ended questions should be used to encourage discussion and challenge underlying assumptions [17]. Check understanding by asking questions and then clarify areas of misunderstanding. Provide feedback when needed. The facilitator should monitor the group dynamic and resolve conflicts should they arise. At the end of the session, elicit reflection and feedback from the group. Include time to summarize key concepts or ask students to summarize the discussion.

Managing Common Problems The facilitator should be prepared to manage common problems that may arise during small group teaching. For example, learners may be reluctant to engage in conversation. The facilitator should assess whether this is due to a lack of preparation or due to conditions of the learning environment. Use open-ended questions and redirect learner questions to the group to increase engagement. Conversely, one or a few students may dominate the discussion [3]. In these instances, the facilitator should use strategies to gain participation from other members of the group.

Small Group Teaching Strategies for Geriatrics Education

Many universities have implemented student-centered small group learning curricula that shift the focus of classroom instruction from knowledge acquisition to application through dialogue and discussion [16]. The most commonly used models are problem-based learning (PBL), case-based learning (CBL), and team-based learning (TBL). Though there are variations between these pedagogical methods, they share several key features. In each, students are presented with a clinical case or scenario with clinical questions or prompts which are discussed in small groups. Students apply prior knowledge or seek out additional information which is then applied to answer questions [1]. Some medical schools have implemented these types of structured curricula to teach geriatrics competencies [18, 19]. Aquifer geriatrics is a series of 26 evidence-based, peer reviewed, online cases which teach geriatrics competencies. The cases can be assigned or adapted for team-based learning at all levels [20].

Other small group teaching strategies can be implemented during small group meetings, resident reports, fellow didactics, or even in the context of a larger group session or lecture. By doing so, a standard didactic can be made more active by applying principles of small group teaching.

Small Group Interactive Strategies

Question/Answer The facilitator poses questions to the group to stimulate discussion.

Example: Ask learners what they want to get out of the session.

Paired Discussion (Think-Pair-Share) A question is posed to the larger group and then students are asked to briefly discuss in teams of two. This strategy can be used to help start a conversation as it encourages participation when the large group is brought back together (Fig. 10.1).

Example: Ask learners to review causes of delirium with a partner.

Breakout Groups Learners are divided into small groups in the context of a larger group meeting. Learners work together to answer a question or perform a task before coming back together as a larger group (Fig. 10.1).

Example: Learners are presented with a clinical vignette for a patient with a complicated medication list and are tasked with prioritizing medications to deprescribe.

Group Round (Go-Around) Each learner is asked to share an answer to an open-ended question. This strategy could be used at the beginning of a session to assess background knowledge or at the end of the session to summarize key points.

Example: Ask learners to share an example of a time they took care of a patient where multimorbidity influenced the treatment recommendation.

Jigsaw Students are divided into small groups. Each group receives a different assignment. The groups are then reformed so that each new group has one student from each original group. The students disseminate the information they learned in the first part of the activity to their new groups (Fig. 10.1).

Example: For a session on comprehensive geriatric assessment, learners are broken into groups that each focus on a practicing a skill such as cognitive assessment (e.g.: mini-cog [21]), mobility assessment (e.g.: timed up-and-go [22]), and functional assessment. The groups are redistributed and in new groups the learners demonstrate each component of the assessment to the members of their new group.

Role Play Students are asked to simulate a case or interaction to develop solutions to a problem, try out new behaviors, and receive feedback [23].

Example: Students practice communication skills while acting out a case involving discussion of goals of care.

3×5 card Students write a response to a prompt on an index card or slip of paper which is then shared with the group or reviewed by the facilitator at a later time. For example, students could be prompted to write a question at the beginning of a session or something they learned at the end.

Example: After a session about goals of care conversations, learners are asked to write one thing they took away from the session or something that they will implement into practice.

Technology Several web-based programs are available that allow learners to engage with educational content using technology. Audience response software can be incorporated into a presentation and allows learners to answer prompts on their personal electronic devices.

Example: Show a list of medications and ask learners to identify high-risk medications using an audience response program.

Games Though a number of different games can be used to encourage active participation in learning, jeopardy-style games in particular are popular in medical education. Jeopardy games can be customized to cover desired topics using templates available for PowerPoint® or web-based software.

Example: A jeopardy-style game reviewing key features of several geriatric syndromes. Geriatric syndromes such as urinary incontinence, falls, weight loss, dementia, and osteoporosis are listed as categories. Questions of increasing difficulty are listed under each category. Learners work in teams to answer questions as a review of important geriatric concepts.

Snowball Learners read or watch a prompt. Then, given 5 min to individually answer 1–3 questions. Next, paired to discuss answers for 5 min. Pairs are joined

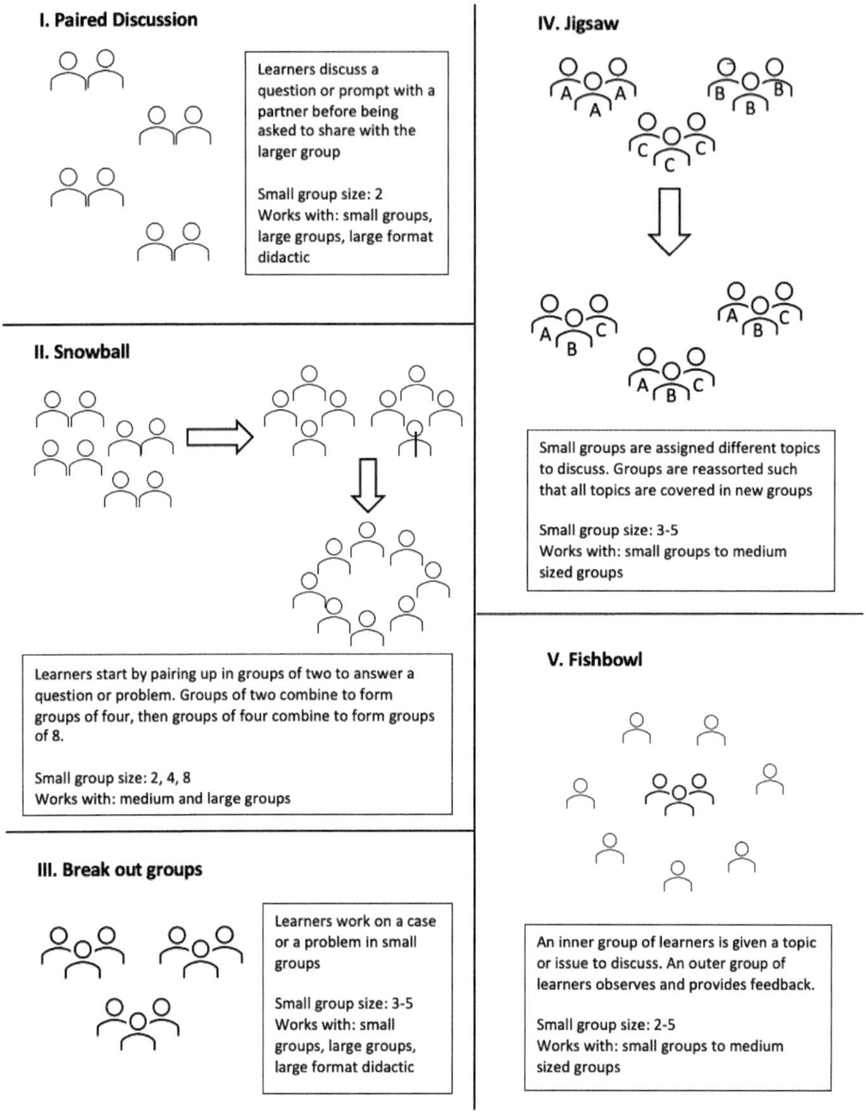

Fig. 10.1 Schematic of selected small group teaching strategies for geriatrics education

together to make groups of four for another 5-min discussion, and then groups of eight, if feasible. The groups of eight report findings and key takeaways back to the larger group [6] (Fig. 10.1). The overall goal is for all learners to have opportunity to participate and promote discussion.

Example: The learners are presented with a complex geriatrics case involving a patient where there is concern for elder abuse and self-neglect. In pairs, learners are asked to define self-neglect and evidence related to the presented case. Pairs are then combined into groups of four to discuss next steps in management including community resources. Finally, groups are again combined and asked to discuss how they would address issues related to patient capacity.

Fishbowl An inner group of learners is given an issue or a topic to discuss. An outer group observes the interactions of the inner group and looks for themes or provides feedback [6] (Fig. 10.1).

Example: A group of learners is asked to role play communication skills in a simulated triad visit where one learner plays a physician, one plays a patient with cognitive impairment, and another is a family member. The outer group observes the visit and identifies important skills used during the simulated interaction.

Video Prompts Short video clips are shown to prompt discussion. This technique may be combined with other teaching strategies such as think-pair-share or audience response systems.

Example: A video clip showing an older adult performing a timed up-and-go. Learners are then asked to comment about features of the gait that they witnessed in the video.

Conclusion

The small group teaching strategies described above may be implemented in a variety of settings with learners of all levels. They are intended to stimulate interaction between learners, which is the central feature of small group teaching. Geriatrics educators may wish to apply these teaching strategies to teach geriatrics principles, including those represented by the Geriatrics 5Ms, to learners at all levels of medical training and for learners in other health disciplines. These strategies may not only be used in true small group settings, but should also be considered as a tool to make teaching large groups of learners more active.

Vignette
After considering various small group teaching strategies, you decide to start your teaching session with a think-pair-share to generate learner engagement at the start of your session. You ask the trainees to discuss with a partner the last patient they evaluated for a fall and the risk factors that may have been present, prior to sharing with the larger group. During your session, you have a trainee demonstrate a timed up-and-go [22]. *At the end of your session, you use a go-around to ask the trainees one thing they will take away from your session and implement into their practice* (Table 10.1).

References

1. van Diggele C, Burgess A, Mellis C. Planning, preparing and structuring a small group teaching session. BMC Med Educ. 2020;20(2):462. https://doi.org/10.1186/s12909-020-02281-4.
2. Walton H. Small group methods in medical teaching. Med Educ. 1997;31(6):459–64. https://doi.org/10.1046/j.1365-2923.1997.00703.x.
3. Burgess A, van Diggele C, Roberts C, Mellis C. Facilitating small group learning in the health professions. BMC Med Educ. 2020;20(2):457. https://doi.org/10.1186/s12909-020-02282-3.
4. Jackson A. Teaching in a small group. In: Presented at: chief resident immersion training. Boston, MA: Boston University School of Medicine; 2012.
5. Mir MM, Jeelani M, Alshahrani MS. A practical approach for successful small group teaching in medical schools with student centered curricula. J Adv Med Educ Prof. 2019;7(3):149–53. https://doi.org/10.30476/JAMP.2019.74911.
6. Jaques D. ABC of learning and teaching in medicine: teaching small groups. BMJ. 2003;326:492–4.
7. Denham AC. Clinical decision-making for older patients with multiple chronic conditions: a case-based exercise for medical students. MedEdPORTAL J Teach Learn Resour. 2016;12:10477. https://doi.org/10.15766/mep_2374-8265.10477.
8. Bagri AS, Tiberius R. Medical student perspectives on geriatrics and geriatric education. J Am Geriatr Soc. 2010;58(10):1994–9. https://doi.org/10.1111/j.1532-5415.2010.03074.x.
9. Fisher AL, O'Keefe EA, Hanlon JT, Studenski SA, Hennon JG, Resnick NM. A brief, intensive, clinically-focused geriatrics course during the third year of medical school. J Am Geriatr Soc. 2009;57(3):524–9. https://doi.org/10.1111/j.1532-5415.2008.02135.x.
10. Strano-Paul L. Effective teaching methods for geriatric competencies. Gerontol Geriatr Educ. 2011;32(4):342–9. https://doi.org/10.1080/02701960.2011.611557.
11. Warshaw GA, Bragg EJ, Brewer DE, Meganathan K, Ho M. The development of academic geriatric medicine: progress toward preparing the Nation's physicians to care for an aging population. J Am Geriatr Soc. 2007;55(12):2075–82. https://doi.org/10.1111/j.1532-5415.2007.01519.x.
12. Harada C. Interprofessional train the trainer workshop: teaching geriatrics to change behavior. MedEdPORTAL. 2013;9:9458. https://doi.org/10.15766/mep_2374-8265.9458.
13. Miller RK, Chippendale RZ, Schwartz AW, Seghal M. Transforming Aging Education for Medical Trainees. Society of General Internal Medicine Annual Meeting, 2021.
14. Sharma N, Lau CS, Doherty I, Harbutt D. How we flipped the medical classroom. Med Teach. 2015;37(4):327–30. https://doi.org/10.3109/0142159X.2014.923821.
15. Haidet P, Levine RE, Parmelee DX, et al. Perspective: guidelines for reporting team-based learning activities in the medical and health sciences education literature. Acad Med. 2012;87(3):292–9. https://doi.org/10.1097/ACM.0b013e318244759e.
16. Koles PG, Stolfi A, Borges NJ, Nelson S, Parmelee DX. The impact of team-based learning on medical students' academic performance. Acad Med. 2010;85(11):1739–45. https://doi.org/10.1097/ACM.0b013e3181f52bed.
17. Muller J, Irby DM. How to lead effective group discussions. Clin Teach. 2005;2:10–5.
18. Yanamadala M, Kaprielian VS, O'Connor Grochowski C, Reed T, Heflin MT. A problem-based learning curriculum in geriatrics for medical students. Gerontol Geriatr Educ. 2018;39(2):122–31. https://doi.org/10.1080/02701960.2016.1152268.
19. Struck BD, Teasdale TA. Development and evaluation, of a longitudinal case-based learning (CBL) experience for a geriatric medicine rotation. Gerontol Geriatr Educ. 2008;28(3):105–14. https://doi.org/10.1300/J021v28n03_08.
20. Sehgal M, Syed Q, Callahan KE, et al. Introducing aquifer geriatrics, the American Geriatrics Society National Online Curriculum. J Am Geriatr Soc. 2019;67(4):811–7. https://doi.org/10.1111/jgs.15813.
21. Borson S, Scanlan J, Brush M, Vitaliano P, Dokmak A. The mini-cog: a cognitive 'vital signs' measure for dementia screening in multi-lingual elderly. Int J Geriatr Psychiatry.

2000;15(11):1021–7. https://doi.org/10.1002/1099-1166(200011)15:11<1021::AID-GPS234>3.0.CO;2-6.
22. Podsiadlo D, Richardson S. The timed "up & go": a test of basic functional mobility for frail elderly persons. J Am Geriatr Soc. 1991;39(2):142–8. https://doi.org/10.1111/j.1532-5415.1991.tb01616.x.
23. Steinert Y. Twelve tips for effective small-group teaching in the health professions. Med Teach. 1996;18(3):203–7.

Chapter 11
Teaching Geriatrics Through Home Visits

Ryan Z. Chippendale, Emily Cetrone, and Megan E. Young

Introduction

Home visits to older adults provide an essential teaching experience and have shown a number of unique benefits for learners of geriatrics [1–3]. Because of their experiential nature, home visits have proven to be an ideal setting for learners to become more adept with geriatric assessments such as medication reconciliation and functional assessments [4–9]. The home visit setting can also promote interprofessional learning because it provides learners the chance to better understand how different professions approach a given patient in the home. Interprofessional teaching on geriatrics home visits can take a variety of forms, including interprofessional preceptors taking learners on home visits as well as pharmacy and medical students participating in home visits together [9–11]. Exposing learners to home care has also been shown to improve attitudes toward caring for chronically ill older adults and enhance interest in practicing home based medicine in the future, potentially growing our geriatrics workforce [6, 12–15].

R. Z. Chippendale (✉) · M. E. Young
Boston University Chobanian & Avedisian School of Medicine, Boston, MA, USA
e-mail: ryan.chippendale@bmc.org; megan.young2@bmc.org

E. Cetrone
University of North Carolina, Chapel Hill, School of Medicine, Chapel Hill, NC, USA
e-mail: ecetrone@unc.edu

A. W. Schwartz (ed.), *Medical Education in Geriatrics*,
https://doi.org/10.1007/978-3-031-32499-4_11

Home visits also provide a robust opportunity to teach competency domains set forth by the Accreditation Council for Graduate Medical Education (ACGME), Liaison Committee on Medical Education (LCME), and other health professional accrediting bodies. Hayashi and Christmas demonstrated, through an extensive literature review, that geriatrics home care experiences can incorporate learning in all six ACGME core competencies for resident learners (patient care, medical knowledge, interpersonal and communication skills, professionalism, systems-based practice, and practice-based learning and improvement) [16]. Similarly, Oates et al. demonstrated that a university-based ambulatory geriatrics medical school clerkship, including home care as a main component, taught principles in nearly all of the Association of American Medical Colleges' (AAMC) core competencies in Geriatrics, including the domains of medication management, cognitive and behavioral disorders, self-care capacity, gait disorders, healthcare planning and promotion, atypical presentation of disease and palliative care [2].

In this chapter, we will elaborate on some of these benefits of teaching geriatrics unique to the home visit setting, as well as provide a roadmap for how to effectively teach learners in the home. We recognize that home visits may be an unfamiliar teaching environment for many learners and educators, so we will provide concrete and practical tips that will help create a successful experience for a wide range of learners, regardless of level or discipline.

Best Practices for Structuring a Geriatrics Home Visit Experience

Orienting the Learners to the Geriatrics Home Visit

Home visits are often an unfamiliar experience for learners and thus proper orientation to the environment and structure of a geriatrics home visit is necessary [1, 3]. Geriatrics practices that have required rotations incorporating home visits for learners routinely include formal group orientations to impart knowledge about unique aspects of the experience. Such orientations may include the following logistical topics: maintaining safety as a trainee when visiting patients in the community; best practices for infection control such as hand hygiene and equipment sanitation; specific environmental instructions in terms of where to place their belongings, how to minimize noise or disruptions, and where to sit in particularly cluttered homes [1, 17]. Additionally, orienting learners to unique educational aspects of the home visit, such as real-time exposure to how the social determinants of health (Fig. 11.1) visibly play into a patient's overall health status (Table 11.1) and how to structure a visit using the Geriatrics 5Ms [18] (Table 11.2) can ensure success for the learner in meeting the experience's goals and objectives [15, 17, 18, 19].

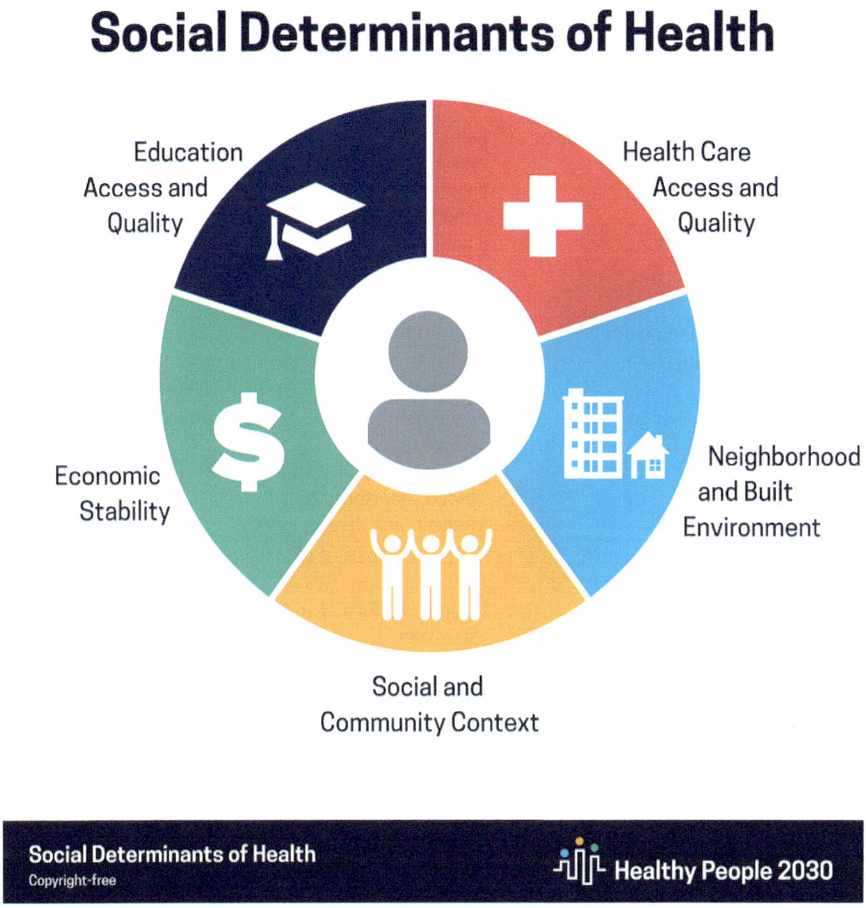

Fig. 11.1 The 5 domains of Social Determinants of Health. Healthy People 2030, U.S. Department of Health and Human Services, Office of Disease Prevention and Health Promotion [20]

Setting Up the Geriatrics Home Visit

Individual providers who are scheduled to bring learners on geriatrics home visits with them should engage in pre-visit planning [1]. This pre-planning can occur prior to the day of visits, asynchronously through secure electronic exchange, or at the start of the session. This crucial step ensures learners are prepared for the unique aspects of the experience. Learners should be assigned distinct roles for the visit. If assigned to lead a visit, they should be informed of this ahead of time so that a chart review can be performed. If multiple learners are present, we recommend assigning each learner specific patients to maximize learning and promote autonomy [1].

Table 11.1 Healthy People 2030 defines the Social Determinants of Health (SDOH) as the conditions in the environment where people are born, live, learn, play, worship and age that affect a wide range of functioning and quality-of-life outcomes and risks

Social determinants of health	Examples commonly observed during geriatrics home visits
Neighborhood and built environment	– Fall risks – Presence of durable medical equipment – Neighborhood safety – Food and medication access
Economic stability	– Unpaid bills visible in the home – Ability to afford medications, home accommodations, health insurance, healthy foods
Education access and quality (including health literacy)	– Safety awareness – Ability to access resources to support function – Ability to understand medical conditions
Health care access and quality	– Presence of assistive devices, durable medical equipment – Access to specialty appointments, home health services, transportation – Medication delivery options
Social and community context	– Access to places of worship or religious community – Social isolation – Presence of formal and informal supports and caregivers

This table demonstrates examples of commonly observed SDOH during home visits [20]

Prior to arrival at the first home, the learner leading the visit (the leading learner) should present a "one-liner" describing the patient to the preceptor and other learners. The leading learner should also be asked to identify how they plan to negotiate the visit agenda based on their pre-reading. The non-leading learners can then be assigned tasks such as performing pertinent geriatric assessments, e.g. fall screening or medication reconciliation, or identifying social determinants of health impacting the patient. This explicit assignment of roles to learners allows for an efficient and effective visit where all members of the team have active learning assignments to enhance engagement. Given the unique environment of the home care setting, preceptors may also use pre-visit planning time to communicate social aspects unique to the patient's care, such as key caregivers to obtain collateral information, family dynamics, or other relevant aspects of the type of visit they are about to perform (e.g. urgent vs. post-hospital vs. routine follow-up visit).

Conducting the Visit with an Older Adult in the Home

Direct Observation

The home care setting allows for a unique opportunity for preceptors to directly observe learners in a deliberate way. Direct observation is known to be a valuable tool for providing behaviorally based feedback to learners [21]. However, there are

Table 11.2 Teaching the Geriatrics 5Ms on home visits

Teaching the Geriatrics 5Ms during home visits	Examples of questions for learners to ask
Mind	• How is the patient's cognition? Is a caregiver present to provide collateral information with patient permission? • Is there evidence of caregiver stress? • Is a personal care attendant or home health aide present? How many hours per week are they assisting the patient? What activities do they perform? • For patients with dementia, what safety measures are in place? Is there access to the stairs? Locked doors? Stove turned off or safety knobs in place if needed?
Mobility	• What is the entrance to their home like? Are there multiple steps? Narrow doors? • What equipment/accessibility do they have in their home? Do they have shower chairs? A raised toilet seat? Grab bars? Assistive devices or a wheelchair? A hospital bed? • What shoes are they wearing? • Do they have a personal emergency response system? Are they wearing it? • Are they able to ambulate so that you can see how they navigate their home environment?
Medications	• Where in the home do they keep their medications? • How are their medications organized? • Do they use pill bottles, medication organizers, prepackaged medications? • What supplements or over the counter (OTC) medications do they have? Any OTC medications with a higher risk of delirium? • Are there any extra pill bottles? Expired medications?
Multicomplexity	• Is their neighborhood safe? • Do they have access to transportation to medical visits? • Are they wearing glasses? Hearing aids? • Do they have enough food in their home? Is their diet appropriate for their medical conditions? • Do they have the incontinence supplies they need? Would they benefit from a commode to prevent incontinence? • Do they have a functioning scale? • What in-home resources are available to them?
Matters Most	• How do they spend their day? • What photographs or stories do they share with you? • Could their home environment be optimized to help them fulfill their goals? • Is their current environment conducive to aging in place? • Are you able to identify a safe and comfortable space to have vulnerable discussions?

Tinetti et al. describe the Geriatrics 5Ms as a communication framework to optimally describe the core competencies of geriatric medicine [18]. This table demonstrates examples of how the Geriatrics 5Ms framework can be applied with learners as a teaching tool on geriatrics home visits

also obstacles, such as time pressures, that preclude direct observation from being done regularly in the clinical setting. When direct observation is not performed optimally, learners can feel uncomfortable and therefore alter their performance [22].

Kogan et al. outline helpful guidelines for direct observation including the importance of clearly discussing expectations and setting goals with the learner prior to the observation [23]. Goal setting may actually help learners feel more comfortable about being observed because it provides them some autonomy about what aspect of their performance will be evaluated. Additionally, setting goals with all learners ahead of the observation helps normalize the experience. Logistically, the faculty observer should situate themselves in the peripheral vision of the patient so that the learner is in the patient's direct view. If the patient starts to direct their comments to the faculty instead of the learner, the observer can redirect their vision toward the learner, which will draw the patient's attention back to them. Direct observation allows preceptors to give specific, behavior-driven, and actionable feedback following the visit (see *Evaluation of the Learner*); it is generally not recommended to give feedback in front of the patient.

Teaching on Geriatrics Home Visits Using the Geriatrics 5Ms Framework

The Geriatrics 5Ms are a powerful way to systematically teach geriatrics principles during home visits [18, 24–26]. Given home care provides such an immersive experience into the life and health of older adults, geriatrics home visits serve as a valuable training environment for teaching around all aspects of Mind, Mobility, Medications, Multicomplexity and Matters Most. Below (Table 11.2) we provide practical examples from the literature and from expert home care faculty of best practices for how to teach the Geriatrics 5Ms on home visits.

Concluding the Geriatrics Home Visit: The Wrap-Up

Debriefing with learners at the conclusion of the visit is an important step to allow them to process and reflect on the unique aspects of caring for older adult patients in their homes. This debrief can occur while transporting between visits (if in privacy) or at the conclusion of the experience in a quiet, safe environment. In line with best practices for debriefing, explicitly creating a non-judgmental space can allow learners to reflect openly on what was experienced [27]. Asking open-ended, self-assessment questions allows for free-flowing conversation. Examples of open-ended questions include: How did it feel to explore the caregiver's stress over caring for her mom as her dementia progresses? (Mind); How do you think you did eliciting the patient's goals during the visit? (Matters Most); How did it feel to perform such a complex medication reconciliation during this transition of care? (Medications, Multicomplexity). If there are multiple learners, soliciting perspectives of how each learner interpreted the experience can be powerful. Potential areas to explore in the debriefing exercise include: impressions of the home environment; the Geriatrics 5Ms framework as a tool to organize a complex visit; the impact of Social Determinants of Health on an individual patient; how the home visit experience may impact the future practice of the learner (which can be powerful regardless of future or current specialty).

Providing individual feedback to learners about their performance is also essential for their growth and development. Giving timely and specific feedback can be challenging if multiple learners are performing home visits together. We recommend asking the leading learner to provide a brief self-assessment at the conclusion of the visit they are leading. The self-assessment can allow learners to identify self-perceived gaps and provide opportunities for preceptors to provide feedback in a non-threatening manner. Engaging other learners in peer feedback is also an opportunity for them to develop an important, potentially new, skill and enhance competency in professionalism while on group home visits [28]. Feedback is further discussed in Chap. 21.

Evaluation of the Learner During a Geriatrics Home Visit

Direct observation of learners in the home allows for the ideal environment to evaluate multiple core educational domains. We will highlight the following specific domains: advanced communication, mobility, interprofessional communication, medication reconciliation, and teamwork using the Geriatrics 5Ms Framework [18].

Mind

Many patients on geriatrics home visits will have a caregiver present, and learners will need to perform third party interviewing—incorporating both the patient and the caregiver. We can observe the learner's ability to obtain collateral information. Furthermore, we can see if learners are able to identify subtle cues in the home that might indicate a patient is having worsening cognitive functioning. For example, we can observe food that has been left out on the counter, laundry, or bills that have piled up, or home delivered meals that have gone uneaten.

Mobility

Performing the physical exam in a patient's kitchen, living room or front porch can be challenging. Faculty can evaluate a learner's ability to be sensitive to the patient's comfort and privacy during the physical exam as they have to alter the environment. For example, if the patient is in the kitchen or living room for the physical exam, learners should find a blanket to use for draping to ensure proper auscultation technique on the skin or may need to move the patient to a different chair or couch in order to achieve optimal positioning for the abdominal exam. If the patient is being seen in a shared living or recreational space (such as an assisted living or an adult day health program), learners should move the patient to their room or a private office. This is also a good opportunity for learners to intentionally evaluate the patient's mobility. We can assess whether or not the learner asks about or looks for assistive devices, observes the patient's gait, and considers partnering with interprofessional teams such as physical and occupational therapy in the home.

Medication Reconciliation

The home provides the perfect setting to perform direct medication reconciliation and evaluate the learner's attention and ability to recognize medication errors, especially during transitions of care [5]. Faculty can evaluate if the learner uses the teach-back method when counseling about medication use and if the learner is mindful of appropriate prescribing practices. The teach-back method is recommended by the Agency for Healthcare Research and Quality as a technique for assessing a patient's understanding of their health information [29].

Multicomplexity

Faculty can also assess whether or not learners can describe the roles and responsibilities of resources available through community agencies such as visiting nurses, home health aides, home care agency case managers, home delivered meals, and adult day health. Furthermore, faculty can evaluate if the learner demonstrates situational awareness and professionalism. Sometimes the learning climate in the home is uncomfortable for the learner (warm temperatures, pets, poverty, neglect or just the unfamiliarity of being outside of a clinic setting), and the ability for the learner to read social cues and maintain their professionalism can be directly observed.

Matters Most

For older patients, particularly for those with cognitive and sensory impairment, learners need to use advanced communication techniques to demonstrate sensitivity and respect, including appropriate body language and thoughtful seating arrangements. Some patients may require the use of an amplification device or telephone interpreter. Additionally, observing learners talk with patients in the home about what matters to them presents an opportunity to evaluate their awareness of their own emotions and attitudes, as well as their coping strategies for managing stress and uncertainty when caring for seriously ill patients. Faculty can evaluate how learners elicit what matters most to an older adult, and work with the patient and team to honor these priorities.

Finally, through simply being in the home environment, we can evaluate learners' ability to incorporate how social determinants of health impact health outcomes and healthcare access for older adults and those who care for them [30].

Teaching Geriatrics Home Care Principles Outside the Home

Many training programs may not have access to traditional home visiting programs to incorporate learners or may have insurmountable barriers to transporting their learners into the home for in-person sessions. Innovative resources have been created to help educators incorporate the principles of geriatrics home visits into health professional curricula despite this. The use of video gaming, simulation, web-based modules, and other novel technologies can allow for curricula to be developed that cover similar domains as home visits, but performed physically outside of the home [31–33]. Blended learning models can also be used when single or minimal home visits can be incorporated into a larger curriculum [34, 35].

Conclusion

As we have described, geriatrics home visits provide an incredibly rich experience for learners to engage in crucial aspects of caring for older adults. Expanding opportunities for home care centered education is essential given it is traditionally rarely incorporated in standardized curricula for health professionals [1]. As the older adult population continues to grow, health care professionals need to be equipped with the expertise to care for these patients in all settings, including at home. Home visits not only expose learners to fundamental core competencies expected in their education, but also help shape a new generation of providers who are competent in caring for multimorbid and seriously ill patients in all sites of care. Geriatrics home visits are an essential component of health care education, regardless of level or discipline of the learner, and this chapter provides tools and strategies necessary to make this a feasible and sustainable environment for teaching.

References

1. Boling P. The physician's role in home health care. Berlin: Springer; 1997.
2. Oates DJ, Norton LE, Russell ML, et al. Multisite geriatrics clerkship for fourth-year medical students: a successful model for teaching the Association of American Medical Colleges' Core

competencies. J Am Geriatr Soc. 2009;57(10):1917–24. https://doi.org/10.1111/J.1532-5415.2009.02449.X.
3. Hayashi J, Christmas C, Durso SC. Educational outcomes from a novel house call curriculum for internal medicine residents: report of a 3-year experience. J Am Geriatr Soc. 2011;59(7):1340–9. https://doi.org/10.1111/J.1532-5415.2011.03471.X.
4. O'Donnell L, Carson L, Forciea MA, et al. What students experienced: a narrative analysis of essays written by first-year medical students participating in a geriatrics home visit. J Am Geriatr Soc. 2013;61(9):1592–7. https://doi.org/10.1111/JGS.12405.
5. Young ME, Demers LB, Parker V, Day H, Chao S. Posthospital home visit as teaching tool for internal medicine residents. Gerontol Geriatr Educ. 2018;41(4):514–21. https://doi.org/10.1080/02701960.2018.1490736.
6. Nagle BJ, Berry A, Gorman L, Dangiolo M. A preliminary qualitative evaluation of an in-home geriatric care elective experience for third-year medical students. Cureus. 2018;10(4):e2415. https://doi.org/10.7759/CUREUS.2415.
7. Tung E, Thomas MR. Use of a geriatric home visit experience to teach medical students the functional status assessment. J Gen Intern Med. 2009;24:244. Published online 2008. https://doi.org/10.1007/s11606-008-0853-0.
8. Denton GD, Rodriguez R, Hemmer PA, Harder J, Short P, Hanson JL. A prospective controlled trial of the influence of a geriatrics home visit program on medical student knowledge, skills, and attitudes towards care of the elderly. J Gen Intern Med. 2009;24(5):599–605. https://doi.org/10.1007/S11606-009-0945-5.
9. Solomon P, Risdon C. Promoting interprofessional learning with medical students in home care settings. Med Teach. 2011;33(5):e236–41.
10. Hatfield CL, Major AB, Purkiss J, LaCour-Chestnut F, Gill AC. No place like home redesign: home-based clinical care as an interprofessional training model for medical and pharmacy students. J Interprof Care. 2020;35(5):744–50. https://doi.org/10.1080/13561820.2020.1801612.
11. Vaughn L, Cross B, Bossaer L, Flores E, Medicine JMF. Undefined. Analysis of an interprofessional home visit assignment. 2014. https://www.stfm.org/Portals/49/Documents/FMPDF/FamilyMedicineVol46Issue7Vaughn522.pdf. Accessed 27 Sept 2021.
12. Yuen JK, Breckman R, Adelman RD, Capello CF, LoFaso V, Reid MC. Reflections of medical students on visiting chronically ill older patients in the home. J Am Geriatr Soc. 2006;54(11):1778–83. https://doi.org/10.1111/J.1532-5415.2006.00918.X.
13. Nothelle SK, Christmas C, Hanyok LA. First-year internal medicine residents' reflections on nonmedical home visits to high-risk patients. Teach Learn Med. 2018;30(1):95–102. https://doi.org/10.1080/10401334.2017.1387552.
14. Roane DM, Tucker J, Eisenstadt E, Gomez M, Kennedy GJ. Assessing the benefits of a geropsychiatric home-visit program for medical students. Acad Psychiatry. 2014;36(3):216–8. https://doi.org/10.1176/APPI.AP.09090156.
15. Goroncy A, Makaroff K, Trybula M, et al. Home visits improve attitudes and self-efficacy: a longitudinal curriculum for residents. J Am Geriatr Soc. 2020;68(4):852–8. https://doi.org/10.1111/JGS.16390.
16. Hayashi J, Christmas C. House calls and the ACGME competencies. Teach Learn Med. 2009;21(2):140–7.
17. Cline M, Pagels P, Gimpel N, Day PG. Utilizing home visits to assess social determinants of health during family medicine residency. PRiMER. 2020;4:31. https://doi.org/10.22454/PRIMER.2020.448665.
18. Tinetti M, Huang A, Molnar F. The geriatrics 5M's: a new way of communicating what we do. J Am Geriatr Soc. 2017;65(9):2115. https://doi.org/10.1111/JGS.14979. Epub 2017 Jun 6. PMID: 28586122.
19. Miller RK, Young M, Chippendale R, Jantea R, Goroncy A, Murdock C, Schwartz AW, Sehgal M. Using the Geriatric 5Ms to teach structural and social determinants of health. J Am Geriatr Soc. 2023;71(12):3967–3972. https://doi.org/10.1111/jgs.18518. Epub 2023 Aug 18. PMID: 37596776.

20. Social Determinants of Health—Healthy People 2030. health.gov. https://health.gov/healthypeople/objectives-and-data/social-determinants-health. Accessed 27 Sept 2021.
21. Fromme HB, Karani R, Downing SM. Direct observation in medical education: a review of the literature and evidence for validity. Mount Sinai J Med. 2009;76(4):365–71. https://doi.org/10.1002/MSJ.20123.
22. LaDonna KA, Hatala R, Lingard L, Voyer S, Watling C. Staging a performance: learners' perceptions about direct observation during residency. Med Educ. 2017;51(5):498–510. https://doi.org/10.1111/MEDU.13232.
23. Kogan JR, Hatala R, Hauer KE, Holmboe E. Guidelines: the do's, don'ts and don't knows of direct observation of clinical skills in medical education. Perspect Med Educ. 2017;6(5):286–305. https://doi.org/10.1007/S40037-017-0376-7.
24. Phillips SC, Hawley CE, Triantafylidis LK, Schwartz AW. Geriatrics 5Ms for primary care workshop. MedEdPORTAL. 2019;15:10814. https://doi.org/10.15766/MEP_2374-8265.10814.
25. Schwartz AW, Hawley CE, Strong JV, et al. A workshop for Interprofessional trainees using the geriatrics 5Ms framework. J Am Geriatr Soc. 2020;68(8):1857–63. https://doi.org/10.1111/JGS.16574.
26. Michener A, Fessler E, Gonzalez M, Miller RK. The 5 M's and more: a new geriatric medical student virtual curriculum during the COVID-19 pandemic. J Am Geriatr Soc. 2020;68(11):E61–3. https://doi.org/10.1111/JGS.16855.
27. Bajaj K, Meguerdichian M, Thoma B, Huang S, Eppich W, Cheng A. The PEARLS healthcare debriefing tool. Acad Med. 2018;93(2):336. https://doi.org/10.1097/ACM.0000000000002035.
28. Lerchenfeldt S, Mi M, Eng M. The utilization of peer feedback during collaborative learning in undergraduate medical education: a systematic review. BMC Med Educ. 2019;19(1):1–10. https://doi.org/10.1186/S12909-019-1755-Z.
29. Use the Teach-Back Method Tool 5. http://www.ahrq.gov/literacy. Accessed 8 Dec 2021.
30. Cetrone E, Young M, Demers L. No place like home: student and faculty perspectives on the value of house calls in medical education. J Am Geriatr Soc. 2021;70:E1–4. https://doi.org/10.1111/JGS.17505.
31. Duque G, Fung S, Mallet L, Posel N, Fleiszer D. Learning while having fun: the use of video gaming to teach geriatric house calls to medical students. J Am Geriatr Soc. 2008;56(7):1328–32. https://doi.org/10.1111/J.1532-5415.2008.01759.X.
32. Kim-Godwin YS, Livsey KR, Ezzell D, Highsmith C. Home visit simulation using a standardized patient. Clin Simul Nurs. 2013;9(2):e55–61. https://doi.org/10.1016/J.ECNS.2011.09.003.
33. Sehgal M, Syed Q, Callahan KE, et al. Introducing aquifer geriatrics, the American Geriatrics Society National Online Curriculum. J Am Geriatr Soc. 2019;67(4):811–7. https://doi.org/10.1111/JGS.15813.
34. Duque G, Demontiero O, Whereat S, et al. Evaluation of a blended learning model in geriatric medicine: a successful learning experience for medical students. Australas J Ageing. 2013;32(2):103–9. https://doi.org/10.1111/J.1741-6612.2012.00620.X.
35. Robertson ML, Schuchman M, Cudjoe TKM, Colburn J. Innovative educational approaches to house calls in the time of COVID-19. J Am Geriatr Soc. 2021;69(8):E20. https://doi.org/10.1111/JGS.17331.

Chapter 12
Teaching Geriatrics in the Hospital: Bedside Geriatrics Teaching

Songprod Jonathan Lorgunpai and Rainier Patrick Soriano

Teaching Geriatrics in the Hospital

Older adults make up about 16% of the population in the USA but represent nearly 40% of hospitalized adults and almost 50% of all health care dollars spent on hospitalization [1, 2]. Hospitalizations and health care spending for older adults are expected to rise as the population continues to age.

A large portion of physicians' medical school education and residency training occurs in acute care settings. The hospital is a very important setting for older adult care and hospitalization often results in complications, including functional, physical, and cognitive decline [3], that are unrelated to the inciting problem prompting hospital admission. The care that older adults receive during a relatively short hospital stay often have long-term impacts. As many of the harmful effects of hospitalization can be avoided or minimized by addressing specific risks that predispose to

S. J. Lorgunpai (✉)
Mount Auburn Hospital, Harvard Medical School, Cambridge, MA, USA
e-mail: Songprod.lorgunpai@mah.harvard.edu

R. P. Soriano
Icahn School of Medicine at Mount Sinai, New York, NY, USA
e-mail: Rainier.soriano@mssm.edu

A. W. Schwartz (ed.), *Medical Education in Geriatrics*,
https://doi.org/10.1007/978-3-031-32499-4_12

poor clinical outcomes, it is imperative that all health care professionals possess and demonstrate skills in the optimal care of these hospitalized older adults.

There are several clinical settings wherein the care of the hospitalized older adult can be taught including medicine services, co-management services (with orthopedics, trauma surgery, psychiatry, or other specialties), geriatric consultation services, and specialized geriatric inpatient units such as acute care of the elderly (ACE) units and geriatric evaluation and management (GEM) units. This chapter emphasizes teaching on the general medicine or geriatric medicine services as these are the more common settings of hospitalized older adults although these concepts can be applied in other settings.

The Bedside Rounds

The medical literature describes various educational programs designed to teach inpatient geriatrics care at all levels of learners, ranging from medical students to practicing physicians [4–7]. Despite all of these various teaching techniques, bedside rounds remain the mainstay of teaching about older adult care in the hospital setting. Table 12.1 provides a general framework in approaching bedside teaching of the hospitalized older adult patient.

Table 12.1 General framework on bedside teaching

Before entering patient's room
• Build rapport with team members
• Assign roles to team members prior to the patient encounter
At the bedside
• Introduce each team member and their roles to the patient and/or family members in the room
• When possible, invite interprofessional team members to collaborate on bedside rounds
• The team member leading the discussion should be positioned at eye level of the patient
• Try to encourage patients to sit up or stand during rounds to promote mobility when possible
• Describe what is about to occur to the patient. Inform them that there may be theoretical teaching discussions that may not be applicable to their illness. The lead discussant should let the patient know about these instances
• Model speaking clearly, loud enough for the patient to hear [8], and using simple language that the patient can understand. Speak in the second person to the patient instead of about the patient in the third person. Avoid language like "talk shop" or language that is not person centered
• Maintain eye contact with patients and learners
• Provide opportunities for patients to ask questions and be involved as teachers
• Summarize what was taught during the encounter to learners and summarize the discussion to patients, including what applies and what does not apply to their management
• Thank the patient for their time and contribution to teaching
After leaving patient's room
• Reflect on patient encounter and provide feedback to learners (see Chap. 21 on providing effective feedback)
• Provide opportunities for learners to ask further questions about what was discussed

The main challenge to teaching geriatrics in the hospital remains to be the time limitations imposed by the nature of the acute care setting [5, 9]. Therefore, teaching key geriatric concepts and modeling high-quality geriatrics care during bedside rounds is a practical and efficient way to educate trainees of all levels. By combining patient care with teaching about geriatrics, learners can observe their teachers model behaviors that focus on the health trajectory of hospitalized older adults. Table 12.2 provides examples of opportunities of tasks and behaviors that demonstrate high-quality geriatrics care at the bedside.

Table 12.2 Modeling high-quality geriatrics care during bedside rounds

Task/behavior	Related domains	Geriatrics 5MS
Review		
Medication administration records	Adverse drug effects and medication errors	Medications
Timing of patient care-related tasks e.g., medication administration, labs, vital sign checks, diagnostic tests	Sleep disturbances, delirium	Medications Mind
Reports from overnight team, nursing, consultants including physical, occupational, and speech therapy if applicable	Immobility, hospital-associated disability, discharge planning	Mind Mobility Multi-complexity
Changes in estimated glomerular filtration rate (eGFR)	Adverse drug effects and medication errors, malnutrition, and dehydration	Medications
Ask about		
Activity level, e.g., times out of bed, number of walks in past day	Immobility	Mobility
Bowel movements	Constipation, malnutrition, immobility	Mind Mobility
Food and fluid intake/urine output	Malnutrition and dehydration, pressure injuries	Mind Mobility
Pain	Delirium, immobility	Mind Mobility
Sleep	Sleep disturbances, delirium	Mind
Examine patient		
Orientation and attention	Delirium	Mind
Skin, focusing on areas of bony prominence	Pressure injuries	Mobility
Presence of tethers (e.g., urinary catheter, intravenous lines, telemonitoring, oxygen nasal cannula)	Urinary retention and incontinence, immobility, delirium	Mind Mobility
Use of bed or chair alarm	Immobility	Mobility

(continued)

Table 12.2 (continued)

Task/behavior	Related domains	Geriatrics 5MS
Examine environment		
Availability of drinking water/oral fluids and dentures	Delirium, malnutrition, and dehydration	Mind
Availability of assistive devices for sensory deficits (e.g., eyeglasses, contact lens, hearing aids, pocket talkers)	Delirium, immobility	Mind Mobility
Availability of assistive devices for mobility (e.g., cane, walker)	Immobility	Mobility
Intervene		
Open window blinds during day	Sleep disturbances, delirium	Mind
Update orientation aids (e.g., whiteboard, monitor) with accurate orientation information	Delirium	Mind
Bring eyeglasses, hearing aids or amplification device, drinking water, dentures to bedside if needed	Delirium, malnutrition, and dehydration	Mind
Invite patient to sit upright or stand during bedside rounds	Immobility, delirium	Mobility Mind
Obtain or confirm collateral information from and provide update to family/caregivers/hospital staff	Discharge planning, hospital-associated disability, goals of care discussions	Mind Matters most Multi-complexity
Schedule goals of care discussions when appropriate	Goals of care discussions	Matters most

Topics in the Care of the Hospitalized Older Adult

Table 12.3 provides a quick reference guide to key geriatric concepts essential in the teaching and modeling of high-quality geriatrics care in the hospital to learners. Each section provides a topic overview and importance followed by its relevance in the hospital setting and concludes with practical teaching behaviors which could be incorporated into and modeled during daily bedside rounds.

- Comprehensive patient assessment
- Delirium
- Immobility
- Hospital-associated disability
- Pressure injuries
- Adverse drug events and medication errors
- Sleep disturbances
- Urinary retention and incontinence
- Constipation
- Malnutrition and dehydration
- Goals of care discussions
- Discharge planning and transitions of care

Table 12.3 Quick reference teaching guide to key geriatric concepts

General assessment of hospitalized older adults	
Teaching rationale	• Obtaining a comprehensive patient assessment for every older adult admitted to the hospital leads to better patient outcomes and to care that is better aligned with patients' goals
Teaching concepts	• During the history and physical exam, speak to older adults clearly, loudly, and in lower pitches, which tend to be more easily understood by older adults as age-related hearing loss typically affects the ability to hear high-pitched noises first • Ensure that an accurate list of medications taken in the outpatient setting is obtained • Review medications thoroughly to ensure each has an appropriate indication for use • In addition to evaluating the complaint that brought the patient to the hospital, assess the patient's baseline and current cognitive and functional abilities (activities of daily living and instrumental activities of daily living), social supports, living situation, and goals of care to obtain a holistic understanding of patients to provide optimal care • Given the high prevalence of cognitive impairment in older adults, it is often necessary to reach out to family members or other caregivers, with patient permission, for additional information
Teaching pearls	• Ask trainees to consider the Geriatrics 5Ms [10], especially on admission and discharge
Delirium	
Teaching rationale	• Delirium, or acute brain failure, is an acute decline in attention and cognition. It is a common, life-threatening, and potentially preventable clinical syndrome among older adults [11] • Many health conditions, including infections and electrolyte abnormalities, can present with or present as delirium (atypical presentation) • Delirium is present in up to 24% of hospitalized older adults on admission, and it develops in up to 56% during the course of hospitalization on the general wards [12] • Delirium arising during hospitalization is associated with prolonged hospital stays, nursing-home placements, increased mortality, and worsening cognitive function [13]

(continued)

Table 12.3 (continued)

Teaching concepts	• Patients with baseline cognitive impairment are at increased risk of delirium • The confusion assessment method (CAM) [14] is the most useful bedside assessment tool to confirm delirium. Diagnosis of delirium is established when patient meets criteria 1, 2, and either 3 or 4: – 1) Acute change in mental status with a fluctuating course AND – 2) Inattention AND – 3) Disorganized thinking OR – 4) Altered level of consciousness • The ultra-brief 2-item screener (UB-2) [15] is a clinician-administered two-item interview that can be administered in less than 1 min. A positive screen (incorrect answer to either of the items below) requires a more thorough diagnostic interview, ideally with the CAM: – "Please tell me the day of the week" – "Please tell me the months of the year backward, say December as your first month" • Although many clinicians think of patients with delirium as being agitated, hyperactive delirium represents only 25% of cases, with the others having hypoactive ("quiet") delirium [13]. Delirium can be present without any outward evidence of agitation • The DELIRIUM mnemonic is a helpful way to remember to assess common contributors to delirium: Drugs, Electrolyte disturbances, Lack of drugs, Infection, Reduced sensory input, Intracranial disorders, Urinary and fecal disorders, and Myocardial and pulmonary disorders [13]. There are often multiple contributors to delirium in each patient, and all identified contributors should be addressed • Implement nonpharmacologic approaches to managing symptoms of delirium in every patient. These approaches include providing reality orientation (to people, place, situation), explanation, and reassurance; reducing isolation and noises; improving hearing and vision; mobilization of the patient; increasing nursing surveillance; maintaining hydration; managing pain; encouraging family members to be at the bedside or requesting bedside sitters if family members are not available; limiting room and staff changes; removing any unnecessary tethers such as intravenous lines and urinary catheters; and coordinating schedules for medication administrations and vital sign checks to allow the patient an uninterrupted period of sleep at night • Reserve pharmacologic approaches to manage symptoms of delirium only when the symptoms would threaten the patients' own safety or the safety of others or would result in the interruption of essential therapy. When medications are used, start at a low dose, and increase the dose slowly as needed. Due to the preferable side effect profile, it is reasonable to start with trazodone. If an additional agent is needed, it is reasonable to add an antipsychotic • Preventing delirium is the most effective strategy for reducing its frequency and complications. Six risk factors targeted in the hospital elder life program, now known as the AGS CoCare: HELP program, decreased delirium incidence and complications [16, 17]: – Orientation and therapeutic activities for cognitive impairment – Early mobilization to avert immobilization – Nonpharmacologic approaches to minimize the use of psychoactive drugs – Interventions to prevent sleep deprivation – Communication methods and adaptive equipment (particularly eyeglasses and hearing aids) for vision and hearing impairment – Early intervention for volume depletion

Table 12.3 (continued)

Teaching pearls	• On daily bedside rounds, have learners assess the presence of delirium using the CAM method or UB-2 screener. If present, have learners assess possible contributing factors using the DELIRIUM mnemonic • On daily bedside rounds, ask learners to confirm that the patient's orientation aids (e.g. whiteboard, monitor) have accurate orientation information that is large enough for them to see, ensure the window blinds are open during the day, encourage the patient to get out of bed and stand during rounds, check that their assistive devices for sensory deficits (e.g. glasses, hearing aids, pocket talkers) are available, and make sure that drinking water is available within reach • Ask learners for potential nonpharmacologic approaches to managing delirium
Immobility	
Teaching rationale	• Immobility contributes to multiple adverse patient outcomes such as increased risk of injurious falls, delirium, aspiration pneumonia, pressure injuries, functional decline, prolonged length of stay, institutionalization, readmissions, increased healthcare costs, and mortality [18] • Hospitalized patients generally spend more than 95% of their time in a bed or chair, even when they are capable of walking independently [19, 20]
Teaching concepts	• It is important for hospitalized patients to ambulate several times a day every day as soon as their medical condition allows. Even patients on ventilators in the intensive care unit have successfully ambulated around the unit [21] • Do not routinely use bed and chair alarms as they substantially restrict patient mobility and have been shown to be ineffective at reducing either falls or injurious falls [22, 23] • The short physical performance battery (SPPB) is a quick and easily administered assessment tool that captures a wide range of functional abilities and can predict future mobility, falls, and disability in activities of daily living [24, 25]
Teaching pearls	• Have learners encourage patients to get out of bed • During rounds, invite patients to sit up or stand during the interview and examination • Have learners ask patients whether they use assistive devices at baseline and have those devices readily accessible to them during hospitalization • Re-evaluate the need for any tethers (e.g., Foley catheters, intravenous lines, telemonitoring, and oxygen nasal cannula) which provide challenges to ambulating • When rounding on a patient who did not get out of bed the previous day, ask trainees to list reasons why immobility should be avoided • When rounding on a patient with concerns for poor balance and lower extremity strength, if appropriate, ask learners to conduct the short physical performance battery and have learners share their observations on different components of the test and deficits identified. When possible, have the team join physical therapists at the bedside when they assess patients' mobility
Hospital-associated disability	
Teaching rationale	• Hospital-associated disability, a new loss of ability to complete one or more activities of daily living (ADLs) without assistance at hospital discharge, is a common complication of hospitalization for older adults • Approximately 50% of disability among older adults occurs in the setting of medical hospitalization [26] • Among hospitalized medical patients over 70 years old, about one-third are discharged with a disability that was not present 2 weeks before admission [27] • Loss of independences with ADL capabilities is associated with multiple adverse outcomes including longer hospital stays, higher readmission rates, nursing-home placement, and higher mortality risk [28, 29]

(continued)

Table 12.3 (continued)

Teaching concepts	• Encourage patients to get out of bed and ambulate several times a day as soon as their medical condition allows • Implement measures to decrease the risk of delirium and ensure adequate nutrition in all patients
Teaching pearls	• Assign trainees to obtain a thorough functional history which includes asking patients or family members about patients' prehospital functioning 2 weeks prior to the acute illness that led to the hospitalization such as typical day-to-day schedule and ability to complete ADLs and IADLs • Have learners obtain physical, occupational, and speech therapy consultations if declines from prehospital function are identified • Have trainees consider patients' prior and current functional abilities in setting up a discharge plan to the most appropriate level of care setting
Pressure injuries	
Teaching rationale	• Pressure injuries (pressure ulcers) are painful, costly, and associated with infections, longer hospitalizations, delayed return of function, and mortality risks • Pressure injuries are common in acute care settings with a median incidence of 15.7% among frail older adults or high-risk individuals [30] • As many as 1 in 16 patients 65 years old or older develop one or more pressure injuries within the first 2 days of hospitalization on a medicine service [30]
Teaching concepts	• Most pressure injuries develop on areas of bony prominence, particularly the sacrum and heels, but can develop in any part of the body, including on the nostrils from nasal cannula use and on the scalp from immobilization with ventilator use • Risk factors for developing pressure injuries include older age, low body weight, physical and cognitive impairment, incontinence, and malnutrition • National Pressure Injury Advisory Panel (NPIAP) stages [31]: – Stage 1: Intact skin with a localized area of non-blanchable erythema – Stage 2: Partial-thickness skin loss with exposed dermis – Stage 3: Full-thickness loss of skin, in which adipose (fat) is visible and granulation tissue is often present – Stage 4: Full-thickness skin and tissue loss with exposed or directly palpable fascia, muscle, tendon, ligament, cartilage, or bone in the ulcer – Unstageable: Full-thickness skin and tissue loss in which the extent of tissue damage within the ulcer cannot be confirmed because it is obscured by slough or eschar – Deep tissue pressure injury: Intact or non-intact skin with localized area of persistent non-blanchable deep red, maroon, purple discoloration, or epidermal separation revealing a dark wound bed or blood-filled blister • Management: Relieve pressure, redistribute pressure with support surfaces, avoid friction, remove necrotic tissue, optimize protein and calorie intake, treat infectious complications as they occur, and control pain
Teaching pearls	• On daily bedside rounds, have learners inspect the skin of at-risk patients, focusing on areas of bony prominence • When pressure injuries are identified, have learners inspect, palpate, and probe for depth at the bedside and come up with the stages of the pressure injuries, what likely contributed to the injuries, and strategies to manage the pressure injuries • Set up a time for learners to assess the pressure injuries with wound consultants when possible • Ask learners to encourage patients to change positions frequency and to get up out of bed and ambulate several times a day

Table 12.3 (continued)

Adverse drug events and medication errors	
Teaching rationale	• Adverse drug events (ADE) and medication errors are common. Intrinsic factors include physiologic decreases in liver and kidney function. Extrinsic factors include being on multiple medications for multiple medical conditions, barriers to medication reconciliation, significant turnover in their medication regimen with many old medications discontinued and new medications introduced during hospitalization • One study found that 49% of hospitalized older adults received at least one potentially inappropriate medication during hospitalization [32] • Serious ADEs include delirium, urinary retention, orthostasis, metabolic derangements, bleeding from anticoagulation, and hypoglycemia • ADEs are associated with increased length of stay, higher costs, and increased risk of death
Teaching concepts	• Conduct thorough medication reconciliation during care transitions, including upon admission and on discharge • Prehospitalization medication lists in the electronic health records are not always accurate. Confirm the medication lists with patient's pharmacists, the patients themselves or with family members for patients who do not manage their own medications. For patients residing in nursing homes or assisted living facilities, request medication lists from these facilities • Ask about herbal and over-the-counter medications • The American Geriatrics Society Beers Criteria for Potentially Inappropriate Medication Use in Older Adults can serve as a starting point for a comprehensive process of identifying and improving medication appropriateness and safety [33]. Medications are included based on having an unfavorable balance of benefits and harms for many older adults compared with alternative treatments. Read the rationale and recommendations statements for each criterion to apply recommendations appropriately • Limit prescribing benzodiazepines, first-generation antihistamines, skeletal muscle relaxants, antipsychotics, and opioids • Deprescribing.org is an online reference tool that supports clinicians in safely reducing or stopping medications for specific drug classes [34, 35] • Medications metabolized by the kidneys should be dosed by the estimated glomerular filtration rate (GFR) instead of the serum creatinine. As older adults often have decreased muscle mass and decreased dietary protein intake, serum creatinine may not be elevated in the presence of decreased kidney function
Teaching pearls	• On daily bedside rounds, have learners evaluate the clinical utility of each medication ordered and its potential for side effects or drug interactions. Ensure that each medication is appropriately dosed based on the most recent eGFR and has an appropriate administration route • Have learners review the medication administration record daily to keep track of which medications are being administered and how frequently, including as needed medications • Ask learners to determine if any medications currently administered intravenously can be converted and orally administered, for patient comfort and to remove the need for a tether that decreases patient's ability to ambulate freely • Ask learners to look up the pre-admission medications and review discrepancies • When a patient is identified as taking a medication that is potentially inappropriate, ask learners to come up with a plan on how the medication could be safely deprescribed

(continued)

Table 12.3 (continued)

Sleep disturbances	
Teaching rationale	• Patients regularly report poor sleep quality and quantity during hospitalization • Multiple factors contribute to this including an unfamiliar sleep setting, conditions related to the acute illness (e.g., pain), environmental noise and light, and the tasks related to providing care (e.g., vital sign checks, venipunctures, diagnostic testing, and medication schedules) • Sleep deprivation is important to prevent, recognize, and address because it is associated with an increased risk of delirium [12]
Teaching concepts	• Non-pharmacological management of sleep disturbance is safe and effective. A protocol using nighttime noise reduction strategies, warm drinks, soothing music, massage treatments, and rescheduled medication administration and measurement of vital signs to avoid sleep interruption significantly reduced the use of sedative-hypnotics in the hospital [16] • Try to avoid benzodiazepines and non-benzodiazepine receptor agonists (e.g., zolpidem, eszopiclone/zopiclone, zaleplon) given their association with cognitive decline, delirium, falls, and respiratory depression in older adults [36–38] • Try to avoid the use of diphenhydramine and other first-generation antihistamines given they are associated with impaired cognition and anticholinergic effects including constipation and urinary retention [39] • When medications are needed, try melatonin given its mild side effect profile, low potential for drug–drug interactions, and potential to improve circadian rhythms. Several studies in hospitalized patients have found improvements in sleep and sleep quality with 1–5 mg of melatonin at night [40, 41] • In hospitals where melatonin is not available, melatonin receptor agonists such as ramelteon are an acceptable alternative, with limited data suggesting they may play a role in preventing delirium in older adult inpatients [42] • When an additional medication is needed, consider trazodone, which is generally better tolerated than benzodiazepines, without the risk for physiologic tolerance or dependence. In a small observational study of hospitalized psychiatric patients, trazodone appeared to be a more effective sleep aid than quetiapine based on patient-reported and nursing-observed sleep outcomes [43]
Teaching pearls	• During daily rounds, have learners ask patients and their nurses about their sleep and review the timing of medication administrations, vital sign checks, and diagnostic testing to optimize sleep • Ask learners to list possible contributors to a patient's sleep disturbance and discuss non-pharmacological approaches that could be tried for the patient
Urinary retention and incontinence	
Teaching rationale	• The most common hospital-acquired infection is urinary tract infection (UTI), which accounts for almost 40% of all nosocomial infections. Most hospital-acquired UTIs are associated with urinary catheters [44] • Up to 25% of hospitalized patients have a urinary catheter placed during their stay [44] • Urinary catheter use should be minimized as it is associated with increased UTI, delirium, immobility (serving as a "one-point restraint"), urethral and meatal injury, scarring, bleeding, pain, and bladder and renal stones (by increasing the risk of urinary tract infections with urea-splitting organisms) [44, 45]

Table 12.3 (continued)

Teaching concepts	• Patients who are unable to void should undergo a thorough evaluation. Medications should be reviewed, especially the use of anticholinergics, calcium channel blockers, and opioids. Patients should also be evaluated for constipation, spinal cord disease, diabetes, vitamin B12 deficiency, benign and malignant prostate diseases (in men), and pelvic organ prolapse (in women) • Appropriate indications for urinary catheter use include [46]: – Inability to void (urinary retention) – Urinary incontinence and (1) stage 3, 4, or unstageable pressure injuries that cannot be kept clear of urinary incontinence despite wound care or (2) nurses find it difficult to provide skin care despite other urinary management strategies – Urine volume measurement when measurement is required to provide treatment and cannot be assessed by other volume and urine collection strategies – Improvement in comfort when (1) acute, severe pain is present with movement or (2) urine collection by catheter addresses patient and family goals in a dying patient – Management of gross hematuria with blood clots in urine • For most patients with urinary retention, start with 1–2 trials of intermittent urethral catheterization while addressing the underlying contributors of the urinary retention. If a patient is still unable to void, it is usually reasonable to keep the urethral catheter in place, assess the need for continued catheter usage daily, and remove the catheter as soon as feasible
Teaching pearls	• On daily bedside rounds, have learners identify the presence of a urinary catheter • If present, ask learners to list the appropriate indications for its continued use. If an appropriate indication does not exist, have the learner arrange for the patient to have a voiding trial without a catheter
Constipation	
Teaching rationale	• Constipation is common in hospitalized older adults due to multiple factors including decreased fluid and fiber intake, decreased mobility, and adverse effects of new medications such as opioids • Constipation can lead to delirium, pain, urinary retention, urinary incontinence, and fecal incontinence [13, 47]
Teaching concepts	• Assess patient's baseline pattern of bowel function on admission and keep track of bowel function throughout hospitalization • Ensure adequate fluid and fiber intake daily. Minimize restrictive diets as possible • Prunes, apples, and whole grains are a good source of high-fiber foods • Encourage regular daily ambulation as soon as safe to do so • Bed pans are usually uncomfortable for most patients and may affect the desire to have bowel movements. Arrange or provide assistance for patients to ambulate to the bathroom • Fiber supplements, also known as bulk-forming laxatives (e.g., psyllium) are safe initial laxatives when needed. Sufficient water must accompany their intake to prevent the supplements from becoming too viscous, which can lead to intestinal obstruction • In patients not responding to fiber supplements, osmotic laxatives (e.g., polyethylene glycol) can be tried. For patients needing additional laxatives, stimulant laxatives (e.g., senna) can be added
Teaching pearls	• On daily bedside rounds, have learners ask patients about their food and fluid intake and bowel movements, encourage fiber intake and mobility, and encourage getting out of bed at mealtimes • When a patient is noted to be constipated on rounds, ask learners to list likely contributors and steps that could be taken for its improvement

(continued)

Table 12.3 (continued)

Malnutrition and dehydration	
Teaching rationale	• Up to 70% of all hospitalized older adults are nutritionally at risk or meet criteria for malnutrition [48] • Poor nutrition status is associated with hospital-acquired infections, longer length of hospital stays, higher readmission rates, increased likelihood of being discharged to an extended care facility, and higher mortality rates [48–50]
Teaching concepts	• The major causes of malnutrition for older hospitalized patients include impaired cognition or delirium; poor appetite, nausea, or constipation; immobility; no access to dentures; difficulty in self-feeding; and severely restricted diet orders • The mini-nutritional assessment (MNA) is a widely validated screening tool for identifying older adults at risk for poor nutrition and is predictive of poor outcomes [51] • There is no need for sodium restriction in patients with hypertension and heart failure when those conditions are well controlled. Salt wasting increases with age, increasing the tendency toward dehydration. Older adults eat less when the food is not tasty • Feeding tubes do not improve the quantity or quality of life in older patients in the final stage of dementia who are no longer able to maintain adequate oral nutrition [52]. Tube-feeding is associated with agitation, increased use of physical and chemical restraints, and worsening pressure ulcers [53]. The American Geriatrics Society's choosing wisely recommendations [53] and guideline on feeding tubes in patients with advanced dementia [54] recommend against their use in most circumstances
Teaching pearls	• On daily bedside rounds, have learners ensure patients have access to dentures and receive any needed assistance with feeding • When concerns of malnutrition arise, ask a learner to conduct the mini-nutritional assessment, share the findings with the team, and consult a nutritionist/dietitian
Goals of care discussions	
Teaching rationale	• An older adult's hospital course may lead to new diagnoses and new prognoses • Hospitalization is often an appropriate event to discuss goals of care with patients and their family members and caregivers, especially when new diagnoses are identified that affect prognosis

Table 12.3 (continued)

Teaching concepts	• Initiate goals of care discussions on admission to determine patients' values, treatment goals, and preferences, including prior documented wishes • Family meetings should be scheduled in advance whenever possible to increase the likelihood that family members or caregivers whom a patient wishes to be present can attend, either in person or virtually • Try to find a quiet room and limit distractions and pagers during the family meeting. Consider asking a team member who is not directly involved with the care of the patient to cover the pagers for learners who will be present at a family meeting • All team members should meet beforehand to ensure that all agree with the clinical situation, prognosis, available options, and recommendations. This helps avoid presenting mixed messages which may confuse patients and family members • Use jargon-free language and validate emotions shown by patients and family members • Present palliative care, including hospice, as a positive, active treatment option for patients with advanced disease, when appropriate • Teach trainees a structured approach to family meetings. Vitaltalk.org provides helpful resources for family meetings. Their 7-steps to a family conference include: (1) Gather for a pre-meeting, (2) introduce everyone and the agenda, (3) explain what is happening, (4) empathize with each person, (5) highlight the patient's voice, (6) plan the next steps together, and (7) reflect post-meeting [55] • Other helpful websites include: – The New England Journal of Medicine videos in clinical medicine series have a helpful video that provides a flexible framework for leading family meetings [56] – Patientprioritiescare.org provides resources that help patients and clinicians focus decision-making and healthcare on patients' own health priorities [57] – ePrognosis.Ucsf.Edu has helpful tools for estimating the mortality risk for hospitalized older adults [58]
Teaching pearls	• Before each family meeting, review structured approaches to family meetings with learner, assign roles, and go over the overall goals and agenda with them • After each family meeting, debrief as a team and share feedback on what went well and what could be improved in future meetings
Discharge planning and transitions of care	
Teaching rationale	• Suboptimal discharge planning is associated with readmissions and worse outcomes for hospitalized older adults • Hospital readmissions from home and skilled nursing facilities occur within 30 days in up to a quarter of older adults [59, 60]

(continued)

Table 12.3 (continued)

Teaching concepts	• Different post-discharge settings available include acute rehabilitation, subacute rehabilitation, assisted living, and independent living settings • Work in conjunction with other health care providers (e.g. social work, case management, nursing, physical therapy, occupational therapy) to recommend appropriate service based on the clinical needs, personal values and social and financial resources of the patient and their families, and the patient's eligibility for community-based services • Discharge summaries should contain core information needed by those assuming care of the patients: a summary of the admitting problems and hospital course, recent and important pending labs, accurately reconciled medication lists including admission medications and all changes, information about advanced directives, baseline and present cognitive and functional status, clinical status, plan of care, scheduled or needed follow-up, hospital physician contact information, social support and contact info, nursing needs, and rehabilitation needs. Consider organizing discharge summaries by the 5Ms
Teaching pearls	• During bedside rounds on the day of discharge, have learners go over the discharge plan with patients and their family members and ask them to share the plan back to the team, to make sure that they understand the plan including follow-up recommendations and when to seek more urgent medical attention • Once a learner has drafted the discharge summary, ask another learner to review it through the perspective of a clinician who is meeting the patient for the first time in the post-discharge setting the patient is being discharged to, to see if any questions arise regarding caring for the patient in the next setting of care and regarding the patient's 5Ms If a patient is readmitted to the hospital, ask learners to list contributors to the readmission and ways to decrease the risk of another readmission in the future

Future Directions

As this chapter illustrates, hospitalization is disruptive for older adults and puts them at risk of many complications and medical errors that occur during transitions of care. Given the many challenges older adults face in the inpatient setting, geriatricians are constantly working on quality improvement and other initiatives to improve the care of hospitalized older adults. One such initiative, the Age-Friendly Health Systems, encourages health systems to reliably provide a set of four evidence-based elements of high-quality care, known as the "4Ms," to all older adults: What Matters, Medication, Mentation, and Mobility. Discussing the challenges older adults face in the inpatient setting could help learners become curious about and motivated to join quality improvement initiatives to improve the care for older adults. Other initiatives include home hospital care, in which hospital-level care is provided in the patient's home. Compared to hospitalization, home hospital care has been associated with improved physical activity, reduced costs of care, reduced risk of delirium, lower rates of admission to long-term care, and increased patient satisfaction, without changes in quality or safety [61–64]. More hospital-level care may be delivered in the home setting in the future, and this shift will undoubtedly have consequences on the teaching of these important geriatric concepts. In the future, learners may need to learn about fitting hospital beds into patients' homes, ordering durable medical equipment, setting up imaging and other tests in patients' homes, training caregivers on how to monitor patients' clinical status, navigating increasingly complex remote monitoring devices, and conducting virtual rounds using telemedicine technologies. Given that older adults will continue to require acute level of care, all health care professionals should be educated and ready to provide high-quality care wherever the acute care site may be.

References

1. https://agingstats.gov/docs/LatestReport/OA20_508_10142020.pdf.
2. https://www.cdc.gov/nchs/data/hus/2019/040-508.pdf.
3. Creditor MC. Hazards of hospitalization of the elderly. Ann Intern Med. 1993;118(3):219–23. https://doi.org/10.7326/0003-4819-118-3-199302010-00011.
4. St Onge J, Ioannidis G, Papaioannou A, McLeod H, Marr S. Impact of a mandatory geriatric medicine clerkship on the care of older acute medical patients: a retrospective cohort study. BMC Med Educ. 2013;13:168. https://doi.org/10.1186/1472-6920-13-168.
5. Karani R, Leipzig RM, Callahan EH, Thomas DC. An unfolding case with a linked objective structured clinical examination (OSCE): a curriculum in inpatient geriatric medicine. J Am Geriatr Soc. 2004;52(7):1191–8. https://doi.org/10.1111/j.1532-5415.2004.52321.x.
6. Podrazik PM, Levine S, Smith S, et al. The curriculum for the hospitalized aging medical patient program: a collaborative faculty development program for hospitalists, general internists, and geriatricians. J Hosp Med. 2008;3(5):384–93. https://doi.org/10.1002/jhm.348.
7. Mazotti L, Moylan A, Murphy E, Harper GM, Johnston CB, Hauer KE. Advancing geriatrics education: an efficient faculty development program for academic hospitalists increases geriatric teaching. J Hosp Med. 2010;5(9):541–6. https://doi.org/10.1002/jhm.791.
8. Aquilina T, Thompson SM, Metcalfe KHM, Hughes H, Sinclair L, Batt F. The involvement of older inpatients in medical student education. Eur Geriatr Med. 2018;9(1):77–82. https://doi.org/10.1007/s41999-017-0023-1.
9. Siegler EL, Capello CF. Creating a teaching geriatric service: ten important lessons. J Am Geriatr Soc. 2005;53(2):327–30. https://doi.org/10.1111/j.1532-5415.2005.53122.x.
10. Tinetti M, Huang A, Molnar F. The Geriatrics 5M's: A new way of communicating what we do. J Am Geriatr Soc. 2017;65(9):2115. https://doi.org/10.1111/jgs.14979. Epub 2017 Jun 6. PMID: 28586122.
11. Mattison MLP. Delirium. Ann Intern Med. 2020;173(7):ITC49–64. https://doi.org/10.7326/AITC202010060.
12. Inouye SK. Delirium in older persons. N Engl J Med. 2006;354(11):1157–65. https://doi.org/10.1056/NEJMra052321.
13. Marcantonio ER. Delirium in hospitalized older adults. N Engl J Med. 2017;377(15):1456–66. https://doi.org/10.1056/NEJMcp1605501.
14. Inouye SK, van Dyck CH, Alessi CA, Balkin S, Siegal AP, Horwitz RI. Clarifying confusion: the confusion assessment method. A new method for detection of delirium. Ann Intern Med. 1990;113(12):941–8. https://doi.org/10.7326/0003-4819-113-12-941.
15. NIDUS-Network for Investigation of Delirium: Unifying Scientists. Instrument: Ultra-Brief 2-item Screener. https://deliriumnetwork.org/wp-content/uploads/2019/05/UB-2.pdf. Accessed 1 Dec 2021.
16. Inouye SK, Bogardus ST, Charpentier PA, et al. A multicomponent intervention to prevent delirium in hospitalized older patients. N Engl J Med. 1999;340(9):669–76. https://doi.org/10.1056/NEJM199903043400901.
17. Inouye S. AGS CoCare: HELP. https://help.agscocare.org/. Accessed 1 Dec 2021.

18. Lorgunpai SJ, Finke B, Burrows I, et al. Mobility action group: using quality improvement methods to create a culture of hospital mobility. J Am Geriatr Soc. 2020;68(10):2373–81. https://doi.org/10.1111/jgs.16699.
19. Brown CJ, Redden DT, Flood KL, Allman RM. The underrecognized epidemic of low mobility during hospitalization of older adults. J Am Geriatr Soc. 2009;57(9):1660–5. https://doi.org/10.1111/j.1532-5415.2009.02393.x.
20. Pedersen MM, Bodilsen AC, Petersen J, et al. Twenty-four-hour mobility during acute hospitalization in older medical patients. J Gerontol A Biol Sci Med Sci. 2013;68(3):331–7. https://doi.org/10.1093/gerona/gls165.
21. Bailey P, Thomsen GE, Spuhler VJ, et al. Early activity is feasible and safe in respiratory failure patients. Crit Care Med. 2007;35(1):139–45. https://doi.org/10.1097/01.CCM.0000251130.69568.87.
22. Shorr RI, Chandler AM, Mion LC, et al. Effects of an intervention to increase bed alarm use to prevent falls in hospitalized patients: a cluster randomized trial. Ann Intern Med. 2012;157(10):692–9. https://doi.org/10.7326/0003-4819-157-10-201211200-00005.
23. Sahota O, Drummond A, Kendrick D, et al. REFINE (REducing falls in in-patieNt elderly) using bed and bedside chair pressure sensors linked to radio-pagers in acute hospital care: a randomised controlled trial. Age Ageing. 2014;43(2):247–53. https://doi.org/10.1093/ageing/aft155.
24. Guralnik JM, Ferrucci L, Pieper CF, et al. Lower extremity function and subsequent disability: consistency across studies, predictive models, and value of gait speed alone compared with the short physical performance battery. J Gerontol A Biol Sci Med Sci. 2000;55(4):M221–31. https://doi.org/10.1093/gerona/55.4.m221.
25. de Rekeneire N, Visser M, Peila R, et al. Is a fall just a fall: correlates of falling in healthy older persons. The health, aging and body composition study. J Am Geriatr Soc. 2003;51(6):841–6. https://doi.org/10.1046/j.1365-2389.2003.51267.x.
26. Gill TM, Allore HG, Holford TR, Guo Z. Hospitalization, restricted activity, and the development of disability among older persons. JAMA. 2004;292(17):2115–24. https://doi.org/10.1001/jama.292.17.2115.
27. Covinsky KE, Pierluissi E, Johnston CB. Hospitalization-associated disability: "she was probably able to ambulate, but I'm not sure". JAMA. 2011;306(16):1782–93. https://doi.org/10.1001/jama.2011.1556.
28. Brown CJ. After three decades of study, hospital-associated disability remains a common problem. J Am Geriatr Soc. 2020;68(3):465–6. https://doi.org/10.1111/jgs.16349.
29. Dharmarajan K, Han L, Gahbauer EA, Leo-Summers LS, Gill TM. Disability and recovery after hospitalization for medical illness among community-living older persons: a prospective cohort study. J Am Geriatr Soc. 2020;68(3):486–95. https://doi.org/10.1111/jgs.16350.
30. Baumgarten M, Margolis DJ, Localio AR, et al. Pressure ulcers among elderly patients early in the hospital stay. J Gerontol A Biol Sci Med Sci. 2006;61(7):749–54. https://doi.org/10.1093/gerona/61.7.749.
31. The National Pressure Injury Advisory Panel. Pressure Injury Stages. https://npiap.com/page/PressureInjuryStages. Accessed 15 Aug 2021.
32. Rothberg MB, Pekow PS, Liu F, et al. Potentially inappropriate medication use in hospitalized elders. J Hosp Med. 2008;3(2):91–102. https://doi.org/10.1002/jhm.290.
33. Panel BtAGSBCUE. American Geriatrics Society 2019 Updated AGS Beers Criteria® for potentially inappropriate medication use in older adults. J Am Geriatr Soc. 2019;67(4):674–94. https://doi.org/10.1111/jgs.15767.
34. Farrell B, Tannenbaum C. The Canadian Deprescribing Network. Deprescribing.org. https://deprescribing.org/.
35. Phung E, Triantafylidis L, Zhang H, Yeh I. New Media, Part 5: online deprescribing tools. J Palliat Med. 2018;21(2):269. https://doi.org/10.1089/jpm.2017.0688.
36. Young JS, Bourgeois JA, Hilty DM, Hardin KA. Sleep in hospitalized medical patients, part 2: behavioral and pharmacological management of sleep disturbances. J Hosp Med. 2009;4(1):50–9. https://doi.org/10.1002/jhm.397.

37. Mahoney JE, Webb MJ, Gray SL. Zolpidem prescribing and adverse drug reactions in hospitalized general medicine patients at a veterans affairs hospital. Am J Geriatr Pharmacother. 2004;2(1):66–74. https://doi.org/10.1016/s1543-5946(04)90008-6.
38. Kolla BP, Lovely JK, Mansukhani MP, Morgenthaler TI. Zolpidem is independently associated with increased risk of inpatient falls. J Hosp Med. 2013;8(1):1–6. https://doi.org/10.1002/jhm.1985.
39. Proctor A, Bianchi MT. Clinical pharmacology in sleep medicine. ISRN Pharmacol. 2012;2012:914168. https://doi.org/10.5402/2012/914168.
40. Shilo L, Dagan Y, Smorjik Y, et al. Effect of melatonin on sleep quality of COPD intensive care patients: a pilot study. Chronobiol Int. 2000;17(1):71–6. https://doi.org/10.1081/cbi-100101033.
41. Andrade C, Srihari BS, Reddy KP, Chandramma L. Melatonin in medically ill patients with insomnia: a double-blind, placebo-controlled study. J Clin Psychiatry. 2001;62(1):41–5. https://doi.org/10.4088/jcp.v62n0109.
42. Hatta K, Kishi Y, Wada K, et al. Preventive effects of ramelteon on delirium: a randomized placebo-controlled trial. JAMA Psychiat. 2014;71(4):397–403. https://doi.org/10.1001/jamapsychiatry.2013.3320.
43. Doroudgar S, Chou TI, Yu J, Trinh K, Pal J, Perry PJ. Evaluation of trazodone and quetiapine for insomnia: an observational study in psychiatric inpatients. Prim Care Companion CNS Disord. 2013;15(6):PCC.13m01558. https://doi.org/10.4088/PCC.13m01558.
44. Saint S, Kowalski CP, Kaufman SR, et al. Preventing hospital-acquired urinary tract infection in the United States: a national study. Clin Infect Dis. 2008;46(2):243–50. https://doi.org/10.1086/524662.
45. Saint S, Lipsky BA, Goold SD. Indwelling urinary catheters: a one-point restraint? Ann Intern Med. 2002;137(2):125–7. https://doi.org/10.7326/0003-4819-137-2-200207160-00012.
46. Meddings J, Saint S, Fowler KE, et al. The Ann Arbor criteria for appropriate urinary catheter use in hospitalized medical patients: results obtained by using the RAND/UCLA appropriateness method. Ann Intern Med. 2015;162(9 Suppl):S1–34. https://doi.org/10.7326/M14-1304.
47. Serrano Falcón B, Barceló López M, Mateos Muñoz B, Álvarez Sánchez A, Rey E. Fecal impaction: a systematic review of its medical complications. BMC Geriatr. 2016;16:4. https://doi.org/10.1186/s12877-015-0162-5.
48. de Luis D, Lopez Guzman A, Nutrition Group of Society of Castilla-Leon (endocrinology DaaN). Nutritional status of adult patients admitted to internal medicine departments in public hospitals in Castilla y Leon, Spain—a multi-center study. Eur J Intern Med. 2006;17(8):556–60. https://doi.org/10.1016/j.ejim.2006.02.030.
49. Sharma Y, Miller M, Kaambwa B, et al. Malnutrition and its association with readmission and death within 7 days and 8-180 days postdischarge in older patients: a prospective observational study. BMJ Open. 2017;7(11):e018443. https://doi.org/10.1136/bmjopen-2017-018443.
50. Charlton K, Nichols C, Bowden S, et al. Poor nutritional status of older subacute patients predicts clinical outcomes and mortality at 18 months of follow-up. Eur J Clin Nutr. 2012;66(11):1224–8. https://doi.org/10.1038/ejcn.2012.130.
51. Vellas B, Guigoz Y, Garry PJ, et al. The mini nutritional assessment (MNA) and its use in grading the nutritional state of elderly patients. Nutrition. 1999;15(2):116–22. https://doi.org/10.1016/s0899-9007(98)00171-3.
52. Gillick MR. Rethinking the role of tube feeding in patients with advanced dementia. N Engl J Med. 2000;342(3):206–10. https://doi.org/10.1056/NEJM200001203420312.
53. American Geriatrics Society. Choosing wisely. Ten things clinicians and patients should question. https://www.choosingwisely.org/societies/american-geriatrics-society. Accessed 2 Feb 2022.
54. Committee AGSECaCPaMoC. American Geriatrics Society feeding tubes in advanced dementia position statement. J Am Geriatr Soc. 2014;62(8):1590–3. https://doi.org/10.1111/jgs.12924.
55. VitalTalk. Family Conference: Bringing family members into the conversation. https://www.vitaltalk.org/guides/family-conference/. Accessed 1 Dec 2021.

56. Widera E, Anderson WG, Santhosh L, McKee K, Smith AK, Frank J. Family meetings on behalf of patients with serious illness. Accessed 1 Dec 2021. https://doi.org/10.1056/NEJMvcm1913056.
57. Tinetti M, Blaum C, Naik A, Dindo L. Patient priorities care. Choosing what matters. Doing what works. https://patientprioritiescare.org/. Accessed 1 Dec 2021.
58. Smith A, Widera E, Lee S, Schonberg M, Schoenborn N, Yourman L. ePrognosis. https://eprognosis.ucsf.edu/. Accessed 1 Dec 2021.
59. Mor V, Intrator O, Feng Z, Grabowski DC. The revolving door of rehospitalization from skilled nursing facilities. Health Aff (Millwood). 2010;29(1):57–64. https://doi.org/10.1377/hlthaff.2009.0629.
60. Jencks SF, Williams MV, Coleman EA. Rehospitalizations among patients in the Medicare fee-for-service program. N Engl J Med. 2009;360(14):1418–28. https://doi.org/10.1056/NEJMsa0803563.
61. Levine DM, Ouchi K, Blanchfield B, et al. Hospital-level care at home for acutely ill adults: a pilot randomized controlled trial. J Gen Intern Med. 2018;33(5):729–36. https://doi.org/10.1007/s11606-018-4307-z.
62. Caplan GA, Coconis J, Board N, Sayers A, Woods J. Does home treatment affect delirium? A randomised controlled trial of rehabilitation of elderly and care at home or usual treatment (the REACH-OUT trial). Age Ageing. 2006;35(1):53–60. https://doi.org/10.1093/ageing/afi206.
63. Isaia G, Astengo MA, Tibaldi V, et al. Delirium in elderly home-treated patients: a prospective study with 6-month follow-up. Age (Dordr). 2009;31(2):109–17. https://doi.org/10.1007/s11357-009-9086-3.
64. Shepperd S, Butler C, Cradduck-Bamford A, et al. Is comprehensive geriatric assessment admission avoidance hospital at home an alternative to hospital admission for older persons?: a randomized trial. Ann Intern Med. 2021;174(7):889–98. https://doi.org/10.7326/M20-5688.

Chapter 13
Teaching Through Inpatient Geriatrics Consultations

Shoshana Streiter

The Challenge of the Geriatrics Clinician Educator

The demands on the time of the geriatrics clinician educator have been increasing on two fronts. As clinicians, geriatricians face the challenge of caring for a growing patient population that is increasing in both size and complexity. And as educators, they must help their trainees gain familiarity with an ever-expanding body of biomedical knowledge while simultaneously guiding them to step into the growing number of roles the geriatrics consultant is expected to fill; that of leader, patient advocate, and health systems innovator, in addition to the traditional roles of clinicians, educators, and researchers [1]. Challenged to make the best use of limited time, geriatricians must seek out creative opportunities for integrating effective and efficient teaching with patient care. This chapter approaches the inpatient geriatrics consultation not only as an opportunity to provide patient care, but as a rich opportunity for teaching and learning.

S. Streiter (✉)
Brigham and Women's Hospital, Harvard Medical School,
Boston, MA, USA
e-mail: sstreiter@bwh.harvard.edu

A. W. Schwartz (ed.), *Medical Education in Geriatrics*,
https://doi.org/10.1007/978-3-031-32499-4_13

Reframing the Geriatrics Consultation as a Teaching Opportunity

Inpatient consultation is a common intervention offered to hospitalized older adults, occurring an average of 2.6 times per admission for Medicare beneficiaries, with at least one specialty consultation called for approximately 90% of admissions [2], with non-teaching teams calling approximately 10% more consultations than teaching teams [3]. Although clinical consultations were created to support patient care and are generally thought of as a tool for optimizing patient care, they also provide an ideal teaching and learning opportunity [4].

Clinical consultations as teaching and learning opportunities are particularly well adapted to the needs of the adult learner. Adults learn effectively when the lessons are relevant, practical, and allow for self-directed education [5]. Principles of geriatrics gain urgency and immediacy for the learner when applied in the context of an individual patient and a clinical question. Additionally, consultations allow learning to happen directly at the bedside, giving teachers the opportunity to model communication and physical exam skills and learners the opportunity to practice the principles they have been taught in real time [6]. Furthermore, because clinical consultations often involve longitudinal follow-up, the geriatrics consultant has the opportunity to observe the rest of the team act on the recommendations, creating an opportunity for feedback. Moreover, clinical consultations present an opportunity to engage with a varied and interprofessional group of learners, as all members of the interdisciplinary care team are potential learners. Finally, the consultation note is likely to be reviewed by future members of the care team, adding another vehicle for dissemination of geriatrics knowledge. Thus, the clinical consultations represent an effective and efficient modality for geriatrics education.

If geriatrics consultations represent an ideal teaching opportunity, why are they not generally thought of as such? A number of barriers exist, including time limitations, logistic barriers of physical workspace and workflow, the perception of the consultant's role as purely clinical [7], and a lack of formal education on the part of trainees and geriatricians on teaching tools and strategies can be applied in a busy clinical setting. Although interest in medical education curricula in geriatrics fellowships has been increasing in recent years, it remains a gap in most geriatric fellowship programs, and formal training in medical education is not an ACGME-required element of the fellowship curriculum [8], although the ability to teach patients, caregivers, and others has been identified as a curricular milestone for geriatrics fellows by the Association of Directors of Geriatric Academic Programs (ADGAP) and American Geriatrics Society (AGS) [9].

Optimizing Teaching and Learning Through Geriatrics Consultation

Although there is limited literature on what makes a geriatrics consultation a high-quality teaching and learning experience, the medical education literature has explored this question with regard to subspecialty consultations in general [10, 11]. Teaching a structured and standardized process for approaching consultations has been shown to result in more effective consultation communication [12, 13]. An example of such a tool is the "5 Cs of Consultation" model, developed by [12] and adapted for the Geriatrics Consultant in Table 13.1.

Several strategies may be more likely to turn a consultation into a productive teaching and learning experience. A well-articulated, focused consultation question has been shown to increase the quality of teaching and learning [4, 14], although Conley et al. found that approximately one in four consultations lack a clear clinical question [15]. Furthermore, in-person communication, despite being limited by logistic challenges such as time constraints and lack of knowledge on the part of the consultant where to find the consulting teams, may enhance the quality of the experience. Face-to-face conversations create an environment conducive to asking questions and are perceived by residents as more likely to generate

Table 13.1 Adapting the 5C's of consultation for geriatrics consults

5 Cs of consultation model[a]	Considerations for the geriatrician
Contact—Consulting and consultant physicians introduce themselves and develop a relationship	Contact—Consider the familiarity of the consulting physician with the role of the geriatrician, including awareness of the CGA (comprehensive geriatric assessment) and expectations regarding the role of the geriatrician in the care plan
Communicate—Concisely describe the clinical story and ask focused questions	Communicate—Include considerations of frailty, function, cognition, and psychosocial support in the clinical formulation
Core question—Have a specific consultation question	Core question—A reason for consultation (e.g. prevention or management of a geriatric syndrome such as delirium or falls) may supplant a focused consultation question
Collaboration—Develop a clinical plan based on conversation between consulting and consultant physicians	Collaboration—Anticipate close collaboration with both other physicians and the broader interprofessional care team, including formal and/or informal caregivers
Close the loop—Ensure that all clinicians understand the plan and maintain communication regarding change in the patient's clinical status	Close the loop—Refine the care plan to align with changing frailty status and patient care goals

[a] *Adapted from* [12]

effective teaching [4]. The need for creating a consulting environment that allows for an easy back and forth with clarifying questions is especially important when consulting between medical specialties, which often communicate with their unique medical languages and culture [14]. In one study, telephone communication between consulting and consultant doctors was shown to be prone to tension and poor communication [16].

Teaching Through Geriatrics Consultations: A Practical Approach

Insights from the medical education literature on how to teach through consultations may be adapted to the geriatrics clinical encounter. Figure 13.1 summarizes a five-step practical approach to turning a geriatrics consultation into a teaching and learning opportunity.

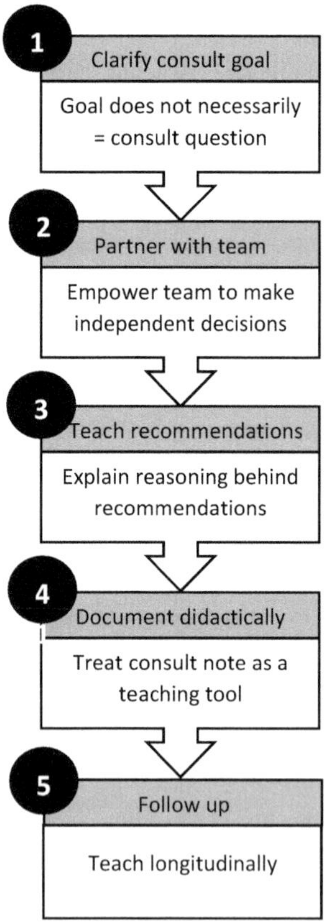

Fig. 13.1 Suggested steps for teaching through geriatrics consultation

Step 1: Clarify the Goal of the Geriatrics Consultation

Case

Ms. D, an 85-year-old woman with a history of moderately advanced vascular dementia, coronary artery disease, congestive heart failure, and diabetes is admitted from her home in the community with shortness of breath. Her admitting exam is suggestive of a congestive heart failure exacerbation. This is her third heart failure exacerbation in the past 6 months and her two prior hospitalizations were complicated by hyperactive delirium. She is fully oriented, calm, and cooperating with care in the Emergency Department. The admitting resident calls to ask for a geriatrics consultation, but admits to not having a specific question, "I'm just worried about her and feel like she could use some extra support."*

**This case represents an amalgam of many patients and is not based on any single individual.*

How a consulting team frames the consultation question has been shown to affect the effectiveness of the consultant interaction, with a well-framed consultation question leading to a better learning experience [4]. Geriatrics, however, is unusual as a medical subspecialty in that it is not organ or disease based [17]. Therefore, rather than addressing focused questions relating to a particular organ or disease, geriatricians often are consulted for assistance managing and optimizing domains of health such as cognition, function, and psychosocial support or managing multisystem-based geriatric syndromes such as delirium or falls. Because of the unique nature of the specialty, rather than pushing the consulting team to narrow down to a particular consultation question, the role of the geriatrician may often be integrated and intertwined in every element of care. Therefore, a more useful way of framing the consultation may be to ask the consulting team what they are hoping geriatrics can contribute by articulating the consultation goal, rather than the consultation question. Although geriatrics consultations certainly can and often do focus on particular questions, they may also be framed not as questions but as goals. The educational advantage of articulating a consultation goal rather than a consultation question is that it implicitly teaches the holistic, multi-domain-based thinking that is integral to geriatrics. A geriatrician clinician educator, approached with the scenario described in case 1 might take advantage of the learning opportunity therein by explaining to the consulting team the holistic nature of geriatrics and reassuring the consulting resident that having a consultation goal is enough. Moreover, this interaction may also be used to educate the consulting resident on the advantage of preventing a complication such as delirium rather than waiting for it to arise and calling a consultation for help managing an already delirious patient.

When clarifying the consultation goal, particular care should be taken not to create the impression that the consultant wishes to avoid performing the consultation, as the perception of "pushback" has been identified as an early barrier to teaching in the consulting process [7]. The geriatrician should make clear to the consulting team that the process of clarifying the consultation goal is for the purpose of providing the most helpful consultation possible.

Step 2: Partner with the Consulting Team

Case, Continued

Ms. D is hospitalized on the inpatient cardiology service, where she is started on IV furosemide and supplemental oxygen. In order to monitor strict ins and outs she has a foley catheter placed. She is also started on telemetry. By hospital day two, her shortness of breath has improved and her oxygen requirement has gone down, although she is still requiring nasal cannula oxygen. On exam, she is now oriented to name only. When asked to say the months of the year in backward order, she is able to say three out of 12 correctly. She does not know that she is in the hospital and periodically becomes agitated with care. Overnight, you learn that she pulled out her foley catheter and had to have it replaced. She continues to pull at her catheter, her telemetry leads, and her IVs. Geriatrics is paged by the medicine team asking for recommendations for pharmacotherapy to manage her agitation and to protect her lines and monitors.

Making recommendations as a geriatrics consultant often involves balancing different risks and clinical situations commonly arise where there is no clear one "right answer." This nuanced process allows for a rich teaching and learning experience, as teams with different expertise share knowledge and develop a care plan in partnership. Rather than making a top-down recommendation, the geriatrics clinician educator may share geriatric care principles with the consulting team and empower them to engage in shared medical decision making in partnership with the patient and/or caregiver(s). This experience will allow the geriatrics consultant to guide learners through progressively more challenging aspects of learning, from the assimilation of knowledge (learning the geriatrics care principles) to their application (applying them to the case of the patient in question) to creative generation of new ideas (engaging in shared medical decision making to generate a care plan tailored to the individual patient in question), a process conducive to a high-quality learning experience [18].

In the case described above, for example, the geriatrics consultant might discuss with the residents the evidence describing the risk of adverse patient outcomes associated with delirium, and how tethers are known to increase the risk of delirium [19, 20]. This risk can then be balanced against the potential advantage of close monitoring for patients with decompensated heart failure. Might there be creative ways to reduce the number of tethers the patient is subjected to? For example, might it be reasonable to replace the detailed information regarding the patient's volume status obtained from the foley catheter with a twice daily ultrasound exam of the inferior vena cava as a proxy for volume status [21, 22]? There will likely be no clear answer in many clinical scenarios, but the process of discussing care principles, balancing competing risks, and generating a care plan allows learning to be effectively and organically integrated into patient care.

Partnership with the consulting team also allows the geriatrician the opportunity to offer experiential learning at the bedside. The geriatrician may choose to model practical skills such as a geriatrics-focused physical exam, cognitive testing, and discussion of advance care planning or may supervise the learner in these skills and provide immediate feedback. Although clinical needs often dictate the mode of communication for the consultation, in-person communication for geriatrics consultations is most likely to result in a good learning experience [23].

When partnering with the team, the geriatrician has the opportunity to both teach and learn from a diverse, interprofessional group, as geriatric patients often require the skills of multiple clinical services. The nurses, nursing aides, physical therapists, occupational therapists, speech and language pathologists, pharmacists, and social workers caring for the patient may all be called into action by the consulting geriatrician as potential teachers, bringing a rich variety of perspectives to the learning experience. In the case described above, a nurse may be able to partner in teaching by describing or modeling for the learner effective ways to communicate with and redirect a patient with delirium.

Step 3: Teach Geriatrics Recommendations

Case, Continued

Although you have worked with the medicine team to mitigate Ms. D's delirium by reducing tethers, eliminating the use of deliriogenic medications, optimizing her sleep-wake cycle, and encouraging non-pharmacologic redirection, she remains confused and agitated. She continues to pull at her IV and has attempted to hit staff. The nursing team is particularly concerned about their ability to maintain safety overnight. They ask you to recommend a plan for pharmacologic management of her hyperactive symptoms, to be used as a last resort to maintain safety if non-pharmacologic strategies prove insufficient.

In the case above, the consulting team has asked a relatively simple question that could be answered with one sentence, giving the name of an agent of choice, a recommended dose and frequency, and instructions regarding monitoring for potential toxicities. In a consultation aimed at providing patient care, making this recommendation would be sufficient. In a consultation aimed at providing patient care *and* teaching, recommendations should be taught, not made. The urgency of the clinical question makes such a case an ideal opportunity for applied learning. The geriatrics consultant should meet with the team, in person if possible, and provide a recommendation while explaining the thought process behind it. Considerations of drug route of administration, half-life, and side effect profile should be discussed with the team, and the reason for the final recommendations should be clarified. This need not be a long encounter, out of respect for the time of a busy clinical team, and can be accomplished in only a few minutes. The geriatrics consultant should ensure the team has the opportunity to ask questions and understands the reasoning behind the recommendation. Fellows may benefit from the use of structured frameworks for incorporating teaching and learning into clinical consultations [7]. Immediately after learning the knowledge behind the recommendation, the team should place relevant orders, allowing for both expeditious patient care and the application of newly acquired learning to help solidify the information for the learner.

Step 4: Document Didactically

Case, Continued

You find a computer and use your standardized geriatrics consultation note template to document your recommendations. You write recommended action items in bold and include a brief explanation of the reasoning behind your recommendations. You include a hyperlink in your note to your hospital's pharmacy intranet page listing medications used for delirium which tabulates the pharmacokinetics, pharmacodynamics, and toxicities of the different agents in the hospital formulary. You include contact information for further questions.

If an inpatient geriatrics consultation represents an abbreviated course in geriatrics, the hospital is the classroom and the consultation note is the textbook. Medical documentation offers an opportunity to integrate enhancement of the teaching experience into patient care. Recommendations should be articulated in clear and simple language, and care should be taken to limit the number of recommendations, as clinically appropriate, which one study has shown leads to increased adherence to consultant geriatrician recommendations [24]. Structuring recommendations according to an evidence based and easy to remember framework such as the "Geriatric 5Ms" [25] may help contextualize learning for the consulting team. Moreover, the consultant should take care to explicate the medical decision making behind the recommendations, including references to the literature as appropriate. Many electronic medical records allow hyperlinks to be inserted into notes, which allows the author to reference supplemental material for clinicians who are interested.

Step 5: Follow-Up

Case, Continued

The following night, around 3 a.m., Ms. D appears agitated and paranoid. She is hitting staff. The night team attempts non-pharmacologic redirection measures, including offering food and drink, turning on soothing music, and asking her son to talk to her on the phone, but they are unsuccessful. The team decides it is necessary to administer a low dose of quetiapine to maintain safety. When you examine her, in partnership with the medical resident, at 8 a.m., she is somnolent and difficult to arouse. You perform a Confusion Assessment Method (CAM) with the resident, and she meets criteria for delirium. You discuss with the resident that this is an expected consequence of quetiapine, and because you have already discussed that this drug has a 6-h half-life, you plan to examine her again later in the day. When you and the resident return to the bedside in the early afternoon, Ms. D is alert and conversant, although not back to her pre-hospital cognitive baseline. You discuss a plan to manage her delirium for the coming night.

Geriatrics consultations are by nature longitudinal, as the geriatrics consultant typically follows the patient throughout a hospital stay. This opportunity for longitudinal learning is an educational advantage, as learners are more likely to retain knowledge that is repeated over spaced time intervals [26]. Following up consultations allows the geriatrics consultant to both confirm that recommendations were implemented as intended, reinforce key teaching points, and use clinical outcomes, whether expected or unexpected, as additional learning opportunities.

Practical strategies for promoting teaching and learning through all stages of the geriatrics consultation process are summarized in Table 13.2.

Next Steps and Future Directions

The literature considering the geriatrics consultation as an opportunity for teaching and learning is scant and numerous questions remain open. What elements of the consultation encounter are most conducive to learning? How do learner attitudes and beliefs about geriatrics impact the educational potential of the consultation encounter? How can a geriatrics consultation note be best constructed to support

Table 13.2 Promoting teaching and learning in geriatrics consults

The consult process	Strategies to teach (not make) recommendations
1. Consulting team calls the consultation	• Clarify the consultation goal • Educate about the role of the geriatrician on the care team • Avoid "pushback"
2. Geriatrics consultant evaluates patient	• Look for opportunities to include team in bedside evaluation • Model geriatric-focused physical exam and communication skills • Observe learner practicing bedside skills and provide supportive feedback
3. Geriatrics consultant provides team with recommendations	• Describe reasoning behind medical decision-making • Engage team in shared decision making • Limit the number of recommendations as clinically appropriate • Guide team in applying knowledge
4. Geriatrics consultant documents recommendations	• Use a standardized format • Keep language clear and simple • Refer to supplemental resources in a convenient way for the learner • Provide contact information for further questions
5. Follow up with patient and team	• Use the clinical trajectory of the patient to reinforce key learning points • Take advantage of spaced learning

learning? What is the potential role of telemedicine consultations and e-consultations as educational opportunities? Furthermore, geriatrics is a dynamic and evolving field, exploring different versions of offering consultative services, including traditional consultations, mobile geriatrics care units, and co-management teams. Further research is needed to elucidate how best to capitalize on the rich educational potential across a range of care models to improve the care of older adults.

References

1. Kuper A, D'Eon M. Rethinking the basis of medical knowledge. Med Educ. 2011;45(1):36–43.
2. Stevens JP, Nyweide D, Maresh S, Zaslavsky A, Shrank W, Md MDH, et al. Variation in inpatient consultation among older adults in the United States. J Gen Intern Med. 2015;30(7):992–9.
3. Kachman M, Carter K, Arora VM, Flores A, Meltzer DO, Martin SK. Describing variability of inpatient consultation practices: physician, patient, and admission factors. J Hosp Med. 2020;15:164–8.
4. Pavitt S, Bogetz A, Blankenburg R. What makes the "perfect" inpatient consultation? A qualitative analysis of resident and fellow perspectives. Acad Med. 2020;95(1):104–10.
5. Knowles MS. The adult learner: a neglected species. Houston, TX: Gulf Pub. Co.; 1973. vii, 198 p.
6. Ho PA, Girgis C, Rustad JK, Noordsy D, Stern TA. Advancing the mission of consultation-liaison psychiatry through innovation in teaching. Psychosomatics. 2019;60(6):539–48.
7. Miloslavsky EM, Mcsparron JI, Richards JB, Puig A, Sullivan AM. Teaching during consultation: factors affecting the resident-fellow teaching interaction. Med Educ. 2015;49(7):717–30.
8. Rivera V, Yukawa M, Aronson L, Widera E. Teaching geriatric fellows how to teach: a needs assessment targeting geriatrics fellowship program directors. J Am Geriatr Soc. 2014;62(12):2377–82.
9. Parks SM, Harper GM, Fernandez H, Sauvigne K, Leipzig RM. American Geriatrics Society/Association of Directors of geriatric academic programs curricular milestones for graduating geriatric fellows. J Am Geriatr Soc. 2014;62(5):930–5.
10. Salerno SM, Hurst FP, Halvorson S, Mercado DL. Principles of effective consultation: an update for the 21st century consultant. Arch Intern Med. 2007;167(3):271–5. https://doi.org/10.1001/archinte.167.3.271. PMID: 17296883.
11. Goldman L, Lee T, Rudd P. Ten commandments for effective consultations. Arch Intern Med. 1983;143(9):1753–5. PMID: 6615097.
12. Kessler CS, Afshar Y, Sardar G, Yudkowsky R, Ankel F, Schwartz A. A prospective, randomized, controlled study demonstrating a novel, effective model of transfer of care between physicians: the 5 Cs of consultation. Acad Emerg Med. 2012;19(8):968–74.
13. Nandiwada DR, Kohli A, Mcnamara M, Smith KJ, Zimmer S, Mcneil M, et al. High-value consults: a curriculum to promote point-of-care, evidence-based recommendations. J Grad Med Educ. 2017;9(5):640–4.
14. Kessler CS, Chan T, Loeb JM, Malka ST. I'm clear, you're clear, we're all clear: improving consultation communication skills in undergraduate medical education. Acad Med. 2013;88(6):753–8.
15. Conley J, Jordan M, Ghali W. Audit of the consultation process on general internal medicine services. BMJ Qual Saf. 2009;18(1):59–62.
16. Wadhwa A, Lingard L. A qualitative study examining tensions in interdoctor telephone consultations. Med Educ. 2006;40(8):759–67.
17. Tinetti M. Mainstream or extinction: can defining who we are save geriatrics? J Am Geriatr Soc. 2016;64(7):1400–4.

18. Bloom BS. Taxonomy of educational objectives; the classification of educational goals. 1st ed. New York: Longmans, Green; 1956.
19. Mattison MLP. Delirium. Ann Intern Med. 2020;173(7). https://doi.org/10.7326/AITC202010060. PMID: 33017552.
20. Inouye SK, Westendorp RG, Saczynski JS. Delirium in elderly people. Lancet. 2014;383(9920):911–22.
21. Krishnan DK, Pawlaczyk B, McCullough PA, Enright S, Kunadi A, Vanhecke TE. Point-of-care, ultraportable echocardiography predicts diuretic response in patients admitted with acute decompensated heart failure. Clin Med Insights Cardiol. 2016;10:201–8.
22. Yavasi O, Unluer EE, Kayayurt K, Ekinci S, Saglam C, Surum N, et al. Monitoring the response to treatment of acute heart failure patients by ultrasonographic inferior vena cava collapsibility index. Am J Emerg Med. 2014;32(5):403–7.
23. Allen CM. A randomized, controlled clinical trial of a geriatric consultation team. JAMA. 1986;255(19):2617.
24. Deschodt M, Jeuris A, Van Grootven B, Van Waerebeek E, Gantois E, Flamaing J, et al. Adherence to recommendations of inpatient geriatric consultation teams: a multicenter observational study. Eur Geriatr Med. 2021;12(1):175–84.
25. Tinetti M, Huang A, Molnar F. The geriatrics 5M's: a new way of communicating what we do. J Am Geriatr Soc. 2017;65(9):2115.
26. Pusic MV, Boutis K, Hatala R, Cook DA. Learning curves in health professions education. Acad Med. 2015;90(8):1034–42.

Chapter 14
Teaching Geriatrics in the Nursing Facility

Laura K. Byerly

Introduction

"I was surprised by how much I liked this experience." This common refrain echoed through the course evaluations of a two-week nursing facility rotation for internal medicine residents [1]. Most came to the facility with few expectations and a sense that, "It'll be like taking care of patients in the hospital," yet walked away repeatedly commenting on how surprised they were by the uniqueness of the nursing facility's patients, available resources, and care teams. One resident remarked at the end of her block, "[Clinicians in nursing facilities] all see patients who are not sick enough to be in the hospital but not safe to be home – that takes a highly skilled physician." This was the resident's first time learning how to care for patients in this "in-between" stage of care.

The nursing facility is a novel healthcare training setting, different from residential care facilities, outpatient care, and inpatient acute care. For clarity, in this chapter, the term "nursing facility" is used to describe the environment that can include both skilled nursing and long-term care units. For situations where only one component of the nursing facility is being referenced, the text will clarify "skilled nursing" or "long-term care."

Within most healthcare training programs, the skilled nursing and long-term care facility models (e.g., "nursing homes") of geriatric care are underutilized as teaching settings [2–4]. Very few medical students have required experience in the nursing facility setting. A 2006 program directors report highlighted that 65% of internal medicine residency programs included some clinical experience in a nursing facility as part of a multi-site rotation, though no studies report *how* or for what duration

L. K. Byerly (✉)
Oregon Health & Science University, Portland, OR, USA
e-mail: byerlyla@ohsu.edu

A. W. Schwartz (ed.), *Medical Education in Geriatrics*,
https://doi.org/10.1007/978-3-031-32499-4_14

those residency programs incorporate the nursing facility [5, 6]. A small Canadian study of family medicine residencies, whose graduates often care for nursing facility patients, indicated that 2 out of 10 training programs had any nursing facility training [7]. This is despite the fact that many trainees' patients frequently discharge to nursing facilities after hospitalization, or present to clinic following a nursing facility admission.

Geriatric patients access all parts of the healthcare continuum—from outpatient primary care, to inpatient admissions and consults, to home-based care—but a frequent transition or end point for older adults within that continuum is the nursing facility [8]. Skilled nursing care has increased in recent years with data suggesting over 26% of hospitalized Medicare patients discharge to skilled facilities [9]. As of 2016, over 1.3 million individuals resided in long-term care nursing facilities; in the same year, 1.6 million Medicare enrollees utilized skilled nursing facility benefits (approximately 5.1% of all Medicare enrollees) [10, 11]. Given the frequency of patient care occurring in the nursing facility, these settings ought to be used more regularly as a teaching site for medical education.

The idea of teaching in nursing facilities is not new. For over three decades, educators noted the opportunities afforded by a nursing facility [4, 6, 12–14]. Kanter, for example, recommended training in nursing facilities for several reasons: (1) patient availability for in-depth history and physical exam training opportunities, (2) interprofessional team modeling, and (3) patient complexity for which incorporating learners as part of rounding would both benefit patients and learners considering effects of multimorbidity [2]. Nursing facilities offer opportunities to learn about the health care system and consider resource limitations intrinsic to the environments. They offer opportunities to focus on "caring" for instead of "curing" patients given the nature of patients cared for, especially in long-term care, and importantly immerse learners in environments where they can acknowledge and reduce existing ageist perspectives. Trainees have also cited the benefits of autonomy offered in nursing facility-based training [2, 15–20].

Caring for older adults in nursing facilities provides opportunities for learners to see both the after-effects of a hospitalization and the diversity of supportive care strategies employed for older adults with significant functional or cognitive needs. Neither of these teaching opportunities occurs within traditional inpatient or outpatient training sites and studies suggest learners and providers value additional training on older adult transitions of care to residential care models [21, 22]. Telehealth models that coach skilled nursing facility care teams to prevent hospital readmission help approximate valuable lessons within the facility, but do not capture the benefit of on-site in-person learning opportunity [23]. Additionally, with increased scrutiny on re-hospitalization, teaching in nursing facilities demonstrates for learners practical ways to improve transitions of care to minimize re-hospitalization and instill a sense of what clinical care is feasible at a nursing facility [24].

In this chapter, we discuss the potential of the nursing facility's skilled nursing and long-term care settings as training sites for both undergraduate and graduate level medical trainees.

The Nursing Facility as Teaching Environment: Opportunities and Challenges

Most providers at some point will have patients who intersect with the nursing facility [8, 25]. Primary care providers follow patients recently discharged from a skilled nursing facility stay, and transition primary care patients to long-term care facilities. Inpatient medicine and surgery providers admit and discharge patients from and to nursing facilities. Both undergraduate and graduate medical trainees must learn about a nursing facility's structure and capabilities—regardless of their future specialty. With the diversity of patient experiences and populations served within the nursing facility, the environment offers unique intrinsic structural and team model opportunities and challenges for educators.

Opportunities Within the Nursing Facility Educational Environment

Interprofessional (IP) Team Structure

Perhaps no clinical environment capitalizes on an IP team as extensively as a nursing facility; educators can capitalize on its authentic opportunity to engage learners in IP education [6, 25–30]. As discussed in Chap. 8 of this text, IP education (or IPE) in healthcare is an opportunity for individuals from two or more professions to learn from, about, and with each other as they care for patients; nursing facilities offer this educational opportunity. The skilled nursing setting primarily exists for patient rehabilitation and nursing care, so most patients engage with at least one therapist, nursing assistant, and licensed nurse on a daily basis. Additionally, all nursing facility patients meet with social service directors, dieticians, recreation therapists, and pharmacists throughout their stays. The medical provider's role is complementary to the rehabilitation and nursing care received at a nursing facility and an on-site IP team provides the learner with a novel educational experience beyond medical care. Learners can shadow rehabilitation, participate in dietician evaluations, and attend care conferences. Table 14.1 highlights ways to engage learners in the IP framework of a nursing facility.

Continuity and Continuum of Care

Skilled nursing facility stays can last up to 100 days based on Medicare reimbursement and payment structures, though tend to be between 2 and 4 weeks, during which time a learner follows the patient from post-hospital discharge to transition to the community. Long-term care patients reside in a nursing facility for months to years, offering additional longitudinal learning opportunities. These longer stays

Table 14.1 Interprofessional team member roles and learning opportunities

Profession	Role within nursing facility	Learning/teaching opportunities for trainees
Medical (MD/DO, PA, NP)	New patient admissions, discharge visits, follow-up (urgent care, monthly or bimonthly Medicare visits)	• Admitting new patients/ discharge visits • Follow up of active medical issues • Advance care planning conversations • Fall assessments and management plans
Nursing (RN, LPN)	Patient care and assessment, wound care, IV and injectable medications, restorative care nursing activities	• Wound care rounds • Weekly patient skin audit exams • Medication administration (e.g., IV, topical treatments) • Restorative care planning
Nursing assistants	Provide daily care for patients, including checking vital signs, ADL care, and ensuring patient safety	• Explanation of transfer equipment (e.g., Hoyer lift) • Meal-time assistance for patients • Communication strategies for dementia related behaviors
Pharmacy	Drug regimen reviews, monitoring for adverse medication events, reviewing psychotropic drugs	• Psychotropic medication review • Medication reconciliation of new patients • Long-term care drug regimen review
Rehabilitation (physical, occupational, speech therapy)	Gross and fine motor rehabilitation, ADL and IADL training, cognitive testing, dysphagia evaluations	• PT/OT evaluations and rehab planning • Cognitive assessments (e.g., ACL, SLUMS) • DME evaluation and training with walker/cane • Caregiver transfer training (e.g., car transfers) • Dysphagia evaluation with thickened liquids/modified textures
Recreation therapy	Provide resident support through activities of choice that foster physical, mental, psychosocial Well-being	• Assess new patients for activity preferences • Engage in facility-based daily rec therapy activities • Assist with development of new activities
Nutrition/dietary services	Weight monitoring, dietary modifications, menu creation, nutritional supplements, tube feed management	• Weight loss/gain evaluations • Counseling on supplement choices • Calculation of tube feed nutrient requirements

(continued)

Table 14.1 (continued)

Profession	Role within nursing facility	Learning/teaching opportunities for trainees
Social services/social work	Financial, social, and community resources planning, care coordination with families	• Care conferences/family meetings • Screening processes/ insurance review • Discharge planning to community
Administration (e.g., director of nursing, executive director)	Admissions processes, quality improvement and monitoring of regulations, infection control protocols	• New patient referral screening meetings • Quality improvement projects and QAPI meetings • Infection control guidelines and review of infection rates

MD/DO Physicians, *PA* Physician assistant, *NP* Nurse practitioner, *RN* Registered nurse, *LPN* Licensed Practical Nurse (also called Licensed Vocational Nurse in some states), *IV* intravenous, *ADL* activities of daily living, *IADL* instrumental activities of daily living, *PT* physical therapy, *OT* occupational therapy, *SLUMS* St. Louis Mental Status Examination, *ACL* Allen Cognitive Level. *DME* durable medical equipment, *QAPI* quality assurance and performance improvement

provide continuity for the on-site learner and opportunities to see a patient improve or decline within the facility. Learners see a patient's recovery and care plan progress outside the level of acute care; this helps fill in the gaps between inpatient and ambulatory care along the care continuum. In general, nursing facility patients are more stable compared to the inpatient setting, which affords learners the chance to look broadly at a patient's care plan, spend more time with their patients, develop communication skills, and engage in care coordination [25].

Quality Improvement/Systems-Based Practice

Accreditation agencies, including the Accreditation Council for Graduate Medical Education, increasingly include guidelines related to quality improvement, patient safety, and systems-based practice [31, 32]. Nursing facilities offer educational opportunities related to quality improvement in systems-based practice due to their own accreditation and licensing bodies [33]. Facilities hold regular Quality Assurance and Process Improvement (QAPI) meetings as well as pharmacy rounds where learners see problem solving related to quality improvement metrics (e.g., falls, antipsychotic use) and how IP teams create opportunities for change. QAPI meetings incorporate nursing facility regulations that guide practice improvement programs, emphasize health care policy, and improve patient quality of life. Rather than relying solely on learners creating de novo quality improvement projects, the nursing home offers learners organic and authentic existing opportunities that can make meaningful clinical care differences for the nursing facility population.

Diversity of Health Needs

All post-hospital roads can lead to the skilled nursing facility, which creates a diverse patient population with many care needs. The skilled nursing facility team admits patients hospitalized for medical, neurological, surgical, and psychiatric diagnoses, who have a "skilled need" (e.g., nursing, physical therapy, occupational therapy, and/or speech therapy). Medical students used to working within one rotation block at a time (e.g., surgery, medicine, neurology) experience the nursing facility as a melting pot where they learn about all medical specialties within the same setting. Residents, and even geriatric medicine fellows, experience the nursing facility as a chance to practice patient care outside of what they would traditionally see on the wards; for example, the internal medicine resident has the opportunity to see the post-op complications of a hip fracture traditionally managed through orthopedic surgery. Nursing facility populations themselves offer opportunities to consider patient equity and disparity issues that affect patient post-skilled rehab stays, or the financial burdens of paying for long-term care.

Challenges Within the Nursing Facility Educational Environment

Transitions of Care/Health System Fragmentation

Patients in nursing facilities come from various outside health care systems, which can challenge the learner accustomed to a specific electronic health record or who cannot access the patient's inpatient or outpatient chart. Additionally, learners may experience frustration if a patient's transition of care from inpatient to nursing facility is confusing or missing critical information. Multiple curricula have focused on safe transitions of care and rotating at the nursing facility provides additional reference points for navigating transitions of care when the transition is across health systems [34, 35]. Seeing the transitions of care process from the perspective of the nursing facility can enlighten the learner to best practices of safe discharging and potentially help them avoid errors when discharging a hospitalized patient themselves.

Informal Daily Structure

Many learners integrate into a highly structured routine in other clinical settings: pre-rounding, rounds, admissions, and sign-out on the wards; pre-charting, clinic visits, precepting, and documentation in the outpatient setting. The nursing facility operates within a less formal structure that can be jarring to learners [18, 25]. Even geriatric medicine fellows doing their longitudinal long-term care rotation may initially struggle with the lack of formal structure. Learners completing a nursing home rotation may frequently ask questions such as, "What time should I see Mrs.

S?" and struggle with the fluid nature to their day. Providing check points for learners throughout the day and week can decrease the learner's cognitive load and help recreate the structure that most other rotations offer, as discussed in the "Tips and Strategies" section below.

Resources Access

Nursing facilities lack the readily available diagnostic tools that learners traditionally utilize within the outpatient and inpatient settings. An EKG, for example, could take hours to be performed and result. Residents and students note the challenge to their typical patient care approach if they are accustomed to creating plans that include, or rely on, rapid test results [17, 18]. Adequate orientation to what can and cannot be done, and in what timeframe, is critical for learners within the nursing facility.

Supervised Educational Time

Nursing facility physicians supervising medical students, residents, and fellows often have other clinical duties that prevent them from being continuously present. This leads to medical learners of any level having the benefits of autonomy, but also the potential for under-supervision [15, 25]. As highlighted in Huls' 2015 focus group analysis, medical students acknowledged benefits of autonomy but also challenges of relying on remote supervision and less ample formal teaching time [17]. Molema's study of family medicine and elderly care residents suggests graduate learners feel similarly [18]. The nursing home challenges the balance between autonomy and supervision; however, there are opportunities and solutions. Utilizing facility advanced practice providers (APPs) for patient care supervision and for formal teaching talks with learners provides both the APP with teaching opportunities and the learner with additional perspectives and on-site supervision. Additionally, engaging learners with the IP team experts provides informal and formal learning opportunities in the absence of an on-site physician supervisor (Table 14.1).

Nursing Facility Teaching Topics and Delivery: Examples and Models

The nursing facility offers educational opportunities within all components of the Geriatrics 5M's framework of geriatric medical education, which highlights key components of geriatric care: mobility, mind, medications, multicomplexity, and what matters most [36]. The following teaching examples apply to both the skilled nursing and long-term care patients of a nursing facility. A consolidated table of existing nursing facility curricula is summarized in Table 14.2.

Table 14.2 Existing nursing facilities-based educational models and curricula

Title	Author	Journal	Year published	Learners	Setting/duration	Goal of activity
Fostering interprofessional geriatric patient care skills for health professions students through a nursing facility-based immersion rotation [30]	Byerly LK, et al.	MedEdPORTAL	2020	Undergraduate medical, pharmacy, physical therapy students	Community Living Center (VA-based nursing facility); 2-week rotation	Interprofessional education and team-based evaluation of falls, polypharmacy/safe prescribing, patient care plans
Creation of an interprofessional clinical experience for healthcare professions trainees in a nursing home setting [27]	Ford C, et al.	Medical Teacher	2013	Undergraduate dental, optometry, nursing, occupational therapy, and social work students; internal medicine interns	Continuing care retirement community; IP training session followed by 1-day activity at facility	"Interprofessional Clinical Experience" providing IP team focused comprehensive care assessments
Interprofessional student teams augmenting service provision in residential aged care [28]	Kent F, et al.	Australasian Journal on Ageing	2016	Undergraduate medical, nursing, occupational therapy, and pharmacy students	Residential aged care facility; one half-day activity	Interprofessional student consultations on long-term care patient care plans
GeriWard Falls: an interprofessional team-based curriculum on falls in the hospitalized older adult [37]	Larson C, et al.	MedEdPORTAL	2016	Undergraduate medical, nursing, pharmacy, physical therapy students	Inpatient hospital wards; one half-day activity. Applicable format for nursing facility	Interprofessional comprehensive fall assessment and prevention
Eating problems in advanced dementia: navigating difficult conversations [43]	Manu ER, et al.	MedEdPORTAL	2020	Residents in internal medicine, medicine-pediatrics, and neurology	Seminar + trigger video-based discussion; one half-day activity. Applicable format for nursing facility	Weight loss in older adults

Unintentional weight loss in older adults: a geriatric interprofessional simulation case series for health care providers [44]	Mulligan R, et al.	MedEdPORTAL	2017	Undergraduate dental, medical, and nursing students	Simulation center at academic medical center; one half-day activity. Applicable format for nursing facility	Interprofessional weight loss assessment in older adults
Education in long-term care for family medicine residents [7]	Oliver D, et al.	Canadian Family Physician	2011	Family medicine residents	Long-term care facility; four half-days per academic year	Immersive case-based experience to prepare residents for future LTC patients
Medical students in residential aged care: a guide [25]	Radford J, et al.	The Clinical Teacher	2020	Undergraduate medical students	Residential aged care facility; 5-day immersive activity	Comprehensive medical assessments of nursing facility patients; formal didactics about older adult care
Teaching aged care facilities: implementing interprofessional prevocational education and practice in residential aged care [39]	Robinson A, et al.	Wicking Dementia Research and Education Centre	2013	Undergraduate medical, nursing, and paramedic students	Long-term care facility; 1-week rotation	Interprofessional assessment and management of dementia in nursing facilities; formal instruction on dementia and end of life care
Demystifying aged care for medical students [35]	Saunders R, et al.	The Clinical Teacher	2017	Undergraduate medical students	Residential aged care facility; one half-day activity	Immersion in facility and interview of patient to foster appreciation for lived experiences of older adults in nursing facilities
Planning for a safe discharge: more than a capacity evaluation [45]	Wong S, et al.	Journal of the American Geriatrics Society	2020	N/A, framework presented for application to learners	Discharge decision-making framework. Applicable format for nursing facility	Tool for patient-centered decision making at time of discharge from acute care

Mobility

Falls are a teachable moment about mobility in the nursing facility. Fall assessments provide a comprehensive way of looking not only at a patient's mobility, but seeing also how mind, medications, and multicomplexity affect risk of falling.

The GeriWard: Falls curriculum, designed for IP inpatient learner teams, provides a 2-h falls evaluation curriculum applicable, and adaptable, to the nursing facility setting [30, 37]. While the activity works well with an IP group of learners who bring various skillsets and perspectives to the activity, solo learners also can complete independent fall assessments. Fall assessment encourages learners to work with a facility's rehabilitation team to understand activity limitations and review adaptive equipment. The GeriWard: Falls curriculum has been adapted to the nursing facility setting by incorporating the following key curricular points, which are outlined on MedEdPORTAL [30]:

1. Formal didactic teaching on falls in the nursing facility independent background reading (as provided in the GeriWard: Falls curriculum) [37].
2. Facility team identifies a patient who has recently fallen in the facility.
3. Learners complete a comprehensive assessment of the fall using a "risk assessment and recommendations" template that includes identification of risk factors related to activity level, assistive devices, environmental hazards, and exam maneuvers such as orthostatic vital signs and the Timed Up and Go [30].
4. Learners present their findings to the facility team.
5. Assessment of learner recommendations by facility team members and learner evaluation of the activity.

Academic training programs have engaged both student and resident learners in the above activities with outcomes suggesting learners both enjoy the activity and feel more confident in conducting falls assessments on their patients. Utilizing falls as a teachable moment related to mobility provides a real-life example of the impact impaired mobility can have on a patient's health and the various strategies used by many professions to try to reduce fall risk. Presenting the fall assessment findings gives learners a chance to both present a complex case and get feedback from the IP team. Additionally, hearing a comprehensive fall assessment helps the facility's IP team to consider a patient's fall history differently [30]. While not all facilities have a fall review team, QAPI meetings frequently discuss fall rates. Learners can utilize the QAPI team meeting as a forum to present at least one fall assessment so that the entire nursing facility team benefits from the learners' assessment and recommendations.

Mind

Nursing facilities offer learners an authentic way to learn about dementia as many patients in long-term care have a dementia diagnosis. The Wicking Teaching Aged Care Facilities Program constructed an IP rotation at a local nursing facility where students created care plans for patients with dementia [38]. During their 1-week rotation, students both learned about dementia in the nursing facility and applied skills to patient care planning. For medical students, focused objectives related to a palliative approach to care of nursing facility patients with dementia and management of dementia related behaviors. This program is replicable with or without an IP group of learners by focusing on the following guideposts:

1. Faculty present a teaching series (see reference for slides) [39]:
   (a) Dementia as a terminal condition.
   (b) Dementia and a palliative approach to care.
   (c) Care for residents with dementia in a residential aged care facility.
2. Learners complete the Dementia Knowledge Assessment Tool Version 2 (D-KAT-2) at start and end of the rotation [40].
3. Learners work in small teams or solo to complete a biopsychosocial comprehensive medical assessment of a patient with dementia.
4. Learners present their assessment to the facility staff at the end of the week.

Medical students completing the program showed a significant improvement in D-KAT-2 scores; medical students noted improved ability to problem solve in complex care situations. However, students did vocalize the challenges inherent in interviewing and assessing patients with dementia and that they had to develop new skills and utilize outside resources (e.g., family caregivers, facility staff) to construct care plans [15]. The experiential learning opportunity, though, is a replicable model for nursing facilities looking to teach about working with, and managing, patients with dementia and dementia related behaviors.

Medications

Many published polypharmacy curricula are applicable to the nursing facility [41, 42]. Within a nursing facility, learners work in tandem with the facility's pharmacy to complete medication reconciliation and review high-risk medications, following guidelines outlined by Centers for Medicare and Medicaid Services. Guidelines particularly relate to psychotropic medications [33]. A formal "Drug Regimen Review" offers a teaching opportunity for consideration of high-risk medications [30]:

1. Pharmacist or medical provider teaches learners about high-risk medications in older adults.
2. Pharmacist identifies a nursing facility patient due for medication list review.
3. Learners review patient medication list for risk and interactions using instructions outlined in MedEdPORTAL. They then interview the patient to discuss drug benefits and risks [30].
4. Learners present findings to the pharmacy team to discuss appropriate medication changes.
5. Learners present findings at patient care conference to develop patient-centered medication plans.

While simple in structure, the process of methodically going through a medication list and reviewing each for potential interactions and effect can help learners understand polypharmacy. Learners showed a significant improvement in knowledge related to making medication changes and appreciated being able to directly interface with, and learn from, the facility pharmacist [30].

Multicomplexity

Unintentional weight loss in a nursing facility demonstrates multicomplexity where weight loss itself is a symptom of the challenging interplay between multiple diagnoses and treatments. Weight loss can relate to poor oral intake from sensory loss or dementia; difficulties swallowing; fluid loss from medications; and social factors related to food resources. Since there is rarely one cause, weight loss offers a chance to consider multicomplexity. Additionally, weight loss involves the IP team and offers teaching opportunities with a facility's dietician not existing in other clinical training settings. Curricula exist, albeit not specifically for nursing facilities, that focus on unintentional weight loss and eating difficulties in older adults [43, 44].

Mulligan created a simulation curriculum on weight loss assessment in older adults. Formal teaching content includes slides focusing on an IP approach to weight loss (e.g. cognitive assessment, oral cavity screening, mobility and function, social determinants of health) that highlight multicomplexity. Mulligan evaluated the curriculum with a pre- and post-knowledge test that showed increased knowledge related to unintentional weight loss. They provide a high-yield unintentional weight loss screening tool relevant in the nursing facility setting (CGWEP Unintentional Weight Loss Screening Tool) [44]. While Mulligan's curriculum includes simulated patient cases, learners should assess patients within the nursing facility who have lost weight. An approach is outlined below:

1. Structured teaching session, such as Mulligan's slide deck, related to unintentional weight loss evaluation facilitated by provider faculty or dietician.
2. Learners assess a nursing facility patient evaluation for weight loss using the CGWEP Unintentional Weight Loss Screening Tool. Consider a long-term care patient for progressive weight loss or skilled nursing facility patient with weight loss from hospital stay or compared to prior outpatient baseline. If no patient is available, use the information from Mulligan's simulation cases to frame discussion.
3. Learners present their findings and causes of weight loss to the facility team or dietician.
4. Learners discuss with the dietician the utility and availability of nutritional supplements for older adults with unintentional weight loss.
5. Consider a "taste test" of supplements and/or a survey of different food and liquid textures/thicknesses to help learners understand what patients experience with diet changes.

Utilizing a weight loss curriculum in the nursing facility provides learners with a hands-on or simulated experience to explore weight loss as a marker of a patient's multicomplexity. Given the various causes of weight loss and challenges associated with weight loss in patients with multiple comorbidities, learners should utilize this exercise to engage in a conversation that goes beyond strictly "calories in" and gets at the multifactorial nature of weight loss.

What Matters Most

There are many avenues in a nursing facility to demonstrate what "Matters Most" to learners. Educators could use this opportunity to talk about health care proxies as well as Portable/Provider/Medical Orders for Life Sustaining Treatment (POLST/MOLST) or other state-specific end of life orders, or delve into the criteria used when transitioning a patient to hospice care. Given the importance of patient preferences and goal setting in the transitions of care process, discharge planning in nursing facilities should include teaching activities focused on the role of patient-centered decision making [8].

Since learners participate in the admission and discharge process of patients, they see the nursing facility as a step along the continuum of patient care. Most undergraduate and graduate learners have likely seen that frequently in healthcare, a gap exists between where a patient wishes to live and what is feasible or safe. For example, many patients wish to return home after their skilled nursing stay, yet the team may not feel home is a safe discharge option. Learners have few opportunities to explore that gap.

Educators can expose learners to the concept of what "matters most" by considering the potential for returning home vs. transitioning to a higher level of care. One potential structure is as follows:

1. Faculty provide both formal teaching related to the various "residential models of care" (e.g., senior communities, assisted living facilities, nursing homes) as well as discharge planning pearls and misconceptions.
2. Utilizing a framework outlined by Wong and colleagues, learners investigate patient preferences, caregiver/family preferences, and IP team recommendations [45].
3. Learners participate in patient care conferences where patients vocalize their goals and IP team members weigh in on their own recommendations and/or the practicalities of the patient's goals.
4. Following the care conference, faculty preceptors debrief learners on their perception of patient and team goal alignment. They also discuss what barriers or opportunities exist to help meet the patient's goals. Faculty guide them through consideration of the following questions:
   (a) What is most important to the patient about the discharge plan?
   (b) What does insurance cover for additional services and what is the potential benefit of additional services for the patient if they return home?
   (c) What family or family-of-choice supports exist for the patient to help meet their goals?

(d) What are the alternative residential models of care to that might better support the patient's needs? (See Chap. 15 of this text on Geriatric Settings of Care).

Through this process, learners not only see the various stakeholders in discharge planning, but also anchor their review of the discharge plan to the patient's goals and perspectives. Since many times, providers focus on the medical conditions affecting discharge planning, this structured approach provides an opportunity for the learner to focus on the patient's preferences in the transitions of care process.

Tips and Strategies for Successful Teaching in Nursing Facilities

The educational opportunities afforded by a nursing facility are vast. Keeping in mind the following practical suggestions can increase the educational yield and learner enjoyment on nursing facility rotations.

1. *Capitalize on existing activities*. Teachable moments regularly and organically occur in a nursing facility. Include learners in team huddles and screening meetings, bring them to pharmacy rounds or quality improvement meetings, or have them present updates on their patients' care plans at care conferences. Engage learners in post-fall assessment with the nursing staff. Work within the nursing facility's activities and the learning opportunities will be authentic and engaging.
2. *Incorporate the IP team as educators*. The facility's IP team can highlight their profession's expertise and how their care plans align and add to the medical plan (Table 14.1) [30, 38]. Having IP team members and learners work together provides supervision and precepting when the faculty provider is not available. We also encourage having multiple health professions students working together within the nursing facility if plausible so that students and residents learn from IP peer groups.
3. *Set flexible schedules with "anchors."* Learners struggle with flexible and fluid schedules if they are not accustomed to that model of training; the nursing facility often adopts a less rigid schedule [25]. Learners need to flex their schedules to see patients around when therapy or nursing is working with a patient and early establishment of this expectation can minimize frustrations. Within that fluid schedule, provide "anchors" for learners: firm precepting times; clearly outlined facility meeting schedules (e.g., care conferences, QAPI) so the learner is present; structured teaching sessions on specific topics at set times. Scheduled anchors decrease the potential for becoming overwhelmed by activities.
4. *Balance structured teaching with patient care experiences*. Many learners come to the nursing facility without significant expertise related to common geriatric syndromes, models of geriatric residential care, and transitions of care. For some, it can be challenging to start seeing complex patients in the skilled nursing or long-term care units. Providing structured teaching sessions on common topics followed by aligning patient care experiences improves their learning experience [25, 30, 38]. Implementing a formal curriculum of teaching topics (e.g.,

falls, polypharmacy, dementia related behaviors) and allocating set times in the schedule for teaching can help learners feel supported and with a foundation of knowledge. Offsite geriatrics faculty can teach remotely through virtual platforms.

Future Directions for Education Within the Nursing Facility

With increasing pressures to find meaningful geriatrics clinical experiences for medical learners, nursing facilities open opportunities for unique and interesting training. The nursing facility offers a variety of future educational opportunities to consider.

For students and residents interested in a longitudinal experience, consider continuity experiences in the long-term care wing. This longitudinal experience is an innate part of geriatric medicine fellowship. Offering weekly preceptorships for medical students within the nursing facility allows the early learner to interact with complex older adults as well as the nursing facility team. Family and internal medicine residency programs should add skilled nursing and/or long-term care experiences as part of their ambulatory continuity clinics; some surgery residencies may also wish to have learners rotate in skilled nursing units to follow post-op courses. Geriatric medicine fellows have required rotations within the nursing facility and can work and teach other learners while obtaining longitudinal exposure to the nursing facility.

Additional GME learners may benefit from spending time in the nursing facility for discrete periods of time. For example, psychiatry residents may benefit from considering dementia related behaviors for both pharmacological and non-pharmacological methods of treatment—the latter of which are prominently featured within the nursing facility. Even emergency medicine residency programs could consider, particularly if they frequently receive nursing facility patients in their emergency rooms, having their learners spend a day at a nursing facility to better understand the environment and potential reasons for transfer to the emergency room. Almost any training program may find a unique opportunity from having their learners spend time in the nursing facility.

With increasing remote teaching technologies, there are growing opportunities for virtual nursing facility rotations. Incorporation of telemedicine into traditional practice breaks down distance and scheduling barriers. Many nursing facilities have laptops/tablets dedicated for patient communication. Learners can "visit" their nursing facility patient remotely, participate in care conferences for their patients, and meet with the IP team while offsite. This experience allows for increased continuity of care and offers teaching opportunities even if a facility needs to quarantine or restrict visitation. Incorporating virtual nursing facility visits also gives patients the opportunity to see their student or resident doctor on a screen and use headphones to help with communication (e.g., volume amplification)—in some ways this might be easier communication for the patient if their facility quarantines require face masks that impede communication (see Chap. 17 on Teaching via Telemedicine).

Finally, there are future opportunities for engaging learners for focused training related to advance care planning and communication skills. A nursing facility provides tangible learning experiences witnessing the important concept of what Flint and colleagues dubbed being "rehabbed to death." [46] Being "rehabbed to death" relates to how many patients spend time in the nursing facility setting within the last year of their life regardless of if such a stay is within their goals. Many patients who are at a nursing facility have had a change in status, either temporary or permanent for long-term care, and would benefit from discussions related to advance care planning and treatment preferences. These conversations take time and practice, especially when learning communication strategies. The nature and length of stay of patient care in a nursing facility offers such time and opportunities.

Conclusion

The nursing facility naturally, and uniquely, represents many of the teaching points relevant to Geriatrics 5M's medical training; it does so in an organic and authentic way that allows the educator to integrate learners into the existing environment rather than creating experiences from scratch. From IP teamwork, to medical complexity, to quality improvement—learners can experience this all through the facility's existing infrastructure and patient population. Published nursing facility experiences suggest that undergraduate and graduate learners both learn within the nursing facility environment and develop a higher appreciation for the IP nature of geriatrics. Using the above examples and guideposts, we encourage educators to utilize nursing facilities for training future providers. Capitalizing on the teachable moments within the nursing facility could help future healthcare professionals improve care for vulnerable older adults across the care continuum.

References

1. Byerly LK, DeLima B, Morgan EA. Program evaluation of a nursing home-based internal medicine rotation for interns. In: American Geriatrics Society Annual Meeting 2020, vol. 68; 2020.
2. Kanter SL. The nursing home as a core site for educating residents and medical students. Acad Med J Assoc Am Med Coll. 2012;87(5):547–8. https://doi.org/10.1097/ACM.0b013e3182557445.
3. Lipsitz LA. The teaching nursing home: an educational and economic resource for geriatric training. Am J Med. 1994;97(4A):24S–6S. https://doi.org/10.1016/0002-9343(94)90204-6.
4. Wiener M, Shamaskin A. The nursing home as a site for teaching medical students. Acad Med J Assoc Am Med Coll. 1990;65(6):412–4. https://doi.org/10.1097/00001888-199006000-00013.
5. Warshaw GA, Bragg EJ, Thomas DC, Ho ML, Brewer DE. Are internal medicine residency programs adequately preparing physicians to care for the baby boomers? A National Survey from the Association of Directors of Geriatric Academic Programs status of Geriatrics Workforce Study. J Am Geriatr Soc. 2006;54(10):1603–9. https://doi.org/10.1111/j.1532-5415.2006.00895.x.

6. Mezey M, Mitty E, Burger SG. Nursing homes as a clinical site for training geriatric health care professionals. J Am Med Dir Assoc. 2009;10(3):196–203. https://doi.org/10.1016/j.jamda.2008.11.002.
7. Oliver D, Emili A, Chan D, Taniguchi A. Education in long-term care for family medicine residents. Can Fam Physician. 2011;57(8):e288–91.
8. Kane RL, et al. JAMA. 2011;305(3):284–93. https://doi.org/10.1001/jama.2010.2015.
9. Werner RM, Konetzka RT. Trends in post–acute care use among medicare beneficiaries: 2000 to 2015. JAMA. 2018;319(15):1616–7. https://doi.org/10.1001/jama.2018.2408.
10. Harris-Kojetin L, Sengupta M, Lendon J, Rome V, Valverde R, Caffrey C. Long-term care providers and services users in the United States, 2015–2016. Vital Health Stat. 2019;3(43).
11. Centers for Medicare & Medicaid Services. Medicare skilled nursing facilities: utilization, program payments, and cost sharing for original Medicare beneficiaries, by type of entitlement, yearly trend. 2020. https://data.cms.gov/summary-statistics-on-use-and-payments/medicare-service-type-reports/medicare-skilled-nursing-facility.
12. Pawlson LG. Clinical medical education in the nursing home: opportunities and limits. J Med Educ. 1982;57(10 Pt 1):787–91. https://doi.org/10.1097/00001888-198210000-00007.
13. Butler RN. The teaching nursing home. JAMA. 1981;245(14):1435–7. https://doi.org/10.1001/jama.245.14.1435.
14. Rosenthal MJ, Marshall CE, Martin SE, Morley JE, Ouslander JG. Nursing home rounds as a format for teaching residents and medical students. J Med Educ. 1987;62(12):975–80. https://doi.org/10.1097/00001888-198712000-00004.
15. Annear MJ, Lea E, Lo A, Tierney L, Robinson A. Encountering aged care: a mixed methods investigation of medical students' clinical placement experiences. BMC Geriatr. 2016;16:38. https://doi.org/10.1186/s12877-016-0211-8.
16. Gugliucci MR, Weiner A. Learning by living: life-altering medical education through nursing home-based experiential learning. Gerontol Geriatr Educ. 2013;34(1):60–77. https://doi.org/10.1080/02701960.2013.749254.
17. Huls M, de Rooij SE, Diepstraten A, Koopmans R, Helmich E. Learning to care for older patients: hospitals and nursing homes as learning environments. Med Educ. 2015;49(3):332–9. https://doi.org/10.1111/medu.12646.
18. Molema F, Koopmans R, Helmich E. The nursing home as a learning environment: dealing with less is learning more. Acad Med J Assoc Am Med Coll. 2014;89(3):497–504. https://doi.org/10.1097/ACM.0000000000000143.
19. Helmich E, Bolhuis S, Prins J, Laan R, Koopmans R. Emotional learning of undergraduate medical students in an early nursing attachment in a hospital or nursing home. Med Teach. 2011;33(11):e593–601. https://doi.org/10.3109/0142159X.2011.610837.
20. Hall P, O'Reilly J, Dojeiji S, Blair R, Harley A. From cure to care: assessing the ethical and professional learning needs of medical learners in a care-based facility. Gerontol Geriatr Educ. 2009;30(4):351–66. https://doi.org/10.1080/02701960903347758.
21. Tanner CE, Eckstrom E, Desai SS, Joseph CL, Ririe MR, Bowen JL, Uncovering frustrations. A qualitative needs assessment of academic general internists as geriatric care providers and teachers. J Gen Intern Med. 2006;21(1):51–5. https://doi.org/10.1111/j.1525-1497.2005.0281.x.
22. Drickamer MA, Levy B, Irwin KS, Rohrbaugh RM. Perceived needs for geriatric education by medical students, internal medicine residents and faculty. J Gen Intern Med. 2006;21(12):1230–4. https://doi.org/10.1111/j.1525-1497.2006.00585.x.
23. Farris G, Sircar M, Bortinger J, et al. Extension for community healthcare outcomes—care transitions: enhancing geriatric care transitions through a multidisciplinary videoconference. J Am Geriatr Soc. 2017;65(3):598–602. https://doi.org/10.1111/jgs.14690.
24. Murray LM, Laditka SB. Care transitions by older adults from nursing homes to hospitals: implications for long-term care practice, geriatrics education, and research. J Am Med Dir Assoc. 2010;11(4):231–8. https://doi.org/10.1016/j.jamda.2009.09.007.
25. Radford J, Dallas A, Ramsay R, Robin E, Todd A. Medical students in residential aged care: a guide. Clin Teach. 2020;17(6):617–23. https://doi.org/10.1111/tct.13168.
26. Sheppard KD, Ford CR, Sawyer P, et al. The interprofessional clinical experience: interprofessional education in the nursing home. J Interprof Care. 2015;29(2):170–2. https://doi.org/10.3109/13561820.2014.942776.

27. Ford CR, Foley KT, Ritchie CS, et al. Creation of an Interprofessional clinical experience for healthcare professions trainees in a nursing home setting. Med Teach. 2013;35(7):544–8. https://doi.org/10.3109/0142159X.2013.787138. Epub 2013 Apr 30. PMID: 23631410.
28. Kent F, Lai F, Beovich B, Dodic M. Interprofessional student teams augmenting service provision in residential aged care. Australas J Ageing. 2016;35:204. https://doi.org/10.1111/ajag.12288.
29. Annear M, Walker K, Lucas P, Lo A, Robinson A. Interprofessional education in aged-care facilities: tensions and opportunities among undergraduate health student cohorts. J Interprof Care. 2016;30:621–35. https://doi.org/10.1080/13561820.2016.1192995.
30. Byerly LK, Floren LC, Yukawa M. Fostering Interprofessional geriatric patient care skills for health professions students through a nursing facility-based immersion rotation. MedEdPORTAL. 2020;16:11059. https://doi.org/10.15766/mep_2374-8265.11059.
31. ACGME Common Program Requirements. Published online July 1, 2017:28.
32. Stratton TD. Legitimizing continuous quality improvement (CQI): navigating rationality in undergraduate medical education. J Gen Intern Med. 2019;34(5):758–61. https://doi.org/10.1007/s11606-019-04875-1.
33. Unroe KT, Ouslander JG, Saliba D. Nursing home regulations redefined: implications for providers. J Am Geriatr Soc. 2018;66(1):191–4. https://doi.org/10.1111/jgs.15128.
34. Eskildsen M, Flacker J. Care transitions workshop for first-year medical students. MedEdPORTAL. 2010;6:7802. https://doi.org/10.15766/mep_2374-8265.7802.
35. Saunders R, Miller K, Dugmore H, Etherton-Beer C. Demystifying aged care for medical students. Clin Teach. 2017;14(2):100–3. https://doi.org/10.1111/tct.12484.
36. Tinetti M, Huang A, Molnar F. The geriatrics 5M's: a new way of communicating what we do. J Am Geriatr Soc. 2017;65(9):2115. https://doi.org/10.1111/jgs.14979.
37. Larson C, O'Brien B, Rennke S. GeriWard falls: an Interprofessional team-based curriculum on falls in the hospitalized older adult. MedEdPORTAL. 2016;12:10410. https://doi.org/10.15766/mep_2374-8265.10410.
38. Robinson A, See C, Lea E, et al. Wicking teaching aged care facilities program: innovative practice. Dementia. 2017;16(5):673–81. https://doi.org/10.1177/1471301215603846.
39. Robinson A, Lea E, Tierney L, et al. Teaching aged care facilities: implementing interprofessional prevocational education and practice in residential aged care. Victoria and Tasmania Dementia Training Study Centre; 2013. http://ecite.utas.edu.au/98537. Accessed 24 Sept 2021.
40. Toye C, Lester L, Popescu A, McInerney F, Andrews S, Robinson AL. Dementia knowledge assessment tool version two: development of a tool to inform preparation for care planning and delivery in families and care staff. Dement Lond Engl. 2014;13(2):248–56. https://doi.org/10.1177/1471301212471960.
41. Hawley CE, Triantafylidis LK, Phillips SC, Schwartz AW. Brown Bag Simulation to Improve Medication Management in Older Adults. MedEdPORTAL. 15:10857. https://doi.org/10.15766/mep_2374-8265.10857.
42. Denson K, Kuester J. Pills, pills, and more pills: a pill box exercise to teach barriers to medication adherence and solutions. MedEdPORTAL. 2015;11. https://doi.org/10.15766/mep_2374-8265.10262.
43. Manu ER, Fitzgerald JT, Mullan PB, Vitale CA. Eating problems in advanced dementia: navigating difficult conversations. MedEdPORTAL. 16:11025. https://doi.org/10.15766/mep_2374-8265.11025.
44. Mulligan R, Gilmer-Scott M, Kouchel D, et al. Unintentional weight loss in older adults: a geriatric interprofessional simulation case series for health care providers. MedEdPORTAL. 13:10631. https://doi.org/10.15766/mep_2374-8265.10631.
45. Wong SP, Sharda N, Zietlow KE, Heflin MT. Planning for a safe discharge: more than a capacity evaluation. J Am Geriatr Soc. 2020;68(4):859–66. https://doi.org/10.1111/jgs.16315.
46. Flint LA, David DJ, Smith AK. Rehabbed to death. N Engl J Med. 2019;380(5):408–9. https://doi.org/10.1056/NEJMp1809354.

Chapter 15
Teaching Geriatrics in Alternative Care Settings (Including Assisted Living Facilities and PACE)

Serena Hsiou-Ling Chao, Ilona M. Kopits, and Judy Kwok

The majority of older adults in the USA are community dwelling, with most living alone (27%) or with a spouse or partner (61%) [1, 2]. For those who are 80 years of age or older, close to 60% report living in single-person households [1]. In 2016, about 1.5% of US community-dwelling older adults lived in residential care communities which include assisted living facilities (ALFs) and similar residences [3, 4]. Others live in the nearly 2000 US continuing care retirement communities (CCRCs) [5]. For comparison, approximately 2% of US older adults (1.2 million in 2019) live in nursing facilities [2]. Participants in Programs of All Inclusive Care of the Elderly (PACE), a health care delivery model for community-dwelling frail elders, may live in all types of community-based housing, and some may require nursing facility stays.

By exposing learners to the variety of places where older adults live, teachers can emphasize how housing and health insurance plan multicomplexity influences healthcare access--and by extension older adults' overall health and well-being. In this chapter we will describe how to teach the Geriatrics 5Ms in residential care communities as well as within the context of PACE. For each care setting, we provide sample cases to illustrate how each of the 5Ms can be taught. These case studies demonstrate the complex care needs of older adults who can no longer live independently in the community without assistance but desire care outside of a nursing facility.

S. H.-L. Chao (✉) · J. Kwok
Cambridge Health Alliance, Harvard Medical School, Cambridge, MA, USA
e-mail: schao@challiance.org; jykwok@challiance.org

I. M. Kopits
Boston University Chobanian & Avedisian School of Medicine, Boston, MA, USA
e-mail: ilona.kopits@bmc.org

A. W. Schwartz (ed.), *Medical Education in Geriatrics*,
https://doi.org/10.1007/978-3-031-32499-4_15

Residential Care Communities

Residential care communities for older adults in the USA include a broad range of living arrangements, provision of assistance with basic activities of daily living (ADLs) and instrumental activities of daily living (IADLs), and access to on-site medical care (Table 15.1). The patients seen in these settings will illustrate to

Table 15.1 Comparison of nursing facilities with residential care communities

	Skilled nursing facility/nursing facility	Assisted living facility (ALF)	Independent living community	Board and care homes/ group homes	Continuing care retirement communities
Description	Provides 24/7 nursing and personal care assistance to those unable to reside in the community. Some offer specialized units for persons with dementia.	Community residential setting that includes private living quarters and bathroom. Some offer specialized units for persons with dementia. Serves less disabled residents than nursing homes.	Provides room and board and some housekeeping. May have social activities and amenities.	Small group living setting with live-in caregivers. More homelike than larger facilities such as ALFs.	Spectrum of residences in one community, usually including independent living, ALF, and nursing facility
ADL assistance	Provides assistance for all ADLs as needed	Minimal to moderate assistance for some basic ADLs	None	Similar to ALF. Some may provide higher level of care similar to nursing facilities (varies by state).	Varies by setting
IADL assistance	Provides assistance for all IADLs as needed	Meals in common dining room, light housekeeping, and laundry	May offer some assistance with goal of minimizing daily responsibilities for carefree lifestyle	Similar to ALF. Some may provide higher level of care similar to nursing facilities (varies by state).	Varies by setting
On site medical care	Yes	Potentially	No	No	Varies by setting

Table 15.1 (continued)

	Skilled nursing facility/nursing facility	Assisted living facility (ALF)	Independent living community	Board and care homes/ group homes	Continuing care retirement communities
Professional on-site staff	RN, LPN, CNA, PT/OT/ SLP, dietitian, physician/APP	Licensed nurse, may or may not be on-site	None	None	Varies by setting
Coverage	Private pay, Medicare A for short-term post-acute care only, Medicaid and long-term care insurance for long-term care costs, health insurance provides coverage for medical visits	Private pay, long-term care insurance, Medicaid (variable, state waivers), health insurance provides coverage for medical visits	Private pay	Private pay, Medicaid (variable, state waivers), health insurance provides coverage for medical visits	Private pay, long-term care insurance, health insurance provides coverage for medical visits

ALF assisted living facility, *ADL* activities of daily living, *IADL* instrumental activities of daily living, *RN* registered nurse, *LPN* licensed practical nurse, *CNA* certified nursing assistant, *PT* physical therapy, *OT* occupational therapy, *SLP* speech language pathology, *APP* advanced practice provider

Adapted from content in [6, 7]

learners the importance of knowing what medical and personal care services are present at each site, so that appropriate management plans can be implemented that meet patients' current needs and goals of care.

Assisted Living Facilities (ALF)

More than 918,000 Americans reside in over 28,000 ALFs or similar residential care communities nationally [3, 4, 8]. In 2018, residential care community residents were predominantly female (67%), non-Hispanic white (89%), and aged 85 and over (55%) [8]. ALFs have great potential to showcase team-based geriatric care to many types and levels of learners [9–12]. These facilities are a residential option for older or disabled adults who need minimal to moderate assistance with some basic ADLs. They provide residents at minimum with a private room or apartment, private bathroom, dining services, housekeeping, and laundry services. Additional supportive services may be available at additional cost.

ALFs are regulated almost exclusively on the state level. Although all states require ALFs to have a licensed nurse on staff, who is not necessarily on site, the training (RN versus LPN) and staffing requirements vary. The primary role of the licensed nurse is to provide oversight of the direct care workers in the provision of personal care to the residents. Licensing, training, and certification requirements of these workers also vary by state [13].

The median monthly cost of an ALF is approximately $4000 per month [14]. The majority of residents privately pay for room and board costs and supportive services. Federal law prohibits Medicaid from covering room and board in residential care settings, but some residents do rely on Medicaid to pay for supportive services with coverage varying by state [6, 14].

ALFs may have medical services on-site but most commonly the residents continue with their primary care providers or enroll in home care medical practices. Some ALFs may provide transportation to medical appointments and/or recreational outings. ALFs not only provide Geriatrics 5Ms learning opportunities similar to those discussed in the teaching geriatrics through Home Visits chapter but also examples of collaborative team-based care involving the staff of an ALF and the primary medical team.

Board and Care Homes

Board and care homes, also known as group homes or adult foster care homes, provide residents similar types of supportive services as ALFs. Unlike ALFs, they typically house fewer than 20 residents. There are no on-site medical or nursing professionals. Group home staff cannot administer medications to residents but may assist them to take medications from prefilled packages if necessary. Residents' access to primary medical care resembles that of ALF residents. The cost of group homes is similar to that of ALFs [15], and most residents pay privately to live here. In some states, Medicaid covers adult foster care services provided in these sites via state waiver programs, but not room and board expenses [6].

Continuing Care Retirement Communities

CCRCs, also known as Life Plan Communities, offer a spectrum of residences, often located on the same campus, that span from independent living to assisted living to nursing facility level of care. In addition to a one-time entrance fee that may exceed $300,000, CCRCs charge residents a monthly fee that typically ranges between $2000 and $4000, depending on the amount and type of supportive services provided [5]. Medicare and Medicaid do not cover the costs associated with

CCRC living. Residents who have purchased long-term care insurance can use it to cover some CCRC costs, depending on the insurance policy terms. For those who must pay out of pocket for CCRC expenses, they may need to sell their homes and other assets in order to pay for CCRC living. People who live in the ALF or nursing facility residence of some CCRCs have access to on-site nursing and medical professional services, some of which are typically covered by health insurance plans.

Programs of All Inclusive Care for the Elderly (PACE)

The goal of the PACE model is to provide coordinated care and services to frail, complex older adults eligible for nursing facility care, allowing them to remain in their homes. The criteria for PACE enrollment include: (1) age greater than 55; (2) living within a PACE organization's service area; (3) living safely in the community; and (4) state eligibility for nursing facility level of care. Ninety percent of PACE participants are dually eligible for both Medicare and Medicaid. Those who are not eligible for Medicaid may pay a sliding scale fee to offset the costs. PACE provides an opportunity for learners to see a capitated model of care delivery where funds can be flexibly used to best serve the participant's goals. PACE organizations receive a monthly capitated payment from both Medicare and Medicaid for each participant. The PACE interdisciplinary team then allocates these funds toward comprehensive care that aligns with the participant's goals, regardless of whether this same service is covered under traditional Medicare fee-for-service plans. Medications, transportation services, and meals are also covered [16].

The interdisciplinary team is key to delivering individualized, coordinated care to each participant. At minimum these teams include nurses, physicians, nurse practitioners, dietitians, social workers, physical and occupational therapists (PT and OT), activity coordinators, van drivers, home health aides, and behavioral health therapists. The team meets regularly to share their assessments and recommendations, allowing for discussion and problem solving to best address each participant's needs. For many learners, PACE presents their first experience with a true team-based approach to clinical care and delivery.

Each PACE organization has a "center" where most care is delivered that consists of a clinical space and an adult day health center. Participants may attend several times a week, allowing them easier access to providers, care delivery, and increased socialization that is crucial for those living alone. These frequent "touches" often can prevent an unnecessary and sometimes harmful stay in the emergency room or hospital. One study from Massachusetts demonstrated that PACE participants' inpatient days, length of stay and number of ED visits were lower than those of a comparable nursing facility cohort [17]. While the goal of the PACE model is to keep participants in the community, some do transition to long-term care in a nursing facility and remain in the PACE organization, with the team continuing to provide the majority of their care. Nursing facility utilization for permanent placement remains low among PACE organizations, at 5% nationwide [18].

As of this year, 32 states and the District of Columbia have PACE organizations totaling 163 nationwide serving approximately 72,000 participants [19]. PACE participants typically have 8 chronic medical conditions (and almost half have dementia) and require assistance with at least three ADLs [20].

Leaders and policy-makers hope to expand access to PACE to Medicare-only older adults and other populations with disabilities. Introduced in 2020, the PACE 2.0 initiative aims to enroll 200,000 participants by 2028 [21]. The initiative makes it imperative that not only geriatricians but also all primary care providers become familiar with the services and systems involved with this care model. Providers will need to know which patients they can refer, and they may maintain their role as PCP while the patient enrolls in the program.

Teaching Geriatrics During a Routine Follow-Up Visit in an ALF

Some medical schools and training programs have incorporated exposure to ALFs into their geriatrics curricula [9–12]. A longitudinal curriculum at Brown University Alpert Medical School pairs first-year students with ALF residents to perform medical interviews and physical examinations [11]. An interprofessional curriculum for students in medicine, nursing, pharmacy, social work and public health has been developed that incorporates screenings and assessments of ALF residents in a variety of geriatrics topics such as fall prevention, medication safety, etc. This program has resulted in additional quality improvement projects in the facility including a transitions of care program following emergency room visits and hospitalization [12].

Creating a curriculum in the ALF setting poses challenges because it is not a typical training setting. Coordination with ALF staff may be needed to ensure that residents are present for visits and are of appropriate cognitive status to participate, but these tasks may be time consuming and compete with other caregiving or administrative responsibilities [9]. Preceptors may need appropriate affiliations or contractual agreements to care for patients in the ALF, so teaching in this setting may be more feasible in facilities with on-site clinicians. Regardless of the challenges, ALF residents benefit from and enjoy the opportunities to interact with learners of all levels. Learners can provide social interaction to isolated ALF residents, provide another set of eyes in the delivery of clinical care, and give the older adults a sense of purpose in contributing to the education of health care providers [9, 12]. Learners cite a greater appreciation for the role of ALFs as a supportive housing environment [11], and they will undoubtedly care for patients residing in this setting as the demand for ALFs grows as the US population ages.

Case 1
Mrs. L is a 91-year-old woman residing in an ALF with diagnoses of mild cognitive impairment (MCI), hypertension, heart failure with reduced ejection fraction, type 2 diabetes mellitus, macular degeneration, stage 4 chronic kidney disease, and osteoarthritis. She ambulates with a 4-wheel walker. She receives the facility's standard package of services (meals, housekeeping, laundry) and assistance with showers three times per week. She self-administers her medications, which are prepackaged by her pharmacy. While her vision is poor, she desires to maintain as much independence as possible and administers her own insulin via pen by listening to the number of clicks. During the early months of the COVID-19 pandemic, communal dining and activities were on hold at the facility and visitors were not allowed. Family had noticed that she seemed confused at times on the phone but attributed this to lapses in memory during a very trying time.

One morning ALF staff found her unconscious lying face down beside her bed when they went to serve her breakfast. She was admitted to the hospital and found to have hyperosmolar hyperglycemic syndrome and decompensated heart failure. The hospital team discovered that Mrs. L last refilled her insulin pen 2 months ago and had not been taking her medications regularly. During the hospitalization, Mrs. L experienced nighttime confusion, and hospital staff observed her closely to prevent her from falling. She was discharged to a skilled nursing facility (SNF) for subacute rehabilitation because she was unable to walk safely due to physical deconditioning. Upon recovery, she returned to her ALF where she is now able to walk very short distances with her walker. At times, she asks the ALF staff to take her to the dining room in a wheelchair due to fatigue.

Teaching in the ALF: Multicomplexity

More than half of ALF residents in the USA are aged 85 and older. The most common medical conditions for these residents are high blood pressure (55%), Alzheimer's disease or other dementias (34%), depression (27%), arthritis (20%), and diabetes (20%) [8]. ALFs provide a fertile teaching ground on how to care for the "oldest old" and frail older adults with complex medical and psychosocial needs in a collaborative manner.

Team-based care is essential in caring for older adults with multicomplexity, and this team can include the ALF staff. While family and loved ones are often part of this team, learners may not realize that the people with the most contact with the patient are often the ALF staff. Because they may have daily interaction with the patient, staff may be the first to recognize acute changes in the patient's health. Collateral information from ALF staff can be incredibly helpful when a patient and/or family cannot give detailed history of the events leading to a patient's acute care presentation.

It is important that clinicians caring for patients residing in ALFs be knowledgeable about the services provided in this setting when formulating treatment plans. A common misunderstanding among clinicians is the role of the ALF-employed or -contracted nursing staff (see below in *Teaching in the ALF: Medications*). In our experience, many clinicians assume that ALF nursing staff will perform similar tasks as nurses in hospitals, nursing facilities, and clinics. However, based on state regulations, ALF nurses may not be allowed to perform vital signs, monitor daily weights, obtain fingerstick glucose readings, etc. Some states designate that only nurses from a certified home health agency (CHHA) may provide skilled nursing services in the ALFs [13]. In Mrs. L's case, state regulations prohibit the nursing staff at her facility from administering insulin to her but ALF nurses in a neighboring state where her son lives are allowed to do so.

Teaching in the ALF: Mobility

By providing care at ALFs, learners will see how the level of care provided at ALFs differs from nursing facilities [10], where residents are generally more disabled and in need of more assistance with ADLs. ALF residents usually have independent mobility, with or without assistive devices. While the decline in function from needing a walker to wheelchair does not necessarily preclude Mrs. L from residing in an ALF, this setting may not be appropriate if the facility lacks staffing levels required to provide her assistance with transfer to and from the wheelchair or to push her wheelchair if she is unable to self-propel. Many states also require that residents be capable of evacuating the facility or moving to an area of safety within the building during an emergency, either independently or with minimal assistance [13]. When a resident is incapable of doing so, a higher level of care may be necessary.

Teaching in the ALF: Medications

Mrs. L may benefit from assistance from the ALF staff to manage her medications. A common misunderstanding for learners is the distinction between assistance with medications and medication administration. They may erroneously assume that nurses at ALFs administer medications to residents, similar to what occurs in a hospital or nursing facility setting. Medication administration typically involves removing the correct dose from a medication container and handing it to a resident or putting it in their mouth, or the direct application of a medication dose (e.g., topical, injectable). In contrast, assistance may include reminders, assistance with opening bottles, centralized storage, and/or record keeping. There is variability in state regulations as to what constitutes assistance with versus administration of medications. State provisions also vary as to who is authorized to assist with or administer medications, with some states permitting unlicensed staff to perform these tasks [13]. Therefore, teachers should prompt learners to ask specific questions regarding how a patient takes medications when performing a medication reconciliation. In Mrs. L's case, state regulation does not permit the ALF staff including nurses to administer injectable medication but may remind her to take self-administered medications.

Teaching in the ALF: Mentation

More than 3 in 10 residents in ALFs or similar residential care communities have a diagnosis of Alzheimer's disease or other dementia [8]. Mrs. L's clinical decline may suggest progression from MCI to dementia and may suggest an increase in care needs. As Mrs. L recuperates, her care team must assess if the ALF can still meet her care needs and/or for additional services to address any unmet need. When there is discordance between level of need and available on-site support, learners should identify how the patient's care can be provided in the least restrictive and most supportive setting. Some ALFs have designated memory care units that provide specialized care and services for residents with dementia. Just as with ALFs in general, the requirements for these units regarding staffing levels, staff training in dementia care, and eligibility vary by state [13].

Teaching in the ALF: What Matters Most

As Mrs. L's health and function have declined, it would be imperative to ensure that advanced care planning is in place. Part of this planning includes confirmation that her care needs can be met at her desired residence. Most states specify in their regulations that ALFs must discharge residents whose health-related needs they cannot meet. Should an ALF resident elect hospice care, some states also have detailed provisions regarding the furnishing of hospice services in the ALF setting. Because ALFs are seen as an attractive option for older adults to remain out of nursing facilities, we must acknowledge that the transition from ALF to a nursing facility can be difficult for the patient and/or family. They may see it as a loss of independence, privacy, and quality of life. A better understanding of ALFs would be beneficial for a clinician to support a patient who may go through such a transition.

Teaching Geriatrics During a Routine Follow-Up Visit at a PACE Center

Several geriatrics fellowship programs and some residency programs utilize PACE as a setting to teach core competencies such as clinical care, medical knowledge, systems-based practice, and communication skills [22]. A learner completing a geriatrics fellowship can fulfill Accreditation Council for Graduate Medical Education (ACGME) requirements for care in several settings within a single PACE rotation [23]. Additionally, PACE team members can teach all types and levels of learners important geriatrics 5Ms principles of care, often through exposing learners to contemporaneous interdisciplinary care collaboration.

In a 2018 survey of directors of ACGME-accredited geriatrics fellowship programs with PACE rotations for trainees (14 out of 48 respondents), a common requirement is for learners to work directly with the interdisciplinary team members in each care setting (home, PACE center, nursing facility, ALF). The learner thus acquires setting-specific knowledge that they can then use to tailor management plans to achieve a participant's goals of care [22]. The following case illustrates this concept.

Case 2

Mrs. P is a 72-year-old woman with hypertension, type 2 diabetes mellitus, anxiety, a remote history of schizophrenia, and osteoarthritis who is now status-post left knee replacement surgery 6 weeks prior to your visit with her at the PACE center. Before her hip surgery, she lived alone in her apartment and received some services to assist with IADL care.

She has been receiving physical therapy (PT) at the PACE center for the past 3 weeks since skilled nursing facility (SNF) discharge. During the session, PT reports that she has worsening pain in the left knee and asks for a medical evaluation. She is seen that same afternoon by the PACE geriatrician and trainee, who revise her pain medication regimen and encourage her to continue with ambulation and therapy. The geriatrician also calls her orthopedics physician, who agrees with the plan. PT continues to work daily with the patient.

Two days later her pain is worse. She asks to see the physician again, who evaluates her together with the PACE rehabilitation staff while she is at the center. Her knee is now warm and erythematous. The geriatrician asks the PACE center staff to check labs on-site. Mrs. P is still able to ambulate, and the PACE team increases her home services so she may return home. The labs reveal an elevated WBC of 16. The patient is able to go to an urgent same-day orthopedic clinic visit, with transportation provided by PACE. She feels discouraged about her possible need for hospitalization, because she only recently returned home from the SNF. She is found to have an infection of the prosthetic joint and is admitted to the hospital for intravenous (IV) antibiotics. She is seen on the inpatient service by the PACE attending physician and geriatric medicine fellow. Three days later, she is transferred to a SNF to continue IV antibiotics, where the PACE attending physician admits her and collaborates with on-site nursing and rehabilitation staff to provide her post-hospital care.

Teaching at PACE: Multicomplexity

The PACE team is uniquely positioned to provide medical management across a patient's multiple transitions from home to hospital to SNF. At Mrs. P's initial hospitalization for her hip repair, the PACE team requested SNF-based rehabilitation for her, despite the trend of discharge to home in orthopedic practice. This was a decision based on what the team knew about her apartment setup, her motivation to participate in therapy, and limitations to how much therapy PACE rehabilitation therapists can provide in the home setting. Because the PACE organization also serves as her health plan, the clinicians were able to make this decision based on their assessments alone without need for further insurance approval.

The PACE rehabilitation team members then communicated regularly with the SNF rehabilitation therapists, while the PACE primary care doctor served as the SNF attending physician of record. Once the patient underwent a successful trial at home and home services were arranged, she was discharged to her apartment. Post-SNF discharge, she maintained daily regular contact with the PACE rehabilitation and primary care (PC) team at the center. The collaboration of these disciplines in real time allowed for prompt identification and management of her subsequent prosthetic joint infection.

In addition to the rehabilitation and PC visits, transportation to appointments with short notice was also available. Lastly, frequent contact with her orthopedic team also made it possible to move quickly when needed. This case illustrates how learners can observe and take part in a well-functioning interdisciplinary team by working with PACE to care for patients across multiple care settings. Team-based care continues to be a vital piece of geriatrics training, and post-graduate training programs often use PACE as a framework to teach these skills [24].

Teaching at PACE: Mobility

Addressing the patient's changing mobility was a key issue in Mrs. P's management. Her goal was to successfully complete rehabilitation after an elective knee replacement in order to regain function. The importance of the PACE rehabilitation team cannot be emphasized enough. Learners have a unique opportunity to see rehabilitation therapists' patient assessments at home and at the center that serve to identify appropriate home care services and durable medical equipment.

Teaching at PACE: Medications

Because PACE providers can follow a patient across multiple care sites, they can ensure that patients receive optimal medication management while avoiding potential hazards of polypharmacy. In Mrs. P's case, the PACE team monitored her pain medication regimen in the inpatient, rehabilitation, and outpatient settings. The PACE physician worked closely with pharmacies to avoid medication errors by completing medication reconciliation at each transition point. The PACE nurse then determined the best way for the patient to receive medications once she returned home, in close collaboration with the physician, to establish a dosing schedule that best suited the patient's needs (e.g. once daily versus multiple times per day administration, PRN vs. scheduled prescriptions).

Teaching at PACE: Mentation

During Mrs. P's stay at the hospital and SNF, the PACE team was able to monitor her mental status. Because of their long-standing relationship with the patient, they noticed subtle changes in her presentation that helped guide next steps in her work-ups and treatment.

Teaching at PACE: What Matters Most

Many PACE patients desire to remain home, even when faced with worsening illness or physical functioning. In this case, Mrs. P's goal was to stay home with improved function after receiving her long-awaited knee replacement. Remaining in her home was a strong incentive for her to perform ADLs and manage her weight. The PACE team was equally invested and able to explore all options to help her achieve this goal, using the expertise of each discipline.

Teaching Geriatrics During a Post-Hospital Discharge Visit in a Group Home

Some learners may not be aware that group homes or ALFs do not offer the same medical follow-up as skilled nursing facilities (SNFs). A post-hospital discharge home visit to a residential community setting such as a group home can highlight the differences in available medical care between these sites [6]. These educational experiences usually involve learners first meeting patients while they are hospitalized followed by performance of a post-hospital discharge home visit [25–28] (Table 15.2).

Table 15.2 Examples of post-hospital visit educational interventions

Intervention	Target learners	Patients	Activities	Learner outcomes
Post-hospital home visit during geriatrics ambulatory rotation [25]	PGY2 and PGY3 internal medicine residents	Recently discharged patients that residents cared for during weekend geriatrics inpatient service coverage	Semi-structured patient and/or family interview to assess their perspective on the hospital discharge Medication reconciliation Review of hospital discharge summary Completion of questionnaire where residents propose potential changes to the discharge plan based on their home visit experience	Self-reported improvement in describing the role that certified home health agencies (CHHA) and nonmedical community services can play in hospital discharge plans
Hospital to home [26, 27]	PGY1 internal medicine resident on a geriatrics rotation	Hospitalized patients about to be discharged home	Pre-discharge and post-hospital home visit patient interviews, both of which are videotaped Videotapes used as teaching triggers during a noon conference session focused on nonmedical aspects of discharge planning	Self-reported increased appreciation for the role of social supports in effective hospital discharge plans, and potential barriers to recovery including environmental challenges
Transition of care rotation (TRACER) [28]	PGY2 internal medicine resident	Recently discharged patients who the residents cared for on an inpatient service	Post-discharge visits in patients' homes, subacute rehabilitation units, or long-term care facilities	Self-reported increased insight into patients' perspectives of the discharge process, level of care fragmentation, and importance of team collaboration

Case 3

Mr. G is an 89-year-old man who was recently hospitalized for acute on chronic systolic heart failure (ejection fraction 25%) and resides in a group home. His other chronic conditions are type 2 diabetes mellitus (A1c 8.7), diabetic retinopathy causing visual impairment, unsteady gait, essential hypertension, hyperlipidemia, and GERD. In the prior 6 months, he has been hospitalized four times, either with acute heart failure or falls. In the hospital, he was treated with intravenous diuretic therapy. He has been discharged home with an increased dose of oral furosemide. The discharge summary also lists pantoprazole; he took omeprazole prior to hospital admission. His other medications were unchanged and include aspirin, lisinopril, metoprolol, metformin, empagliflozin, and rosuvastatin.

He is feeling fatigued and short of breath when he ambulates from his bedroom to the dining room. He is discouraged about his worsening health status. He tells the clinician that he does not want to go back to the hospital again. He wants to focus on doing the things he enjoys with the people he loves. To this end, he would like his dyspnea to improve. He is not concerned about his diabetes management.

Post-Hospital Visit Teaching in a Group Home: Multicomplexity

On such a visit, one could ask learners to assess if discharge back to the group home was clinically appropriate. If the patient's medical or functional needs exceed what a group home can support, then the hospital team should have discussed the option of SNF transfer with the patient. Because group homes lack on-site nursing professionals, this type of patient would not be receiving daily nursing assessments, as would be available in a SNF. If the patient's function has declined below a level that group home staff can manage, supplemental informal caregiving support from the patient's family members or others would be necessary, if available. Alternatively, the patient may qualify for home health aide services provided by a certified home health agency (CHHA) if he also has skilled needs.

Hospital teams should connect a patient residing in a group home to home-based skilled services for which he is eligible. If the patient warrants nursing assessment, due to changes in medication regimen such as in Mr. G's case, then the patient should be referred to a CHHA, also called visiting nurse agencies (VNA) in some regions of the USA. Medicare A reimburses these skilled visits as long as the patient is deemed to be homebound by a referring medical provider [29], defined as the inability to leave one's home without assistance due to illness or injury. Typically, VNAs only provide 2–3 nursing visits per week, although some agencies have the staffing capacity to provide daily nursing visits if clinically indicated (i.e. wound care). This Medicare A benefit was designed to be temporary in duration; therefore, skilled nursing visits will typically stop once the patient's medical conditions have stabilized, as will home health aide services provided by the agency.

In Mr. G's case, his increased weakness and dyspnea on exertion would make it difficult for him to travel to his primary care clinic for nursing visits. Therefore, one could refer him to VNA for home skilled nursing visits to monitor his response to the new heart failure regimen.

Post-Hospital Visit Teaching in a Group Home: Mobility

Older adults who are homebound and living in group homes who have not returned to their previous baseline functional status would be eligible for home-based physical therapy (PT) and occupational therapy (OT) sessions. Just as with home skilled nursing visits, Medicare A would reimburse these treatments on a temporary basis, until the patient has either returned to their baseline status or achieved stability [29]. Mr. G would be eligible for such home-based PT and OT.

Post-Hospital Visit Teaching in a Group Home: Medications

One key teaching point to emphasize on a post-hospital group home visit is the importance of accurate medication reconciliation. Medication-related rehospitalization is common, with published rates as high as 64% [30]. Transitions of care from the hospital to another site of care create high risk for medication adverse events in older adults [31].

One adverse event that can be seen is duplication of medications from the same drug class, because hospital pharmacy formularies sometimes lack patients' home medications. Therefore, the patient can be unintentionally given a prescription for an alternative medication from the same drug class upon hospital discharge, leading to potential confusion or medication error.

Should residents need assistance with taking medications, group home staff can assist in this task only if medications are located in prefilled packages. If a medication dosage has been changed during a hospitalization, the medication package at the group home will not contain the updated dosage unless the hospital providers contacted the pharmacy prior to discharge to place a new order. In this situation, a pharmacy would create a new prefilled medication package to deliver to the group home, and a pharmacy courier would remove the old prefilled medication package.

In Mr. G's case, the teacher and learner need to call the pharmacy to stop pantoprazole, because he is already receiving omeprazole in his prefilled medication packages. They also need to inform the pharmacy about the increased furosemide dosage and confirm that the pharmacy will be sending a courier to the group home to replace the old medication package with a new one.

Post-Hospital Visit Teaching in a Group Home: Mentation

A post-hospital home visit is an important time to assess patients for delirium. For a group home resident, delirium precipitated by recent acute illness may affect his ability to participate in daily activities, which in turn should prompt discussion about whether he requires more caregiving support than can be provided by the group home staff. In Mr. G's case, the teacher and learner should perform delirium screening with validated tools such as the Confusion Assessment Method (CAM) [32].

Post-Hospital Visit Teaching in a Group Home: What Matters Most

If a patient with multiple chronic conditions has had multiple hospitalizations within the prior 6 months, it would be important to readdress his care preferences on a post-hospital home visit. Patients with frequent rehospitalizations in the setting of cancer and/or CHF and associated with ADL impairments have particularly high 1-year mortality [33, 34].

When a patient is deciding whether new therapies should be started, he will be weighing several factors, including what hopes he has for the months ahead, what tradeoffs he is willing to accept to achieve his goals of care, and his estimated life expectancy [35]. Teachers and learners can utilize the American Geriatrics Society-recommended principles of care for older adults with multiple chronic conditions framework [36] to assist the patient in making treatment decisions. This framework centers management decisions on the patient's priorities for achieving the highest possible quality of life while accounting for his anticipated health trajectory and the risks versus benefits of therapies. They can also use the Patient Priorities Care framework [37], which is further discussed in Chap. 20.

In Mr. G's case, the teacher and learner should validate the patient's belief that his health is declining. Using the frameworks mentioned above, confirm his care preferences, identify what tradeoffs he is willing to accept, and adjust his treatment plans accordingly. Invite his family and other health care team members to participate in this discussion as he wishes. Confirm that he would not want to intensify his diabetes medication regimen. Insulin would not be feasible, given that he does not have adequate vision to self-administer insulin injections and group home staff cannot administer medications via injection. Finally, discuss with the patient if a transition to a palliative approach, or perhaps to a nursing facility where more nursing and personal care assistance are available, aligns with his current care preferences. Readdress advance directives and update the Physician Orders for Life Sustaining Treatment form (POLST) to reflect his wishes.

Discussion

Residential care communities and PACE are unique places to teach all levels and types of learners about geriatrics, and particularly well suited to emphasize the geriatrics 5Ms. Seeing patients in these settings offers teachers opportunities to highlight the variability in medical and personal care support services inherent to each setting. This adds another layer of multicomplexity that healthcare providers must account for when developing management plans with older patients. Such variability necessitates healthcare providers to clearly identify the patients' top care priorities, engage a multidisciplinary team, and connect patients to additional community-based medical and nonmedical services that will help patients achieve their goals of care. Students and post-graduate trainees should learn in these settings if available, so that they will be prepared to provide high-quality person-centered care to older adults across the healthcare continuum.

References

1. Housing America's older adults 2019. Joint Center for Housing Studies of Harvard University. 2019. https://www.jchs.harvard.edu/housing-americas-older-adults-2019. Accessed 27 Sept 2021.
2. 2020 Profile of Older Americans. The Administration for Community Living, U.S. Department of Health and Human Services. May 2021. https://acl.gov/aging-and-disability-in-america/data-and-research/profile-older-americans. Accessed 18 Feb 2022.
3. Centers for Disease Control and Prevention: FastStats on Residential Care Communities. 2019. https://www.cdc.gov/nchs/fastats/residential-care-communities.htm. Accessed 27 Sept 2021.
4. Harris-Kojetin L, Sengupta M, Park-Lee E, Valverde R, Caffrey C, Rome V, Lendon J. Long-Term Care Providers and services users in the United States: data from the National Study of Long-Term Care Providers, 2013–2014. Vital Health Stat 3. (38):x-xii; 1–105.
5. How continuing care retirement communities work. AARP. 2019. https://www.aarp.org/caregiving/basics/info-2017/continuing-care-retirement-communities.html. Accessed 28 Sept 2021.
6. Kane RL. Finding the right level of posthospital care: "We didn't realize there was any other option for him". JAMA. 2011;305(3):284–93. https://doi.org/10.1001/jama.2010.2015. PMID: 21245184.
7. Markowitz A. Finding the Right Long-Term Care for Your Loved One. AARP. 2020. https://www.aarp.org/caregiving/basics/info-2020/long-term-care/?.html. Accessed 15 Oct 2021.
8. Caffrey C, Sengupta M, Melekin A. Residential care community resident characteristics: United States, 2018. NCHS Data Brief, no 404. Hyattsville, MD: National Center for Health Statistics; 2021. Accessed 14 Oct 2021. https://doi.org/10.15620/cdc:103826.external.icon.
9. Pruchnicki A, Janeski J, Mitchell E, Fetten E. Teaching at an assisted living facility. Care Manag J. 2008;9(4):186–91. https://doi.org/10.1891/1521-0987.9.4.186.
10. Saffel-Shrier S, Gunning K, Van Hala S, Farrell T, Lehmann W, Egger M, Miniclier N. Residency redesign to accommodate trends in geriatrics: an RC-FM variance to establish a patient-centered medical home in an assisted living facility. Fam Med. 2012;44(2):128–31.
11. Tong IL, Dodd KA, Warrier SS, Pugliese LJ, McMackin NY, Taylor JS. An assisted living facility curriculum to introduce geriatrics to first-year medical students. Gerontol Geriatr Educ. 2015;36(1):79–95. Epub 2014 Oct 6. https://doi.org/10.1080/02701960.2014.954041.
12. Lee J, Cioltan H, Goldsmith P, Heasley B, Dermody M, Fain M, Mohler J. An assisted living interprofessional education and practice geriatric screening clinic (IPEP-GSC): a description and evaluation. Gerontol Geriatr Educ. 2021;42(2):166–77. Epub 2018 Apr 13. https://doi.org/10.1080/02701960.2018.1463222.
13. Carder P, O'Keeffe J, O'Keeffe C. Compendium of residential care and assisted living regulations and policy: 2015 Edition. 2015. https://aspe.hhs.gov/reports/compendium-residential-care-assisted-living-regulations-policy-2015-edition-0. Accessed 9 Mar 2022.

14. Assisted living facilities: weighing the options. AARP. 2019. https://www.aarp.org/caregiving/basics/info-2017/assisted-living-options.html. Accessed 8 Oct 2021.
15. Abrahms S. Group homes an alternative for seniors who can't age in place. AARP. 2020. https://www.aarp.org/caregiving/basics/info-2020/group-homes.html. Accessed 28 Sept 2021.
16. Understanding the PACE Model of Care. National PACE Association. https://www.npaonline.org/start-pace-program/understanding-pace-model-care. Accessed 28 Sept 2021.
17. PACE Evaluation summary. Division of Health Care Finance and Policy, Executive Office of Elder Affairs. 2005. https://archives.lib.state.ma.us/handle/2452/70646. Accessed 30 Sept 2021.
18. Segelman M, Szydlowski J, Kinosian B, McNabney M, Raziano DB, Eng C, van Reenen C, Temkin-Greener H. Hospitalizations in the program of all-inclusive care for the elderly. J Am Geriatr Soc. 2014;62(2):320–4. Epub 2014 Jan 13. https://doi.org/10.1111/jgs.12637.
19. https://www.npaonline.org/find-a-pace-program#:~:text=Find%20a%20PACE%20Program%20Near,72%2C000%20participants%20across%20the%20country.&text=Start%20with%20a%20state%20search,search%20to%20refine%20the%20results. Accessed 3 May 2024.
20. Williams CT, Chandrasekaran S. Program All Inclusive Care of the Elderly (PACE) [Updated 2023 Oct 28]. In: StatPearls [Internet]. Treasure Island (FL): StatPearls Publishing; 2024. Available from: https://www.ncbi.nlm.nih.gov/books/NBK597375/.
21. https://www.westhealth.org/publications/asa-lets-pick-up-the-pace-expanding-the-reach-of-the-gold-standard-program-of-all-inclusive-care-for-the-elderly/. Accessed 3 May 2024.
22. McNabney MK, Suh TT, Sellers V, Wilner D. Aligning geriatric medicine fellowships with the program of all-inclusive care for the elderly (PACE). Gerontol Geriatr Educ. 2021;42(1):2–12. Epub 2018 Dec 18. https://doi.org/10.1080/02701960.2018.1532891.
23. Tanabe MK. PACE rotation enhances geriatric medicine fellowship training. J Am Geriatr Soc. 2004;52(5):853–4. https://doi.org/10.1111/j.1532-5415.2004.52230_13.x.
24. Keough ME, Field TS, Gurwitz JH. A model of community-based interdisciplinary team training in the care of the frail elderly. Acad Med. 2002;77(9):936. https://doi.org/10.1097/00001888-200209000-00041.
25. Young ME, Demers LB, Parker V, Day H, Chao S. Posthospital home visit as teaching tool for internal medicine residents. Gerontol Geriatr Educ. 2020;41(4):514–21. Epub 2018 Jul 18. https://doi.org/10.1080/02701960.2018.1490736.
26. Matter CA, Speice JA, McCann R, Mendelson DA, McCormick K, Friedman S, Medina-Walpole A, Clark NS. Hospital to home: improving internal medicine residents' understanding of the needs of older persons after a hospital stay. Acad Med. 2003;78(8):793–7. https://doi.org/10.1097/00001888-200308000-00009.
27. DeCaporale-Ryan LN, Cornell A, McCann RM, McCormick K, Speice J. Hospital to home: a geriatric educational program on effective discharge planning. Gerontol Geriatr Educ. 2014;35(4):369–79. Epub 2014 Jan 6. https://doi.org/10.1080/02701960.2013.858332.
28. Meade LB, Hall SL, Kleppel RW, Hinchey KT. TRACER: an 'eye-opener' to the patient experience across the transition of care in an internal medicine resident program. J Community Hosp Intern Med Perspect. 2015;5(2):26230. PMID: 25846349; PMCID: PMC4387321. https://doi.org/10.3402/jchimp.v5.26230.
29. Home Health services. In: Your Medicare Coverage. U.S. Centers for Medicare and Medicaid Services. https://www.medicare.gov/coverage/home-health-services. Accessed 30 Sept 2021.
30. El Morabet N, Uitvlugt EB, van den Bemt BJF, van den Bemt PMLA, Janssen MJA, Karapinar-Çarkit F. Prevalence and preventability of drug-related hospital readmissions: a systematic review. J Am Geriatr Soc. 2018;66(3):602–8. Epub 2018 Feb 22. https://doi.org/10.1111/jgs.15244.
31. Marcum ZA, Handler SM, Boyce R, Gellad W, Hanlon JT. Medication misadventures in the elderly: a year in review. Am J Geriatr Pharmacother. 2010;8(1):77–83. PMID: 20226395; PMCID: PMC2904235. https://doi.org/10.1016/j.amjopharm.2010.02.002.

32. Inouye SK, van Dyck CH, Alessi CA, Balkin S, Siegal AP, Horwitz RI. Clarifying confusion: the confusion assessment method. A new method for detection of delirium. Ann Intern Med. 1990;113(12):941–8. https://doi.org/10.7326/0003-4819-113-12-941.
33. Walter LC, Brand RJ, Counsell SR, Palmer RM, Landefeld CS, Fortinsky RH, Covinsky KE. Development and validation of a prognostic index for 1-year mortality in older adults after hospitalization. JAMA. 2001;285(23):2987–94. https://doi.org/10.1001/jama.285.23.2987.
34. Levine SK, Sachs GA, Jin L, Meltzer D. A prognostic model for 1-year mortality in older adults after hospital discharge. Am J Med. 2007;120(5):455–60. https://doi.org/10.1016/j.amjmed.2006.09.021.
35. Bernacki R, Hutchings M, Vick J, Smith G, Paladino J, Lipsitz S, Gawande AA, Block SD. Development of the serious illness care program: a randomised controlled trial of a palliative care communication intervention. BMJ Open. 2015;5(10):e009032. PMID: 26443662; PMCID: PMC4606432. https://doi.org/10.1136/bmjopen-2015-009032.
36. Boyd C, Smith CD, Masoudi FA, Blaum CS, Dodson JA, Green AR, Kelley A, Matlock D, Ouellet J, Rich MW, Schoenborn NL, Tinetti ME. Decision making for older adults with multiple chronic conditions: executive summary for the American Geriatrics Society guiding principles on the care of older adults with multimorbidity. J Am Geriatr Soc. 2019;67(4):665–73. Epub 2019 Mar 10. https://doi.org/10.1111/jgs.15809.
37. Tinetti ME, Naik AD, Dindo L, Costello DM, Esterson J, Geda M, Rosen J, Hernandez-Bigos K, Smith CD, Ouellet GM, Kang G, Lee Y, Blaum C. Association of patient priorities-aligned decision-making with patient outcomes and ambulatory health care burden among older adults with multiple chronic conditions: a nonrandomized clinical trial. JAMA Intern Med. 2019;179(12):1688–97. Epub ahead of print. PMID: 31589281; PMCID: PMC6784811. https://doi.org/10.1001/jamainternmed.2019.4235.

Chapter 16
Teaching Geriatrics in the Online Classroom

Alexandra E. Petrakos, Travis W. Crook, and Maria C. Duggan

Learning Objectives

By the end of this chapter, the reader will be able to:

- Describe the value of teaching geriatrics in the online classroom.
- Describe challenges to teaching and learning geriatrics in the online classroom.
- Apply the basic principles of adult learning theory in designing a lesson plan for use in the online classroom.
- Identify strategies to adapt in-person instructional modalities for teaching geriatrics in the online classroom.
- Describe the current applications and tools used to host and augment online geriatrics learning experiences.
- Prepare for an online, synchronous teaching session in a way that will minimize distractions and interruptions.
- Actively engage learners during an online session.

A. E. Petrakos (✉)
Vanderbilt University School of Medicine, Nashville, TN, USA

Feinberg School of Medicine, Northwestern University,
Chicago, IL, USA
e-mail: alexandra.petrakos@nm.org

T. W. Crook
Vanderbilt University School of Medicine, Nashville, TN, USA

M. C. Duggan
Tennessee Valley Veterans Affairs Geriatric Research, Education and Clinical Center,
Vanderbilt University School of Medicine, Nashville, TN, USA

A. W. Schwartz (ed.), *Medical Education in Geriatrics*,
https://doi.org/10.1007/978-3-031-32499-4_16

Introduction

As the population of older adults grows and geriatricians remain in high demand, geriatrics specialists are increasingly called upon to educate other providers and trainees on evidence-based care of older adults [1]. Teaching in an online classroom is a way for the geriatric specialist to reach a broader audience while minimizing costs and ideally without sacrificing the quality of the educational experience [2, 3].

While the online classroom encompasses both synchronous and asynchronous learning, this chapter will discuss synchronous online learning only; online resources for teaching geriatrics asynchronously are discussed in Chap. 24. With synchronous online learning, learners are taught in a virtual classroom and interact with teachers in real time. With asynchronous online learning, learners review pre-generated learning material without live teacher interaction. For the purposes of this chapter, "online classroom" and "online learning" will refer exclusively to a virtual, synchronous learning environment.

The transition from in-person learning to online learning requires forethought and preparation. As with most change, it is important to acknowledge and prepare for potential challenges that may hinder geriatric education in the online classroom. Teachers should maintain the classic concepts of adult learning theory in order to optimize learner retention [4], appropriately select the online teaching modality and tools to convey their lesson and prepare for the technical and technological aspects of the online classroom. Finally, teachers should adhere to best practices specific to the online classroom to maximize learner participation and engagement.

This chapter will describe the value, the challenges, and the best practices of teaching geriatrics in the online classroom.

Value of Teaching Geriatrics in the Online Classroom

Online medical education, both synchronous and asynchronous, has been growing steadily for years [5]. The online classroom allows learners from disparate geographical locations to engage in active learning in real time and maintain interaction with their teachers and peers. Several studies conducted within the field of non-medical secondary education have shown online learning to be as effective as in-person learning, as evidenced by stable exam grades and grade point averages ([2]; Signor 2003).

Online teaching can also increase learner access to material and reduce education costs. A survey of university students revealed that many learners found online learning more beneficial than in-person classes because learners could hear their teacher better and view the presentation slides more easily [6]. Additionally, online teaching reduces the need for classroom reservation and travel, making it a more cost-effective option [2, 6]. The impact of this can be quite broad, from medical students not needing to commute or rent housing near school, to national conference attendees learning up-to-date geriatrics practices from the comfort of their home-offices, as was the case during the American Geriatrics Society Virtual Annual Meeting 2021.

The value of teaching in the online classroom is particularly relevant for the field of geriatrics, where so few geriatricians exist. Recent education models in geriatrics have demonstrated how online teaching can reach non-specialist providers. In San Antonio, Texas, geriatricians reached broader audiences by live-streaming their Geriatrics Grand Rounds via Facebook Live; over 2 years these live-streamed conferences reached participants from over 26 states and 28 countries [7]. Other academic institutions have used Twitter (e.g. @GeriMedJC and @GeriJC Twitter accounts) to host regular geriatric journal clubs with a short live component. Within its first year, @GeriMedJC had 541 followers from six continents, while @GeriJC had 144 followers within its initial 3-month rollout with 178 tweets in journal club discussion [8, 9].

Outside of social media, Project ECHO (Extension for Community Healthcare Outcomes)—a model of medical education that uses video-conferencing to increase rural access to subspecialty services [10]—has been adapted by several academic institutions to increase community access to geriatrics learning. These regular interactive teleconferences are hosted by interdisciplinary geriatrics providers who teach community providers, including primary care providers, resident physicians, and nursing facility staff, how to better care for older patients. Attendees of geriatrics-themed ECHO sessions self-reported improved geriatrics self-efficacy and increased geriatrics-specific knowledge, with 65% reporting intention to change their practice [11–13]. These results highlight the success of these educational initiatives in teaching geriatrics principles online.

The onset of the COVID-19 pandemic in early 2020 sparked a new urgency in transitioning in-person teaching to the online classroom, especially within medical education, which led to positive outcomes and lasting innovation. A systematic review of the effectiveness of online education during the COVID-19 pandemic revealed many strengths of interactive online teaching methods, including providing wider access to teachers who are content experts, peer mentoring for education and psychological support, and even meaningful, remote patient interactions [14]. One example of innovation in the online classroom triggered by the pandemic is GERIAtrics Fellows Learning Online and Together (GERI-A-FLOAT), an "educational series that uses virtual meetings to deepen knowledge of geriatric medicine and to convene fellows from across the country for networking and peer support" [15]. GERI-A-FLOAT was developed in the early days of the pandemic after the potential risks of in-person teaching became evident. Since its inception, these interactive webinars have reached a wide audience including participants from almost 30 states and 10 countries, with sessions taught by geriatric subspecialty experts from numerous academic medical institutions. The GERI-A-FLOAT model demonstrates the many benefits of online teaching: it increases learner access to information, standardizes learning through high-quality expert teaching, decreases educator and learner burden and cost, and provides the additional advantages of professional networking and peer support. Additionally, it is a translatable model that can be applied in other specialties and fields to rapidly develop new, quality curriculum.

Challenges of Teaching in the Online Classroom

As with most advances in education and technology, the transition from in-person to online teaching comes with potential difficulty. Various challenges and barriers to teaching in an online classroom have been identified and can be described in four main categories: limitations in scope, technology challenges, challenges from educator perspective, and challenges from learner perspective.

Although many teaching modalities can be adapted for use in the virtual setting (see Table 16.1), the scope of online learning has limits. Certain hands-on or procedural components of geriatrics curricula are more conducive to in-person teaching.

Table 16.1 Medical education teaching modalities and modifications for online use in teaching geriatrics

Teaching modality	Advantages	Disadvantages	Modifications for online use	Online examples in geriatric medical education
Readings	Available, provides groundwork, evidence-based, can be accessed at optimal time	Passive, teacher-centered, can easily overload learner, unlikely to result in long-term knowledge	Electronic documents or PDFs	Electronic textbooks like geriatrics review syllabus [16], online journal articles, medical databases
Lecture	Provides groundwork, presentation software widely available, evidence-based, can be recorded and reviewed later	Passive, teacher-centered, danger of cognitive overload, limited attention span of learners, learning can be superficial	Screen share on virtual platform	Virtual medical grand rounds [7], house staff noon conference
Discussion groups	Participatory, develop social skills	Often require prior preparation by learner, require facilitation to ensure learners are engaged	Breakout rooms, shared word docs, online discussion boards	GERI-A-FLOAT [15], virtual geriatrics journal club [8, 9]
Q&A panels	Participatory, can be learner-centered	Effectiveness can vary depending on learner participation	Chat box for queuing questions	Geriatrics fellowship application Q&A sessions

Table 16.1 (continued)

Teaching modality	Advantages	Disadvantages	Modifications for online use	Online examples in geriatric medical education
Review	Active, participatory	Teacher-centered	Jeopardy [17], Kahoot [18], Quizlet [19], PollEverywhere [20]	Geriatrics board review sessions
Case discussions	Embeds learning in context of real patient, objectives adjusted "on the fly," learner-centered	Not always available, good for auditory learners, team members may have disparate experience and knowledge	Breakout rooms, QR codes for handouts [21, 22]	MM&I conference, Aquifer Geriatrics [23], monthly audio Most Difficult Case Conference [24]
Demonstration/ modeling	Modeling a skill can incorporate other "hidden" objectives, like patient-centered care and professionalism	Passive, teacher-centered	Breakout rooms, Quizlet [19], PollEverywhere images [25]	Learner observation of telehealth encounters, demonstration of interview or physical exam skills with SP
Role play	Active, participatory, cost-effective, learners appreciate different perspectives	Learner may be resistant, time-consuming to set up scenarios and debrief	Breakout rooms, video or audio recording for reviewing and feedback	Practice performing capacity assessments or patient priorities care conversations [26]
Standardized patient	Active, participatory, SPs can be trained to give feedback	Teacher-centered, learner may be resistant	Recorded video session for reviewing and feedback	Virtual geriatrics OSCE [27], virtual geriatric assessment with sensory-impairing devices (i.e.: earplugs, glasses with tape) during virtual session
Writing	Active, participatory, can facilitate habits or reflection, deepens learning	Learner may be resistant, time-intensive, especially if delivering feedback	Shared Google Docs [28], muted video session	Writing workshop to promote wellness

(continued)

Table 16.1 (continued)

Teaching modality	Advantages	Disadvantages	Modifications for online use	Online examples in geriatric medical education
Learning projects	Active, participatory, learners can set goals, address higher-order skills of analysis and synthesis	Learner resources needed, time-intensive, high faculty:learner ratio required if plan for mentoring	Breakout rooms, Padlet [29], Miro [30]	QI project on 4Ms, learner presentations
Experiential	Contextual, deepens prior learning experiences, addresses hidden curriculum	Without appropriate debrief can reinforce negative learning	Video session	Participate in actual telehealth encounter with preceptor supervision
Self-assessment	Promotes self-directed and lifelong learning	Requires mentoring for optimum effectiveness	Video session with pre-provided shared assessment documents	Annual review with geriatrics fellowship director or geriatrics division chair

Adapted from Skeff and Stratos [31]. *Methods for Teaching Medicine*. ACP Press, American College of Physicians

GERI-A-FLOAT Geriatric Fellows Learning Online And Together, *Q&A* question and answer, *QR* quick response, *MM&I* morbidity, mortality and improvement, *SP* standardized patient, *OSCE* Objective Structured Clinical Examination, *QI* quality improvement, *4Ms* Framework of Age-Friendly Health Systems, per the Institute for Healthcare Improvement, which includes mobility, mentation, medications, matters most

For example, learning to diagnose active rheumatoid arthritis by palpating the bogginess of inflamed hand joints is best achieved through bedside exam; teaching how to debride a necrotic sacral pressure injury is best accomplished via supervised bedside procedure. In the online classroom, teachers should only develop lesson plans with learning objectives that can be adequately met in the virtual setting. For topics that are more effectively taught in person, teachers should seek out opportunities for face-to-face learning.

Challenges with technology affect both learners and educators and include problems with hardware, software, and internet connection. Hardware issues may include not having a webcam or microphone, whereas software issues could include not having the appropriate program or correct version installed. The two most important issues related to internet connection are unreliability of the connection and variable learner access to internet connectivity. Multiple studies and reviews have indicated that unreliable internet connection can be a hinderance in online teaching [32, 33]. An arguably more pressing issue is unequal access to internet in remote areas or within less advantaged learner populations.

Educators face their own unique set of challenges in pursuing online teaching. Limitations in technical knowledge, insufficient time to learn new skills, and an institutional culture that is unsupportive of adapting new practices can all make a transition to online teaching difficult [32, 33]. Moreover, teaching geriatrics in an online classroom requires a heightened ability for multitasking, as educators must manage their own screensharing, monitor the chat, and keep an eye on the dashboard. This can be challenging for educators at institutions with minimal expert guidance available, inadequate faculty development programs, and lack of funding for applications and tools to host their online classroom [32].

Lastly, the online educational experience for learners can be impacted by decreased learner engagement and low learner motivation and expectations [33]. Keeping learners engaged can be particularly challenging in the online classroom [14]. Distance created by the screen interface, being muted by default and occasionally by internet latency can make learners feel disconnected from the class, and thus less engaged and less motivated to learn. This distance also makes it easier for learners to be distracted by their unique surroundings, family [34, 35], and other applications on their devices without the pressure from neighboring peers or a circulating teacher to maintain attention. Additionally, in order to participate verbally, learners need to actively unmute themselves, which creates another barrier to participation that may decrease learner engagement. Finally, learners accustomed to in-person learning may expect to learn less in the online classroom or think that teachers will have lower expectations of them; this may result in learners applying themselves less. While these barriers may seem daunting, the following section will aim to present tips and tricks that teachers can utilize in their online geriatrics classroom to address the above learner issues.

Best Practices: Online Lesson Development

Effective online teaching requires adequate preparation. This section will cover tips to developing the online lesson before the teaching occurs.

Adult Learning Theory

When preparing a lesson for the online classroom, a teacher should apply the basic concepts of adult learning theory to keep the lesson appropriate, relevant, and engaging. Teachers should keep in mind the following four concepts of adult learning theory: (1) adult learning builds on the learner's prior experiences, (2) adult learning should be relevant and immediately applicable to the learner, (3) adults learn best through problem-solving, and (4) adults want to be involved in their educational experiences [4].

First, in order to build on learners' prior experiences, the teacher should identify learners' current understanding of the topic at hand. This can be done with a pre-session survey or a needs assessment. The teachers can then present new information that immediately relates to the learners' existing understanding. This approach is called building on the zone of proximal development [36], and it is a practice that promotes teaching new content that is attainable to the learner, rather than content that is rudimentary or overly challenging and can decrease learner interest.

Second, content should also be relevant and applicable to the learner. Lesson relevance and applicability are easily expressed through learning goals and objectives, which can be developed using the revision of Bloom's Taxonomy [37] and should be outlined and referenced at the start of the lesson. To determine whether the learning objectives were achieved, teachers should prepare evaluations to solicit learner feedback post-session, most easily captured using web-based surveys with the link placed in the chat and/or using a QR code that learners can scan with smartphones [21].

And third and fourth, adult learning theory promotes teaching through problem-solving and using other ways to actively involve the learner in the lesson [4]. Teachers should lay the groundwork for learner participation by incorporating questions and activities directly into their lesson plan. These questions and activities serve as scheduled opportunities to task learners to actively apply their prior knowledge and critical thinking during the session [38]. For example, in planning an interactive lecture about different settings of care, the teacher may focus the lesson on a patient case about 82-year-old Mrs. D who developed hip pain after falling and can no longer ambulate. The teacher can keep learners engaged by asking a series of multiple-choice questions, like "Would Mrs. D be best cared for at home, in the clinic, or in the hospital?" followed later by, "Is Mrs. D now best suited for post-acute rehab at home, at a skilled nursing facility, at an inpatient rehab, or at a long-term acute care facility?" The teacher can use polling or word cloud tools embedded into their lecture to gather responses. Alternatively, teachers can prepare a variety of different question types to provoke more thought and discussion, like "What kind of potential complications do you foresee for Mrs. D now that she is admitted to the hospital?" The teacher could also actively engage the learner by incorporating a game into the session, like the virtual Geriatrics Escape Room that was developed at the University of California San Diego to teach core geriatrics principles to medical residents [39], or the gamification-based intervention to teach polypharmacy concepts to postgraduate physicians developed at the European Academy for the Medicine of Ageing [40]. Further interactive techniques will be discussed later in this chapter.

Instructional Modalities and Online Teaching Tools

Lesson development should consider teaching modalities and online tools for use in the online classroom. The teaching modality and online tools should be selected early in lesson development to align with learning goals and objectives [31] and to augment the delivery of the material [41].

Most medical education teaching modalities can be adjusted for use to teach geriatrics in the online setting. Table 16.1 reviews common medical education teaching modalities with suggestions on how to modify for online use and examples of when this might be appropriate in geriatrics education. The transition from in-person teaching to the online classroom requires understanding of both how to modify the lesson for virtual use and which platforms and tools to use. A few of these modalities are particularly useful for modification to the virtual setting, either due to frequent use in geriatrics education, such as interactive lectures and discussion groups, or due to the potential for applying to telemedicine, like physical exam workshops and standardized patient interactions. With increasing incidence of telemedicine clinician–patient visits [42], it is important for trainees to practice their clinical skills in a virtual setting in order to ensure competency. For example, a virtual workshop on geriatric assessment can include review of history-taking to assess for geriatric syndromes as well as cognitive and falls assessments. Teaching via telemedicine is addressed in detail in Chap. 17.

In addition to the many online teaching modalities, there are numerous programs and tools that can be used to host the online classroom and to promote interactivity and collaboration during an online lesson. Table 16.2 lists a variety of online

Table 16.2 Online platforms and tools for use in the virtual classroom

Category	Application/ tool examples	Features	Best use	Examples for geriatric medical education
Unified communications	Zoom GoToConnect Microsoft teams	Video, audio, and chat communications. Screen share, annotation, breakout room functionality	Virtual learning with a flexibility of different active learning activities and participation/ engagement	Host interactive sessions like GERI-A-FLOAT [15] and Project ECHO [11]
Classroom/ learning platforms	Google classroom Blackboard learn WebEx	Same as above, plus learning management system to integrate curriculum and grading	E-learning platforms used for housing all components of an educational experience including assignments, assessments, and evaluations	Host and house geriatrics curriculum for medical students
Video conference	Skype FaceTime WhatsApp Facebook Live	Video and audio communication, +/− chat feature	Meetings, shorter learning, or didactics meant to be recorded and disseminated to a larger, passive audience	Host one-on-one feedback with students or residents on completion of geriatrics rotation Live-stream geriatrics grand rounds via Facebook Live [7]

(continued)

Table 16.2 (continued)

Category	Application/ tool examples	Features	Best use	Examples for geriatric medical education
Tools for interactivity	AHA slides PollEverywhere Slido	Live polls, Q&A, quizzes, real-time charts and feedback, word clouds	In the moment, active, virtual participation that can be embedded periodically throughout a lesson	Embed multiple-choice image-based questions in a geriatric dermatology talk
Tools for collaboration	Padlet Miro Canva	Virtual bulletin board/canvas with embedded communication capabilities	Small group breakouts with large group collaboration, facilitates deliverables, peer teaching, etc.	Medical students posting reflections on virtual messaging board as part of an anti-ageism curriculum [43]
Games platforms	Quizlet Socrative Kahoot Goosechase	Quizzes, polls, embedded feedback Real-world scavenger hunts	Active participation that can allow for testing of knowledge, identifying topics that warrant more discussion, or identifying struggling students	Test learner comprehension with end-of-rotation quiz on identification and treatment of geriatric syndromes

Please note that, as with most technological devices, these types of platforms and tools are likely to be ever-evolving and may become obsolete in the near future. These platforms and tools listed are current as of the time of publication

GERI-A-FLOAT Geriatric Fellows Learning Online And Together, *ECHO* Extension for Community Healthcare Outcomes

programs and tools, as well as their respective features, that are available for use in virtual geriatric education. While it may be tempting to rush to incorporate many online tools because they are often fun to use, using online tools inappropriately or too often can detract from the lesson and leave learning objectives unmet. Determining the most effective and efficient way of disseminating the content to the learners based on the context and learning goals should drive the selection of appropriate tools.

Prepare the Online Classroom

To ensure learners are prepared for the online classroom, teachers should conduct a technological needs assessment upfront to determine if all participants have adequate hardware, software, and internet access [44]. If any learners lack the required technology, accommodation should be attempted by program leadership. This may be as simple as helping the learner gain access to a local library or by installing internet at the learner's residence, as was sometimes the case with remote learning during the COVID-19 pandemic [45].

Teachers must be attentive to aspects related to unique needs of learners. Any activities planned should be easily accessible to all learners. An online classroom should be inclusive and offer accommodations for learners with disabilities. Teachers should avoid assumptions relating to the digital literacy skills of their learners by providing detailed guidance and troubleshooting instructions to learners in advance [44, 46]. Depending on the size of the group and the complexity of the online session, teachers may want to provide participants with a tutorial on what to expect and how to use the features of the online application. For example, participants registered for the Virtual AGS Annual Meeting 2021 could access a *Frequently Asked Questions* webpage and various tutorial videos demonstrating how to join and participate during the online sessions. Given that online learners may be geographically dispersed, teachers should ensure communication of the correct time zone to ensure timely participation.

In addition to preparing their learners for the online classroom, the teacher should prepare to host an online session by following these steps:

- Become familiar with the audiovisual communication program and any other electronic tools that will be used during the lesson.
- Test and ensure adequate internet connectivity; consider using a hardwired ethernet cable.
- Test camera and microphone.
- Ensure minimal backlighting and a simple backdrop to avoid distraction.
- Complete a full practice run and correct any glitches prior to the session.
- Mute email notifications and silence phones/pagers if possible.
- Put a do-not-disturb sign on the door and/or notify other occupants of the teaching space to avoid disrupting the teaching session.
- Password-protect the virtual meeting to prevent uninvited participants from interrupting and have a plan in place on how to manage intruders if the session is breached [14].
- Consider inviting a technical support person to the first few online sessions to serve as the contact for technical issues; this allows the teacher to focus on the lesson content and learners.
- Develop and test a back-up plan for each component of the technology used during the session (e.g. *What if my microphone breaks? What if my computer dies? What if the online tool does not work? What if learners cannot access the online whiteboard?)*

Best Practices: Interactive Online Teaching

Promoting learner participation can be achieved by using best practices for interactive online learning, described below and summarized in Fig. 16.1.

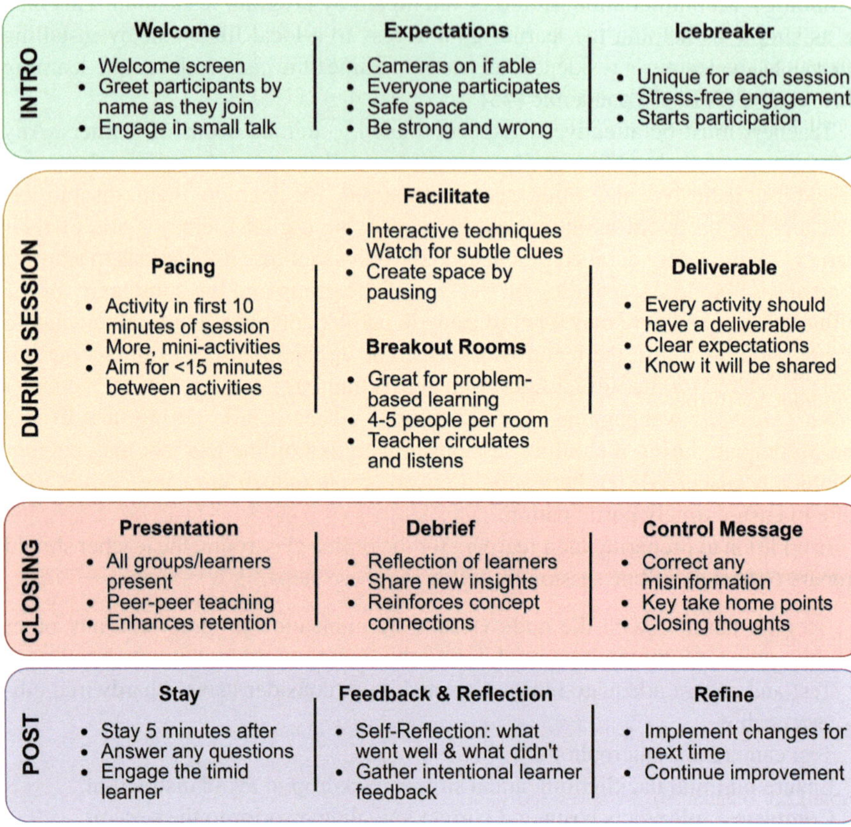

Fig. 16.1 Best practices for interactive online geriatrics learning. Flowsheet summarizing the best practices that teachers should use to optimize learner engagement and class flow for an online, synchronous teaching session

Session Introduction: Welcome, Expectations, and Icebreaker

The teacher should welcome learner participation by creating a comfortable and supportive online learning environment. This is especially important with online learning as compared to the in-person classroom due to the distance barrier that online learning creates and difficulty generating a sense of connection both between teacher and participants and among participants. As participants join the session, it can be helpful to have a "welcome" screen shared so participants feel like they are entering a classroom. Alternatively, the facilitator can maintain a dashboard or gallery view with cameras on, so that session attendees can see their peers and converse casually prior to the start of the lesson.

To promote a session with high learner interaction, teachers must set the expectation for participation which can be done in a variety of ways. The teacher may want to inform learners before the session in writing and at the start of the session verbally that all attendees are expected to give full attention and active participation throughout the session. It may be helpful to specifically encourage that learners perform some, or all, of the following, as is relevant to the learners' needs and type of course being taught:

- Close other browser windows and put away distracting devices.
- Turn on cameras if safe and able. ("If safe and able" is key as this makes room for the learner who doesn't have a safe home environment or is juggling child-care, for example, and may help combat zoom fatigue.)
- Consider using the "raise hand" tool for questions.
- Contribute thoughts and questions via the chat function.
- Remain muted when not speaking to minimize distracting sounds; unmute microphone to speak.
- Engage fully in any planned activities.

Private chat messages between learners may be distracting, or may foster community-building between learners, depending on the situation. Most applications allow teachers to disable the private chat feature, which can be done in advance if appropriate. Whatever ground rules the teacher chooses to establish upfront will give learners a clear understanding of expected online classroom etiquette and appropriate behavior and can be referred to later as a reminder to learners if issues arise.

During the introduction, the facilitator can ask easy-to-answer "icebreaker" questions that will encourage learners to speak up early in a low-pressure environment. The icebreaker method not only humanizes the learning experience but also helps to reduce learner inhibitions and thus results in easier participation later [47]. Icebreaker questions can serve additional purposes (e.g. assessing learners' knowledge on the session topic, determining personal learning goals among students, or allowing teacher and learners to get to know each other better).

Finally, troubleshooting any teacher or learner technical issues upfront during the introduction can minimize potential interruptions or barriers to participation as the session progresses.

Teaching During Session: Facilitate, Pacing, Breakout Rooms, and Ensuring Deliverables

Although much learner interaction is planned, some learner participation will be spontaneous and should be mediated by the teacher using interactive techniques. These techniques are best employed when all participants have their cameras on and teachers have their interface in dashboard view with learners visible so that teachers may directly engage with individual learners by name. Utilizing dashboard view, teachers may notice pre-participatory behavior. For example, a microphone symbol that goes unmuted and then re-muted may represent a learner that wants to contribute but needs more of an invitation. Due to the need to unmute or type thoughts into the chat or simply due to connection latency, there can be a delay in question response; the teacher should allow participants ample time to reply [48]. A simple way to prevent rushing is to take a sip of water after asking a question. While singling out students by asking knowledge-based questions that they may not know creates an uncomfortable learning environment, calling on individuals for defined participation can raise the pressure just enough to effectively keep learners engaged [49] and may be necessary to increase participation in the online classroom. Examples of defined participation include asking an individual to read a passage, to give an opinion, or to answer a general question with assurance that "there is no wrong answer." Alternatively, if the learners divide into "think-pair-share" groups, where learners think independently about a question and discuss their preliminary thoughts with a partner or small group, the learner can then be asked directly to share their partner's or group's ideas, which may relieve some of the stress of being called on [50]. It can also be helpful to have students post discussion question responses to a message board *prior* to the session so the teacher can select participants with particularly thoughtful contributions to expand on their comments during class; this can alleviate stress as students may simply repeat what they had already posted; this is known as "warm calling." Additionally, teachers can practice the "around the room" method, engaging one learner after another, or poll the classroom by raise of hands. For more timid learners, it is important to offer the option to submit responses via the private chat function. These techniques can significantly increase learner participation and thus improve the effectiveness of the lesson.

Teachers should schedule their planned activities appropriately, include short breaks, and reserve time for transitioning between activities. Foundational studies of synchronous in-person education demonstrated that a 50-min lecture followed by a 10-min break resulted in adequate learning, as measured by test scores [51], whereas more recent studies have shown that modern-day students have a 10–15 min attention span with decreasing rates of retention beyond 15 min [52]. While online lectures have been less studied to date, educators do know that the attention span during virtual sessions is even shorter, and quick (1-min) breaks may be required as often as every 7 min to maintain learner engagement [53, 54]. Generally, a 50-min online session should have two to three activities, the first of which should be scheduled within the first 10 min of the session in order to maintain the learner engagement that was established with the initial icebreaker and prevent waning attention. This type of lesson plan with short activities and frequent breaks has been described as high intensity interval training for the virtual classroom [55].

Breakout rooms are excellent tools to use for small group work, including problem-based learning, and require active monitoring by teachers. Consistent with the principles of adult learning theory, studies in medical education have demonstrated that students learn well through problem- or case-based learning [56]. Problem-based learning is often achieved through use of the flipped classroom, where learners independently study pre-session materials and come to class prepared to apply what they have learned through a problem set within a small group. This technique can be easily adapted to the online classroom by use of breakout rooms. Breakout rooms provide the ideal setting for learners to work on the deliverable for any given lesson.

Using breakout rooms may seem intimidating at first, but the following strategies can help teachers streamline their breakout room experience. Teachers should assign groups of no more than five learners, since larger groups make it more difficult for each member to participate [57], and provide written instructions and expectations for group work in addition to giving a verbal explanation. Turning the camera off during breakout room sessions allows the teacher to act as a non-intrusive facilitator, moving from room to room to listen in and take notes that will serve as talking and teaching points later when the whole class is reconvened. With the teacher's camera turned off students may be more likely to continue working without being distracted by their teacher's presence. The teacher can generally only be in one breakout room and thus can only observe one group at a time; providing a shared online word document via the chat (prior to participants entering breakout rooms) or utilizing a whiteboard program so that learners can document their work during breakout groups is one way to allow the facilitator to keep closer tabs on multiple groups' progress at once. Finally, teachers can use broadcasts to communicate messages to all groups, for example, to notify groups of session time remaining so participants can wrap up accordingly.

Having a deliverable, or a product that learners develop throughout the lesson and share at the end of the session, is a kind of problem-based learning that can help teach important content in a way that learners will retain. The deliverable focuses the teacher and learners on key learning objectives, gives a defined goal for participants to work toward, and ensures active participation as learners create the deliverable in small groups and later as learners share their discoveries in large group.

Closing and Post-Session: Learner Presentations, Control Message, and Gather Feedback

Once the full group is back together, learners can share with their peers what they discovered or accomplished during the breakout session. The teacher, who took notes about individual group activity while circling through each room, should prompt specific small group members to share the insightful comments they made during small group discussion.

During the last 5 min of the session, teachers should review the biggest take-home points from the lesson as well as answer any remaining questions from learners. With abundant learner participation and peer-peer teaching, some concepts may be taught incompletely or somewhat incorrectly. Teachers should use this time to correct misinformation and fill in any gaps, emphasizing the most important learning objectives. Teachers should acknowledge good group discussion and thank learners for their engagement, as this can reinforce positive online classroom habits.

After the session, teachers should remain available to learners and should reflect and gather feedback on the lesson to ultimately refine the session for future use. It is important to intentionally reserve a few minutes for *after* the session to answer individual questions, as this may be the only time to engage with more introverted learners. Teachers should provide evaluation forms to learners to solicit feedback on whether learning objectives were met, what learners liked and why, as well as what could be improved about the lesson. This is also the time for teachers themselves to reflect on what went well, what did not go well, and why. Using learner feedback and self-reflection, teachers can modify and improve their lesson to be more effective for future sessions.

Conclusion

Medical educators will be increasingly tasked with teaching geriatrics concepts in an online classroom. Despite the challenges of teaching in an online classroom, teaching in this setting can lead to a wide reach of learners and can be efficient and cost-effective, ultimately spreading geriatric competence more effectively from a small group of geriatrics educators. The best practices, teaching modalities, applications, and tools discussed in this chapter can help educators to prepare and equip themselves for effective teaching in the online classroom in order to improve the health and well-being of older adults.Institution Where Research PerformedVanderbilt University Medical Center, Nashville, Tennessee.

Financial Support Maria Duggan receives salary support from the Department of Veteran Affairs Office of Academic Affiliations.

Conflicts of Interest and Sources of Funding Alexandra E. Petrakos, Travis W. Crook, and Maria C. Duggan have no conflicts of interest to disclose.

References

1. Callahan KE, Tumosa N, Leipzig RM. Big ‘G’ and little ‘g’ geriatrics education for physicians. J Am Geriatr Soc. 2017;65(10):2313–7. https://doi.org/10.1111/jgs.14996.
2. Francescucci A, Rohani L. Exclusively synchronous online (VIRI) learning: the impact on student performance and engagement outcomes. J Mark Educ. 2018;41(1):60–9. https://doi.org/10.1177/0273475318818864.
3. Signor L. Virtual lectures versus face-to-face lectures: A four-year study exploring the impact on students’ results. In G.T. Crisp D, Scholten I, Barker S, Baron J (Ed.). Adelaide, Australia: ASCILITE. 2003. pp. 700–3.
4. Knowles MS. The modern practice of adult education: from pedagogy to andragogy (revised and updated). Chicago: Association Press; Follett Pub. Co.; 1980.
5. Ruiz JG, Mintzer MJ, Leipzig RM. The impact of E-learning in medical education. Acad Med. 2006;81(3):207–12. https://doi.org/10.1097/00001888-200603000-00002.
6. Darius PSH, Gundabattini E, Solomon DG. A survey on the effectiveness of online teaching–learning methods for university and college students. J Inst Eng Ser B. 2021;102:1325. https://doi.org/10.1007/s40031-021-00581-x.

7. Powers BB, Hartmann P, Welch M, Ross J. Expanding the reach of geriatrics grand rounds using Facebook live. J Am Geriatr Soc. 2019;67(10):E4–6. https://doi.org/10.1111/jgs.16185.
8. Gardhouse AI, Budd L, Yang SYC, Wong CL. #GeriMedJC: the twitter complement to the traditional-format geriatric medicine journal Club. J Am Geriatr Soc. 2017;65(6):1347–51. https://doi.org/10.1111/jgs.14920.
9. Manocha G, Morton C, Chapman E, Pellecer D, Zeitlow K. Strengthening collaborations for geriatrics knowledge: Twitter Journal Club for Geriatrics Fellows. Innov Aging. 2021;5:765. https://doi.org/10.1093/geroni/igab046.2811.
10. Arora S, Geppert CM, Kalishman S, Dion D, Pullara F, Bjeletich B, Simpson G, Alverson DC, Moore LB, Kuhl D, Scaletti JV. Academic health center management of chronic diseases through knowledge networks: project ECHO. Acad Med. 2007;82(2):154–60. https://doi.org/10.1097/ACM.0b013e31802d8f68.
11. Bennett KA, Ong T, Verrall AM, Vitiello MV, Marcum ZA, Phelan EA. Project ECHO-geriatrics: training future primary care providers to meet the needs of older adults. J Grad Med Educ. 2018;10(3):311–5. https://doi.org/10.4300/JGME-D-17-01022.1.
12. Gleason LJ, Martinchek M, Long M, Rapier N, Hamlish T, Johnson D, Thompson K. An innovative model using telementoring to provide geriatrics education for nurses and social workers at skilled nursing facilities. Geriatr Nurs. 2019;40(5):517–21. https://doi.org/10.1016/j.gerinurse.2019.03.018.
13. Jafari P, Kostas T, Levine S, Martinchek M, Johnson D, Graupner J, Thompson K. ECHO-Chicago geriatrics: using telementoring to "geriatricize" the primary care workforce. Gerontol Geriatr Educ. 2020;41(3):333–41. https://doi.org/10.1080/02701960.2019.1572005.
14. Wilcha RJ. Effectiveness of virtual medical teaching during the COVID-19 crisis: systematic review. JMIR Med Educ. 2020;6(2):e20963. https://doi.org/10.2196/20963.
15. Duggan MC, Goroncy A, Christmas C, Chippendale R. Staying afloat in the COVID-19 storm: GERIAtrics fellows learning online and together (GERI-A-FLOAT). J Am Geriatr Soc. 2020;68(10):E54–6. https://doi.org/10.1111/jgs.16755.
16. GeriatricsCareOnline.org. https://geriatricscareonline.org/ProductAbstract/geriatrics-review-syllabus-11th-edition/B057/.
17. Byrne R. Twelve tools for creating end-of-year review activities. 2019. https://www.freetech4teachers.com/search/label/Jeopardy.
18. Kahoot.com. https://kahoot.com/.
19. Quizlet.com.
20. PollEverywhere.com/app.
21. QR-Code-Generator.com.
22. Wolber A. How to make a QR code: 5 ways to generate QR codes. 2022. https://www.techrepublic.com/article/how-to-create-qr-codes-5-methods/.
23. Aquifer Geriatrics. 2022. https://aquifer.org/courses/aquifer-geriatrics/.
24. Danto-Nocton ES, Simpson D, Rasansky M, Pascarella LC, Malone ML. Strength in numbers: a National Monthly Case Conference Series for fellows. J Am Geriatr Soc. 2018;66(7):1404–8. https://doi.org/10.1111/jgs.15448.
25. Poll Everywhere Updates. https://blog.polleverywhere.com/instruction-image/.
26. PatientPrioritiesCare.org.
27. Dawson CM, Schwartz AW, Farrell SE. A telehealth clinical skills education adaptation. Clin Teach. 2020;17(4):437–9. https://doi.org/10.1111/tct.13223.
28. Docs.google.com.
29. Padlet.com.
30. Miro.com.
31. Skeff K, Stratos G. Methods for teaching medicine. Minneapolis, MN: ACP Press, American College of Physicians; 2010.
32. O'Doherty D, Dromey M, Lougheed J, Hannigan A, Last J, McGrath D. Barriers and solutions to online learning in medical education - an integrative review. BMC Med Educ. 2018;18(1):130. https://doi.org/10.1186/s12909-018-1240-0.

33. Regmi K, Jones L. A systematic review of the factors—enablers and barriers—affecting e-learning in health sciences education. BMC Med Educ. 2020;20(1):91. https://doi.org/10.1186/s12909-020-02007-6.
34. Dost S, Hossain A, Shehab M, Abdelwahed A, Al-Nusair L. Perceptions of medical students towards online teaching during the COVID-19 pandemic: a national cross-sectional survey of 2721 UK medical students. BMJ Open. 2020;10(11):e042378. https://doi.org/10.1136/bmjopen-2020-042378.
35. Kaur H, Singh A, Mahajan S, Lal M, Singh G, Kaur P. Assessment of barriers and motivators to online learning among medical undergraduates of Punjab. J Educ Health Promot. 2021;10:123. https://doi.org/10.4103/jehp.jehp_682_20.
36. Vygotskiĭ LS, Cole M. Mind in society: the development of higher psychological processes. Cambridge, MA: Harvard University Press; 1978.
37. Anderson LW, Krathwohl DR, Bloom BS. A taxonomy for learning, teaching, and assessing: a revision of Bloom's taxonomy of educational objectives. Complete ed. London: Longman; 2001.
38. Samson P. Fostering student engagement: creative problem-solving in small group facilitations. In: Collected essays on learning and teaching, vol. 8; 2015. https://files.eric.ed.gov/fulltext/EJ1069715.pdf.
39. Devlin S, Guan J, Reichstadt J, Sladek E, Gupta R. The University of California San Diego Geriatrics Escape Room: a didactic innovation. J Am Geriatr Soc. 2021;69(1):E1–3. https://doi.org/10.1111/jgs.16913.
40. Schlogl M, Roller-Wirnsberger RE, Hernes SS, Perkisas S, Bakken MS, Miot S, Balci C, Dani M, Pajulammi H, Piaggi P, Drenth-van Maanen C, Singler K. Teaching geriatric medicine through gamification: a tool for enhancing postgraduate education in geriatric medicine. Aging Clin Exp Res. 2022;34(2):455–63. https://doi.org/10.1007/s40520-021-01933-9.
41. Crook T. Innovative teaching at a distance: Using technology to engage learners at a distance [Lecture video recording]; 2020.
42. CDC. Telehealth and telemedicine; 2020.
43. Chow S, Javier N, Kelley A, Ramaswamy R. Feasibility and impact of an ageism curriculum for medical students in a Geriatrics Clerkship. In: Annual meeting of the American Geriatrics Society, Orlando, Florida, USA; 2022.
44. Besche H, Schwartz AW, Cockrill B. Ensuring equitable access to remote learning during the COVID-19 pandemic. Acad Med. 2021;96(5):e19–20. https://doi.org/10.1097/ACM.0000000000003854.
45. Staff K. COVID-19 April 7 updates: Williamson County extends stay-at-home order; abortion ban upheld. KUT. 2020;90(5).
46. Luke K. Twelve tips for using synchronous virtual classroom technologies in medical education. MedEdPublish. 2021;10:66. https://doi.org/10.15694/mep.2021.000066.1.
47. Chlup DT, Collins TE. Breaking the ice: using ice-breakers and re-energizers with adult learners. Adult Learn. 2010;21(3–4):34–9. https://doi.org/10.1177/104515951002100305.
48. Turner T, Palazzi D, Ward M, Lorin M. The Clinician-Educator's Handbook. Baylor College of Medicine. 2008. https://media.bcm.edu/documents/2014/84/clinicianedhandbook.pdf.
49. Rudland JR, Golding C, Wilkinson TJ. The stress paradox: how stress can be good for learning. Med Educ. 2020;54(1):40–5. https://doi.org/10.1111/medu.13830.
50. Shen D. Pair and share. 2022. https://ablconnect.harvard.edu/pair-and-share-research.
51. Cooke ML. Academic and industrial efficiency: a report to the Carnegie foundation for the advancement of teaching; 1910.
52. Bradbury NA. Attention span during lectures: 8 seconds, 10 minutes, or more? Adv Physiol Educ. 2016;40(4):509–13. https://doi.org/10.1152/advan.00109.2016.
53. Boyette M. RLI survey: bite-size learning is hot at ASTD conference, but execution is lagging back on the home front; 2014.
54. Kerres M. Microlearning as a challenge for instructional design. In: Didactics of microlearning: concepts, discourses and examples. Munster: Waxmann; 2007. p. 98–109.

55. Ringel R, Tarallo B, Green L. 5 steps to stay focused when teaching online. 2020. https://hbsp.harvard.edu/inspiring-minds/5-steps-to-stay-focused-when-teaching-online.
56. McLean SF. Case-based learning and its application in medical and health-care fields: a review of worldwide literature. J Med Educ Curric Dev. 2016;3:JMECD.S20377. https://doi.org/10.4137/JMECD.S20377.
57. Watson A. What's the ideal size for online discussion groups? Learning & the Brain; 2020.

Chapter 17
Teaching Geriatrics in Video Telemedicine

Becky B. Powers and Lauren R. Moo

Introduction

As the landscape of medicine changes it is important that learners develop clinical skills not only in general telemedicine but also in its application in geriatrics. The term telemedicine is broad and encompasses multiple forms of technology. This technology not only includes video visits but also remote monitoring (e.g., vital signs, ECGs), e-Health (using the internet to disseminate health information), store and forward transmission of data (e.g., images, X-rays), e-consults (asynchronous chart reviews and communication to other health professionals), and telephone visits. Telemedicine is a subset of telemedicine that is practiced by healthcare professionals, including physicians, who use technology to evaluate and treat a patient in another location. Most frequently this is done via video visits and telephone visits (Fig. 17.1). While all of these modalities play an important role in the care of older adults and geriatrics education, this chapter will focus primarily on video telemedicine in geriatrics.

Case Example: Telemedicine Modalities

*At a patient's last in-person visit, you asked a patient with congestive heart failure to get a chest X-ray and increase their diuretic. A follow-up **video visit** was scheduled. During this visit, a learner reviews daily blood pressure and weight data obtained by*

B. B. Powers (✉)
San Antonio Veterans Affairs Geriatric Research Education and Clinical Center, University of Texas Health San Antonio, San Antonio, TX, USA
e-mail: powersb3@uthscsa.edu

L. R. Moo
New England Geriatric Research Education and Clinical Center at Veterans Affairs Bedford Healthcare System, Massachusetts General Hospital, Harvard Medical School, Boston, MA, USA

A. W. Schwartz (ed.), *Medical Education in Geriatrics*,
https://doi.org/10.1007/978-3-031-32499-4_17

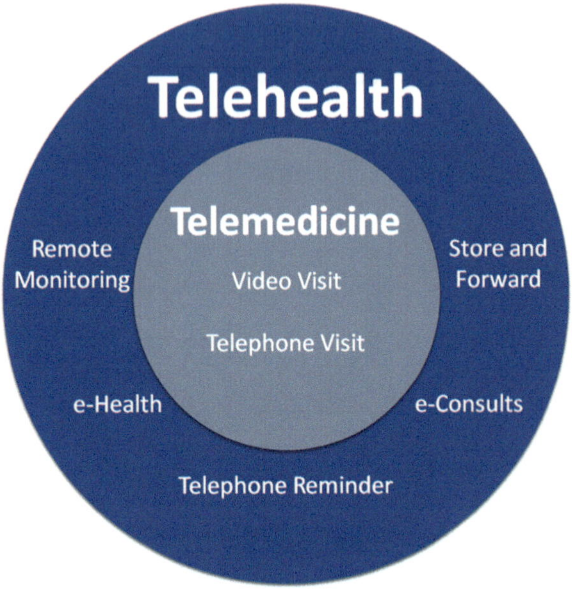

Fig. 17.1 Telemedicine is the broad use of technology in patient care. It does not require intervention or medical decision making. Telemedicine is a subset of telemedicine where medical professionals use technology to synchronously evaluate and treat patients in a different location. Learners should understand the role of all telemedicine modalities, but this chapter focuses on video telemedicine

remote monitoring *and the chest X-ray that was read by a remote radiologist through* ***store and forward*** *technology. The team pharmacist had previously completed a* ***telephone visit*** *for medication reconciliation which is also reviewed prior to initiating the video call. During the video visit, you note that the patient has persistent mild edema despite increasing diuretic use and place an* ***e-consult*** *to cardiology requesting that they review the chart and make medication recommendations.*

Importance of Telemedicine in Patient Care of Older Adults

Telemedicine brings a number of benefits to the aging population. It allows for the provision of care to older adults who lack access to local geriatric specialists, have poor mobility, or have transportation issues [1, 2]. Video telemedicine can also allow family members involved in the older adult's care to participate in video visits even if they are not co-located with the patient. Video telemedicine also has the benefit of mimicking a home visit allowing the clinician to better understand their socio-economic context [3, 4].

Importance of Telemedicine in Geriatrics Education

During the COVID pandemic there has been increasing use of telemedicine technologies and increasing use of internet technology across all age groups [5]. As a result a larger number of older adults are comfortable using technology. Learners need to know how to use telemedicine because as the patient population ages, technology uptake will be even more common [6]. Telemedicine is expanding to all age groups;

however, older adult patients may be more vulnerable to barriers and challenges than the younger population [7, 8]. These challenges may include access to technology, access to broadband, and not being digital natives. Younger learners who are likely to be digital natives, i.e. grew up with the presence of digital technology and the internet, may not appreciate the experiential, generational, and cognitive issues that some older patients may face when trying to navigate telemedicine platforms.

Learners who may already have experience in using telemedicine may not yet have experience or competence in delivering *geriatric* care via telemedicine. For example, virtual visit communication strategies such as looking into the camera to simulate eye contact is not only good webside manner, but may be particularly critical for patients who may be hard of hearing and rely partly on lip reading. Additionally, geriatric care is frequently provided by interprofessional teams which require increased advance planning regarding division of activities and virtual handoffs. These and other issues magnify the need for training to achieve competence in geriatric virtual care. Educators can reference competencies for video telemedicine with older adults for assistance with evaluation and assessment of learners in this care setting [9].

Workflow for Teaching Telemedicine to Geriatric Learners

Clinically, video telemedicine is often used as a surrogate for in-person care; however, there are unique differences when practicing and teaching in this clinical setting [10]. Clinical and educational considerations in holding a video visit can be likened to staging a play or television show of a patient interaction. The "plot" or clinical interaction is the main focus, but what goes unseen are the many subtle supporting actions that set up the "show" for success.

Behind the Scenes: Preparing for Video Visits

Video telemedicine visits may require more pre-planning than traditional in-person visits. The first step is to ensure that a video telemedicine visit is indicated for the patient and that the patient is willing to be seen via video. Additional considerations include equipment, scheduling, and backup plans.

Equipment

All visit participants including clinicians, learners, patients, and caregivers must have access to devices that have webcams, microphones, and internet access. Certain patients may need additional equipment. For example, patients with hearing impairment may need external speakers or headphones to allow for adequate amplification; patients with visual impairments may need a large screen; and patients being seen for mobility or home safety assessments may need a portable device like a tablet or smartphone. Additionally, all visit participants must know how to use the platform and be able to access the visit.

Scheduling

Extra considerations need to be made when scheduling appointments. For patients who struggle with technology, appointments should be made when someone is available for technical support such as a family member or neighbor. Additionally, telemedicine visits offer the opportunity to include more people than who can attend in-person. When scheduling, the patient should identify who should be included in the visit so all important participants are given access.

Backup Plans

Before conducting visits, clinicians and learners must have a backup plan for how to contact the patient if the connection fails. Additionally, a plan should be in place on how to communicate to the patient if the team is running late. This plan could include transitioning to a telephone visit or notifying the patient via telephone, text, or email of changings in schedules.

Cast of Characters: Incorporating Learners and Family Members

Video telemedicine visits can be as simple as a patient speaking directly to a learner and preceptor. However, as in many aspects of geriatrics, team-based care is frequently necessary. Coordinating virtual teams may require more extensive preplanning than for in-person teams, but by eliminating the need for co-location it is possible to include members who otherwise would not be able to participate. In this way, telemedicine modalities may easily lend themselves to clinical interprofessional education as learners from different professions do not need to be co-located to care for patients contemporaneously.

Potential Care Team Members

Learner(s), physicians, other health professionals, telemedicine support, or scheduling support. These members may be individually located, co-located with each other, or co-located with the patient.

Potential Patient Participants

Patients, informal and formal caregivers, family, friends, or acquaintances who are only there to help with technology may all be participating in the visit. These players must be identified along with their relationship to the patient.

Orchestrating the Dialogue

Video telemedicine is an opportunity to demonstrate to learners the complexity of bringing together care teams for older adults. Teams should be well defined with a well-defined process for roles, handoffs, and communication that includes learners. Additionally, as learners may not be co-located, they must be more explicitly introduced to all team members and to the patient with their roles clearly identified.

Chat functions that are present in most telemedicine platforms are powerful tools for just-in-time teaching. Learners can send questions to their preceptors via chat without having to stop the conversation with patients. Preceptors can send learners reminders, references, and forms to use during the visit (e.g. cognitive, depression, or functional screening). Team members can also be contacted to relay logistical information or for warm-handoffs.

Lights, Camera, Action: Setting the Stage for Successful Communication

Webside Manner is the way in which a clinician interacts with patients during virtual visits; it is the telemedicine equivalent of bedside manner [11]. Learners must be reminded that most geriatric patients are not digital natives, and communication styles must be adjusted accordingly.

Body Language

Learners are less able to rely on body language for conversational cues such as giving instructions or ensuring a patient is included in a conversation when caregivers are present. Additionally, they must be aware of their presence on the camera. When speaking with non-digital natives, actions such as leaning back in their chair or looking at an EMR on a secondary screen may falsely convey disinterest and lead to communication breakdown. Leaning in a little closer to the camera can indicate more attentive listening.

Environment

Sensory and cognitive impairment frequently occur in the geriatric population and can interfere with virtual visits. To minimize the impact of these conditions on the visit, learners should be coached to manage their virtual environment. Adequate lighting is important for patients with low vision; therefore, learners should ensure they are not sitting in a dark room, in shadow, or in front of a window which causes glare. For patients with hearing impairment, learners should ensure that their microphone is working well and that they are in an area with low ambient noise. Additionally, the background should be professional and free of distracting clutter.

Computer Management

Eye contact is an important way to build trust and a therapeutic relationship. Many non-digital natives struggle when clinicians look away from the camera whether it is to type, look at the patient image at the bottom of the screen, or check the EMR on the second screen. Ways to manage this include making the video window smaller and putting it directly underneath the camera so that when you are looking at the patient you are also looking at the camera. Learners can also be coached to verbalize when they look away at an EMR to help patients understand why the learner is no longer looking at the patient or visible in the frame.

On Location

Unlike traditional clinical settings, in telemedicine visits patients, caregivers, preceptors, and learners may all be in different locations. This leads to challenges and opportunities for clinical care and education.

Before the visit begins, the location of all participants must be known.

Patients

Patients may not be located in their primary place of residence during a telemedicine visit. Patients could be in their home, a family member's home, a long term care facility, assisted living facility, subacute nursing facility, outpatient clinic, inpatient, a car, in a rural location, etc. All of these locations give clinical information. Some locations, such as subacute nursing facilities, allow learners to obtain additional clinical information or assistance with exams. Learners should be prepared to incorporate these nuances into their assessments. Additionally, knowing a patient's exact location and telephone number is essential in case of emergency.

Learners and Preceptors

Learners and preceptors may not always be at the same site during telemedicine visits. Locations can range from being in the same room, being in the same site but separate rooms, the learner or preceptor being located with the patient while the other is in a remote site, or both being in separate remote sites. Interprofessional team members may be involved in the visit, for example, a nurse or social worker in a long term care facility or a pharmacist assisting with the visit from a remote site. Additionally, learners from remote locations may also be shadowing by watching the visit remotely. The opportunity for team members, learners, and preceptors to be located separately or together allows for a large range in precepting techniques.

Communicating the Plan

The people present with patients on telemedicine visits may not always be the caregivers, but rather someone who is able to help with technology. When communicating follow-up plans, this should be clarified and caregivers brought into the conversation. Additionally, unlike in-person visits, patients cannot be given a written list of instructions. Patients and caregivers should be asked how they would like to receive this information (patient portal, traditional mail, etc.).

Models of Precepting

Telemedicine brings strengths and challenges to clinical learning and with careful planning it can be a robust learning environment. Many challenges can be overcome by choosing a precepting model that best fits the clinical scenario and learner type. Considerations when choosing a precepting model include the level of learner, presence of interprofessional teams, physical locations, patient preference, and the ratio of learners to preceptors. Given the many potential locations of older patients, including not just private homes and in-patient units but also assisted living facilities and rehabilitation hospitals, consideration of the locations of learners, patients, and preceptors is particularly important. Table 17.1 includes some potential

Table 17.1 Models for precepting geriatrics telemedicine based on location of learners, preceptors, and patients

Locations	Direct supervision	Indirect supervision	Patient discussion
Learner and preceptor co-located, patient at remote location	• After introductions, preceptor sits off camera to encourage direct patient–learner engagement	• Preceptor can drop in on multiple virtual visits • Preceptor can be called into virtual visit via message from learner	• Learner presents case to preceptor outside video visit or places patient in virtual waiting room • Learner and preceptor discuss patient on camera, possibly on mute
Learner, preceptor, and patient all at different locations	• Preceptor logged into virtual visit throughout	• Preceptor can be called into virtual visit via message from learner • Preceptor joins visit only for wrap-up	• Preceptor can join end of visit for virtual bedside presentation • Preceptor and learner discuss patient after visit
Learner or preceptor (not both) co-located with the patient	• Preceptor can virtually observe in-person learners • Remote learners can observe master clinicians co-located with patients	• Preceptors can supervise learners at multiple locations	• Preceptor can summarize patient for remote learners • Learners and preceptors can communicate via messaging or telephone

Choice of model depends on the learner's stage (e.g. resident versus fellow) and regulatory requirements approaches. Clinical scenarios and resources vary by site, and educators are encouraged to "mix-and-match" aspects that fit their clinical and educational needs. No matter what model is chosen, educators must ensure that roles, expectations, and communication strategies are well defined prior to the virtual visit.

Other Precepting Considerations

Communication During Visits

Lines of communication between learners, preceptor, and patient must be even more clear in a virtual setting. Many learners are digital natives and may be unaware of the difficulties some patients may experience using telemedicine modalities. These learners can be coached to be able to explain the use of video platform to their patients and to ensure they explain how different aspects of the visit will take place (e.g., virtual waiting rooms, preceptor logging in and out, chat functions). The virtual format allows for sharing of resources such as links, articles, and assessment tools with both patients and learners. Additionally, preceptors need to be very clear with their expectations regarding learner communication prior all visits.

Time Management

Unlike in-person visits where patients can see longer lines, or stick their heads into the hallway and ask questions, patients have no feedback about delays in virtual care. Without this feedback, patients can think they have been forgotten or that they are using technology incorrectly. Learners should be coached about the extra importance of being on time for virtual visits, and in clinic methods on how to handle virtual visits when running late.

Others Visit Participants

Patients are frequently seen with caregivers, either with them in the visit or at a distance and calling in separately. Learners may need to speak to caregivers without the patient and can be coached through those interactions. Additionally, many telemedicine visits are done using interprofessional teams which may also consist of learners from multiple levels. In addition to ensuring adequate communication about handoffs within the team, consideration should also be paid to who is precepting the learners, when the precepting will take place, and if the precepting will be in a group or individualized.

Epilogue: Wrapping up the Visit

The ending of a video telemedicine session is more abrupt than the ending of a typical office visit. In a telemedicine visit, when the window closes, the session is over. However, in an office visit, when the clinician leaves the room the patient will still interact with other staff members before leaving the office. Often this interaction includes asking clarifying questions, collecting paperwork, arranging for testing, and arranging a follow-up appointment. Although office support may be a part of the video telemedicine care team, there is no "front desk" to cue patients about paperwork, testing, and follow-ups. Assessments and plans must be explicit and understood by all involved. This added complexity lends itself to teaching learners of all levels about transitions of care.

Plan Communication

Interprofessional Team Handoffs

If a patient is scheduled to see another member of the interprofessional team, learners need to know in advance who that person is, how to alert them that the patient is ready, and how to pass on pertinent information. This is a learning opportunity that may not be available in-person if the interprofessional team is not typically a part of the in-person team.

Implementation and Logistics

After a telemedicine visit, more thoughtful planning is required to arrange for the many activities normally done in the clinic or in close proximity to the clinic (e.g., phlebotomy, scheduling follow-up appointments, filling out forms, referrals, vaccines, chest X-rays, and ECGs). Learners must be introduced not just in the virtual clinic procedures to arrange for these needs, but more importantly they must know how to explain these procedures to their patients. The need to be explicit about this process in video telemedicine visits helps demonstrate to learners the complexities that older patients may face when navigating the healthcare system.

Utilizing Other Telemedicine Modalities

The post-visit planning is also an opportunity to showcase how other forms of telemedicine can be used to assist the patient such as remote monitoring for vital signs, store and forward technology for labs and X-rays, and e-consults with other providers.

Follow-Up

Just as clinical learners need to be able to triage patients in-person to the appropriate levels of care, they also need to be taught how to triage virtual patients for their follow-up. Learners should be asked to determine if patients are stable enough for a repeat telemedicine visit for follow-up, if their condition requires an in-person visit for follow-up, or if they are more acutely ill and need to proceed to the emergency room for follow-up. Learners also need to be able to communicate to the patient the plan for follow-up. When clinically necessary, learners need to include caregivers in the plan.

Teaching Via Telemedicine: Geriatrics 5Ms Case Examples

The above sections discussed teaching the logistics of telemedicine with older adults. The cases below illustrate opportunities to teach clinical geriatrics content during telemedicine visits.

Case Example: Mind and Medications
Ms. J is a 74-year-old retired high school math teacher who lives alone and volunteers with the local home building charity. Her son and daughter-in-law, who live 20 miles away, accompany her to the video visit and express concerns that Ms. J has been forgetful, repeating stories, and has called them a few times to ask how to get home from previously familiar nearby shops. Ms. J dismisses their concerns and appears surprised to hear that she has ever called them lost. Her family reports this denial and their responses lead to anger and frustration in Ms. J.

During the visit, your learner reviews her medications, including over the counter and new medications prescribed by other clinicians, and takes a careful history regarding the time course of her cognitive and mood symptoms. Your learner listens closely to the patient and family's accounts paying attention to other dementia warning signs, does a thorough review of systems looking for possible signs of infection or other causes for delirium, and inquires about past psychiatric history and current sleep and behavioral history. To determine whether any cognitive decline has impacted her level of function, your learner also asks about instrumental and basic activities of daily living.

Mental status examination includes unscored assessment of MS. J's ability to relate medical details, converse about current events, word finding difficulties, repeating questions, and ability to name common objects you hold up to the camera. Deciding a standardized assessment is warranted, your learner asks Ms. J to go get a piece of paper and pencil while he opens up a prepared PowerPoint presentation that has the visual stimuli from standard assessments, such as the MoCA, SLUMS, or ACE-R and displays it by sharing via the video conferencing platform's chare screen feature. For tasks such as writing or clock drawing, he asks her to hold the drawings up to the camera.

When asked about her medications, Ms. J says she thinks she was started on a new medication recently, but cannot recall the name or which doctor prescribed it. Her son asks her if the new medication is with the others on the kitchen counter where she usually keeps her pill bottles and the learner asks her to bring over all the bottles there. The learner then conducts a medication reconciliation and discovers she has bottles of both lorazepam prn and trazodone prn, written by different prescribers, and she is unable to say when she last took either.

After wrapping up the visit, you ask the learner to list things they learned about the patient during the video visit that they might not otherwise know. For example:

1. Although it was the patient's laptop they used for the video visit, the daughter-in-law was the one managing the technology suggesting a decline in her ability to perform complex tasks or learn new things.
2. Teaching award trophies displayed on the mantle behind remind us that she was an accomplished teacher and help put her current cognitive state in perspective.
3. She has a days of the week pill organizer but the pills from Monday morning and Wednesday evening were not taken suggesting poor adherence.
4. Touring the home allows visualization of prn medications and those requiring special storage, such as insulin, beyond what would typically be possible in a clinic setting.
5. A more complete understanding of the patient's supplements, herbal remedies, nutraceuticals is possible as they can bring the bottles or other containers to the video visit.

Case Example: Mobility, Multicomplexity, and Matters Most

Mr. P is an 81-year-old former plumber with a history of HTN, IDDM, prostate CA, and sciatica. He reports that he fell last week when he got out of bed to urinate, with minor injury to his left shoulder and forearm as he hit the bedside table.

During the video visit, your learner takes a thorough recent history including asking about any recent illnesses or medication changes. When questioned about his recent blood sugar readings, Mr. P mentions that the values are transmitted to the clinic daily and the learner is then able to find them in the electronic medical record and confirm that they have been in a good range. When asked about his blood pressure readings, he offers to go retrieve his blood pressure log from the bedroom, the learner notes that he uses both arms to push up from his chair, reports he feels dizzy upon standing, leans on the corner of the counter and the door jamb as he leaves the room, and seems to be favoring his left leg. When he returns, he mentions that he has had increasing pain in his lower back that shoots down his left leg. Suspecting sciatica, you suggest the learner have Mr. P attempt a slump test by asking him to clasp his hands behind his back, tuck his chin and slump forward, and then to lift first his right then left leg straight out while flexing his toes up toward the ceiling. When lifting the left leg increases his back pain, plans are made to order spine imaging.

He has the blood pressure cuff you provided him at his last visit and an empty log booklet. He mentions that he has not been motivated to use it or to do household chores since his girlfriend moved out 6 months ago. The learner notices a picture of children playing on a beach taped to the refrigerator. He beams and tells you they are his grandchildren, but that he has not seen them in years because his kids no longer talk to him.

After wrapping up the visit, you ask the learner to list things they learned about the patient during the video visit that they might not otherwise know. For example:

1. The home appears quite cluttered, with stacks of magazines in the corners and scatter rugs visible in the hallway, all of which represent trip hazards.
2. A walker visible in the background seems to be used to store clothes suggesting he has been prescribed but has not been using an assistive device. Gait assessment was possible just through observation of the patient standing and walking in his home as he usually would.
3. With proper patient instruction, maneuvers performed during the visit allowed diagnosis of a condition traditionally requiring direct physical examination.
4. His self-care appears to have declined in the context of fraying social supports.
5. Cues from a patient's home can help stimulate conversations about what matters most to a patient, and patients may be more relaxed having these conversations in their own homes.

Overarching Benefits, Challenges, and Adaptations When Teaching Geriatrics Via Telemedicine

Common concerns regarding performing telemedicine visits with older adults include challenges performing physical exam maneuvers and challenges with patients' technological abilities. However, there are many benefits of telemedicine in these areas as well as adaptations that may help overcome real and perceived challenges.

Benefits

Telemedicine can benefit many learners who would not otherwise have an opportunity to do in-person home visits a chance for that richer, more personal experience. It may also allow them to do home visits with patients they would not otherwise get to see, such as to follow-up after hospital discharge for a patient who lives far away from the medical center. To teach using telemedicine, both learners and teachers need to be able to describe and discuss the benefits, challenges, and adaptations necessary to complete video telemedicine visits with older adults. This includes an understanding that successful video visits often require some adaptations and real time creative problem solving including around things such as unexpected technology glitches and interruptions in the home environment. Preceptors themselves need to be comfortable providing patient care via telemedicine to appropriately model best practices for their learners.

Challenges

While in-person, hands on assessment in the clinic is still the gold standard for most physical examination elements, there are a few areas for which a home observation may give you more information, such as being able to watch patients stand up from a favorite chair and walk around in their own home. Clearly, there are inevitable limitations related to lack of specialized equipment in the home such that otoscopic, fundoscopic, and pelvic examinations, for example, are not generally feasible via home video visits. And other assessments that depend on tactile feedback, such as the assessment of crepitus or cogwheeling is not possible.

Adaptations

However, with a little creativity, and by employing patient-generated data, patient or family assistance, and use of household items, many systems can be assessed via video telemedicine. In fact, partly prompted by the sudden need to do more telemedicine encounters during the early stages of the COVID-19 pandemic, many medical specialty societies published guidelines for telemedicine examinations including, for example, tele-audiology, tele-neurology, tele-physical therapy, and tele-dermatology. Many of these tele-adaptations involve a combination of having the patient themselves or a family member assist with physical examination maneuvers, such as joint or abdominal palpation, checking for pitting edema, and holding body parts up to the camera (or moving the camera to display body parts). Many also advise creative use of household objects such as cans of known weight for strength testing, a cool item from the refrigerator for sensory testing, and the use of pencil and paper to aid in cognitive assessment. In other words, learners should be taught a combination of pre-planning and dynamic problem solving based on the particular patient and assessment of their environment allows for a more complete assessment than might have originally been imagined. While a telemedicine based examination is generally not better than an in-person examination, it is definitely better than nothing and often more than adequate for diagnosis and management.

Older Adults Interfacing with Telemedicine

Benefits

While many older adults do not currently have video-capable devices that they know how to use, the percentage that do is steadily increasing [12]. Telemedicine allows clinicians to reach older patients who could not otherwise easily access in-person or specialty care due to rurality, limited mobility, etc. Telemedicine also allows caregivers who otherwise would not be available to participate.

Challenges

Common sensory impairments in older adults such as hearing and vision difficulties may limit interactions virtually more than in person. Cognitive impairment may limit both the ability to operate the technology and the ability to understand how to engage with clinicians through video. Even those without frank cognitive impairment may also have limited technology literacy and comfort accessing and navigating the virtual environment. Older adults may experience the digital divide meaning a lack of access to technology, video-capable equipment, and having a higher likelihood of living in a region without broadband or cellular access [8, 13, 14].

Adaptations

Sensory: Hearing impairment can potentially be overcome by advising patients to use headphones or external speakers that can adjust the volume to a higher level. Pocket talkers can be used to allow the patient to receive amplified sound while the caregiver hears at a normal level. Clinicians should sit somewhere with low levels of background noise and ensure that they are facing the camera and not backlit to allow for lip reading. Lighting on the clinician's side should be oriented so the clinician is clearly visible without glare (cataracts), shadowing (macular degeneration), or backlighting (to allow for better nonverbal communication). If closed captioning is available on the platform, patients should be instructed how to use it, although some find it distracting. For visual impairment, patients should be encouraged to use a device with a large screen rather than on a small device like a smartphone. If displaying anything on the screen such as stimuli for mental status exams, ensure that a large font is used.

Cognitive: For patients with cognitive impairment ensure there is someone accompanying them on the visit for assistance with technology. Be alert that this person may not be necessary or appropriate to serve as an informant in cognitive or medical assessments. If there are options to employ a platform with a simple user interface such as one where the patient does not need to check email or login and just answers an incoming video call at the appointed time. Patients may benefit from having a practice session before the visit to teach them how to use their device and the video interface.

Digital Divide: At times the digital divide is prohibitive and a phone visit or in-person visit is needed. However, if the barrier is lack of a device, patients can be encouraged to reach out to family, friends, and neighbors to borrow devices capable of broadband connection within the patient's home. Be alert to local programs that distribute devices for telemedicine use or give access to shared community-based video telemedicine equipment (Walmart, VFW).

Coming Attractions in Geriatric Telemedicine Education

All learners need to be able to provide telemedicine care. Even if they are not going to be geriatricians, they will be interacting with older adult patients and need to establish competency in video telemedicine with older adults. As technology continues to improve and evolve both learners and preceptors need to continue to adapt and improve their skills with telemedicine.

Opportunities

Proficiency in telemedicine and embrace of teleconferencing as a modality for teaching geriatrics may afford the field the opportunity to expand into new arenas, which in turn may increase access to geriatrics training.

Virtual Fellowships/Rotations: Through tele-geriatrics, learners from locations at a distance from established training sites might offer virtual geriatrics fellowships or quality geriatrics training to medicine or family practice residency programs that do not have strong geriatrics curricula [15].

Telemedicine Sim Labs: The development of simulation laboratories that allow for the teaching of best practices in telemedicine would allow for the incorporation of older adult patients with common geriatric syndromes including those that require adaptations for successful telemedicine encounters. For example, having a simulated patient be one with low tech literacy and partial hearing loss would encourage learners to employ best practices for clear communication during a video visit, skills applicable to all specialties.

Access to Diverse Patient Populations: Telemedicine allows learners access to older adult populations that they would otherwise not encounter. For example, learners could expand their clinical experiences to care for patients in rural areas, Indian Health Services, or jails. Additionally telemedicine opens opportunities for clinical care in non-traditional care sites like Meals on Wheels, senior centers, or at local Area Agencies on Aging.

Access to Diverse Preceptors: When preceptors are not required to be co-located with learners, it is more feasible to bring in faculty from other departments or locations to serve as master clinicians. Depending on educational needs, these could be clinicians from other disciplines or from other professions.

Non-Traditional Learners: Telemedicine can extend the reach of geriatrics education to learners of all levels. Non-traditional learners may be more easily included on telemedicine visits than in-person visits. Pre-clinical students and other observers can be incorporated by sitting out of view of the camera or by signing in from another location. Patients must still be alerted to their presence and agree to the observation. Care should be taken to not include too many virtual observers as frequently their image would appear to be the same size as the clinician's thus interfering with the patient interaction. Additionally, observation or recording of these visits whether with real patients or standardized patients could be used in training of learners up to the CME level.

Interprofessional Education: By bridging gaps in distance, telemedicine may create unique possibilities for interprofessional education. Students who would normally never interact can be brought together to care for patients and learn from each other. Opportunities for creativity abound and can include serial individual visits with group discussions, group visits, or learning conferences following patient interactions.

Conclusion

As patients who readily utilize telemedicine care age, geriatrics telemedicine skills will become increasingly important. Learners who may already have experience in using telemedicine may not yet have experience or competence in delivering *geriatric* care via telemedicine, yielding an opportunity for geriatrics educators. Teaching the medical content of geriatrics over telemedicine is very similar to teaching geriatrics in person, and these visits can be conceptualized as virtual home visits. With a little creativity and adaptation, geriatrics educators can utilize this emerging care modality to teach core geriatrics concepts and improve the health of older adults.

References

1. Raj M, Iott B, Anthony D, Platt J. Family caregivers' experiences with telehealth during COVID-19: insights from Michigan. Ann Fam Med. 2022;20(1):69–71.
2. Gately ME, Tickle-Degnen L, McLaren JE, Ward N, Ladin K, Moo LR. Factors influencing barriers and facilitators to in-home video telehealth for dementia management. Clin Gerontol. 2022;45(4):1020–33.
3. Moo LR. Home video visits: two-dimensional view of the geriatric 5 M's. J Am Geriatr Soc. 2020;68(11):2425–7.
4. Record JD, Ziegelstein RC, Christmas C, Rand CS, Hanyok LA. Delivering personalized care at a distance: how telemedicine can Foster getting to know the patient as a person. J Pers Med. 2021;11(2):137. https://doi.org/10.3390/jpm11020137.
5. Choi NG, DiNitto DM, Marti CN, Choi BY. Telehealth use among older adults during COVID-19: associations with sociodemographic and health characteristics, technology device ownership, and technology learning. J Appl Gerontol. 2022;41(3):600–9.
6. Nearing KA, Lum HD, Dang S, et al. National geriatric network rapidly addresses trainee telehealth needs in response to COVID-19. J Am Geriatr Soc. 2020;68(9):1907–12.
7. Rodriguez JA, Betancourt JR. Differences in the use of telephone and video telemedicine visits during the COVID-19 pandemic. Am J Physiol Renal Physiol. Published online 2021. https://search.ebscohost.com/login.aspx?direct=true&profile=ehost&scope=site&authtype=crawler&jrnl=10880224&AN=148273804&h=GFk8zyiBAR0%2BELohzJYRyxkKlweCu6k%2F0RhrP8aiEJvU5ort7LNU98CYXzcXMpgcjk%2FivW29ADqIRTWqvofiWQ%3D%3D&crl=c.
8. Frydman JL, Gelfman LP, Goldstein NE, Kelley AS, Ankuda CK. The digital divide: do older adults with serious illness access telemedicine? J Gen Intern Med. 2022;37(4):984–6.

9. Powers BB, Van Zuilen RM, Schwartz AW, Dang S, McLaren JE, Hoang-Gia D, Moo LR. Competencies for video telemedicine with older adult patients. J Am Geriatr Soc. 2023;71(4):1283–1290. 10.1111/jgs.18246. Epub 2023 Mar 23. PMID: 36951209.
10. Hovaguimian A, Joshi A, Onorato S, Schwartz AW, Frankl S. Twelve tips for clinical teaching with telemedicine visits. Med Teach. 2021;8:1–7.
11. Onorato S, Joshi A, Schwartz AW. Lights, camera, action: optimizing virtual video visits to provide high-quality care. J Gen Intern Med. 2021;36(6):1751–4. https://doi.org/10.1007/s11606-020-06278-z. Epub 2020 Oct 27. PMID: 33111243; PMCID: PMC7592130.
12. PewInst_2017.05.17_Older-Americans-Tech_FINAL.pdf.
13. Eberly LA, Khatana SAM, Nathan AS, et al. Telemedicine outpatient cardiovascular care during the COVID-19 pandemic: bridging or opening the digital divide? Circulation. 2020;142(5):510–2.
14. McCullough J, Ganju KK, Ellimoottil C. Does telemedicine transcend disparities or create a digital divide? In: Evidence from the COVID-19 pandemic; 2021. https://doi.org/10.2139/ssrn.3834445.
15. Powers BB, Hartmann P, Welch M, Ross J. Expanding the reach of geriatrics grand rounds using Facebook live. J Am Geriatr Soc. 2019;67(10):E4–6.

Part IV
Selected Topics in Teaching Geriatrics

Chapter 18
Diversity, Equity, and Inclusion in Geriatrics Education

Jade Connor and Daniele Ölveczky

Introduction

The population of older adults in the United States (US) is becoming increasingly more heterogeneous, with more older adults identifying with non-White racial and ethnic groups, lesbian, gay, bisexual, transgender, and queer/questioning (LGBTQ+) communities, and immigrant communities. In 2019, about one-fourth of people 65 years and older were people of color, and this is projected to increase by 115% by 2040 [1]. An estimated 7% of older adults identify as LGBTQ+ [2]. Beyond these subgroups, older adults encompass a range of lived experiences, abilities, and healthcare practices. With this growing diversity among the population of older adults in the US, issues of diversity, equity, and inclusion (DEI) have become increasingly more relevant for geriatric medical education.

Diversity refers to the variation in the individuals in a given setting. In medicine, diversity can be viewed from many levels (e.g., in patient populations, among healthcare trainees and professionals, within the leadership of institutions) and axes of difference (e.g., race, gender, sexual orientation, place of origin, language, socio-economic status, etc.). *Inclusion* describes how diversity is incorporated in

J. Connor
Harvard Medical School, Massachusetts General Hospital, Boston, MA, USA
e-mail: Jade_connor@hms.harvard.edu

D. Ölveczky (✉)
Beth Israel Deaconess Medical Center, Harvard Medical School, Boston, MA, USA
e-mail: dolveczk@bidmc.harvard.edu

A. W. Schwartz (ed.), *Medical Education in Geriatrics*,
https://doi.org/10.1007/978-3-031-32499-4_18

organizations. The lens of inclusion asks: How is the diversity of the group reflected in the organization's values, priorities, and practices? Do organizational activities integrate the perspectives and lived experiences of individuals in the group? Are all members of the group able to contribute and enact change at every level? How are members supported in their work? How are individuals protected from bias, discrimination, and retaliation? *Equity* is the principle that all individuals should have the same opportunities. Equity is a process that is rooted in justice and respect for persons, incorporating their identities. It requires intentional awareness and investigation of difference, commitment to change, redistributive and reparative action, and constant evaluation of progress.

In this chapter, we will provide context about health disparities in geriatrics populations in the US, give an overview of the status of DEI in geriatrics medical education, describe best practices for integrating DEI themes in geriatrics medical education, and offer insights into the future of geriatrics education from a DEI perspective.

Health Disparities and Aging

Health disparities in older adulthood span many axes of identity and dimensions of healthcare (Table 18.1). The difference in life expectancy between White and Black populations at age 65 was more than 2 years in 2020 [9]. Although women live longer than men, they are more likely to live in poverty, to live alone, and are less likely to receive home care services [1]. About 9% of older adults live at or below

Table 18.1 Examples of health disparities in older age

Geriatrics health disparity	Axis of disparity	Proposed causes of disparity	Structural drivers of disparity
Immunization rates (e.g., influenza, pneumococcus, COVID-19) [3, 4]	Race, ethnicity, English proficiency	Low health literacy, limited interactions with healthcare providers	Racism, socioeconomic status (SES), health insurance coverage, geographic location, lack of interpreter services
Advanced care planning [5, 6]	Race, ethnicity, English proficiency	Low health literacy, patient distrust of health system, provider/patient discomfort with conversation	Racism, historical injustices, SES, health insurance coverage, lack of interpreter services
Access to home care services [7]	Gender	Lack of financial resources, gender roles in caregiving	Sexism, SES, employer-based insurance programs, health insurance coverage
Drug and alcohol use [8]	Sexual orientation	Distrust of health system, allostatic load due to trauma, stigma, and discrimination	Heteronormativity, homophobia, historical injustices, SES

the poverty line, with the highest rates of poverty among Hispanic and Black women living alone (32.1% and 31.7%, respectively) [1]. Lesbian, gay, and bisexual individuals are more likely to have a disability than their heterosexual counterparts [8]. Although data on the health and care of transgender older adults are limited, transgender people have even worse access to healthcare and poorer health outcomes [10]. Beyond racial, gender, and sexual identity, other factors including disability, primary language, incarceration history, and experience of discrimination also portend worse health outcomes [11].

These health disparities have been well documented in the literature, and there have been growing calls for a shift in the research focus from documenting health disparities to investigating the origins and drivers of these differential outcomes [12]. Research thus far has elucidated some of the drivers of these disparities in specific instances (Table 18.1).

Many frameworks have been constructed to conceptualize how health disparities are created, perpetuated, and mitigated. One such framework is the Life Course Theory, first introduced by Elder in 1975 and subsequently applied to health disparities by Braveman and Barclay [13]. The Life Course Theory describes how one's health is shaped by the physical, psychosocial, and environmental factors introduced at different points in one's life that compound and interact as one ages. These factors range from biological (like teratogen exposure in utero) to structural (such as poverty), and they can modulate one's risk of adverse health outcomes later in life. The biological and structural exposures are related by the concept of allostatic load, which describes the biological effects of chronic stress over time [14]. Allostatic load is the mechanism by which structural forces such as prejudice, discrimination, and stigma are embodied at the genetic and cellular level and has been associated with conditions like cardiovascular disease, diabetes, and cancer [14]. Taken together, the Life Course perspective on health disparities emphasizes the accumulation of health exposures over time, the bidirectional influence of biological and structural factors, and the intergenerational nature of disparities.

Another framework for analyzing health disparities is the Health Equity Promotion Model put forth by Fredriksen-Goldsen et al. (2014) and first applied to LGBTQ+ health disparities [15]. This model describes how individuals' experience of internalized, interpersonal, and structural bias affects their biological, psychological, behavioral, and social functioning, which in turn manifests in differential mental and physical health outcomes throughout their lives [15]. The Health Equity Promotion Model takes a lifespan perspective while emphasizing the unique ways in which intersecting identities affect these pathways. These two frameworks—and others like them—are useful tools in deconstructing the health disparities observed in older adulthood. Moreover, both frameworks highlight the necessity of multilevel and multidimensional interventions to tackle disparities.

One such intervention is the education of health professionals. Training current and future health professionals to describe, investigate, and intervene on health inequities has been advocated for by several governmental, healthcare, and professional organizations. However, many barriers exist to enacting adequate education in these topics. There is a dual deficit in a robust geriatrics workforce as well as a robust healthcare workforce well-versed in health disparities (one can imagine the limited number of faculty at medical institutions with the experience required to teach about the unique ways that health inequities affect a geriatric population) [16]. Furthermore, there is limited research on health disparities within the field of geriatrics, perpetuated by the lack of research infrastructure and support of the study of these topics [12]. At an institutional level, academic medicine has historically placed less value on DEI work, often failing to support or promote trainees and faculty who engage in this work [17]. Many medical institutions do not include health equity in their missions, do not employ individuals that reflect the diversity of the nation or of their own patient populations, and fail to consistently practice inclusion. Lastly, social forces like White supremacy, sexism, heteronormativity, and xenophobia pervade the field of medicine and uphold oppressive structures [18]. All of these factors hinder the integration of DEI themes into medical curricula in geriatrics.

Current State of DEI in Geriatrics Medical Education

Much of the medical education on DEI issues in the field of geriatrics has focused on cultural competency. *Cultural competency* in medical education refers to the attitudes, knowledge, and skills needed to care for the diversity of social and cultural contexts in which patients live [19]. Cultural competency (and related approaches like cross-cultural care and cultural humility) was adopted by medical institutions in response to the growing evidence base and awareness of health disparities and the effect of provider bias in exacerbating them [19]. In undergraduate medical education, the Liaison Committee on Medical Education (LCME) has included cultural competency as a required educational component for medical students since 2000 [20]. The American Geriatrics Society (AGS) put forth a curriculum in 2006 on ethnogeriatric education, emphasizing specific elements of cultural competency required to care for diverse older populations [21]. This curriculum even includes modules on elders from various ethnic groups in the US, highlighting the cultural beliefs, behaviors, and health needs of these populations [22].

In graduate medical education, cultural competency is also a common program requirement for residencies and fellowships in the US from the Accreditation Council for Graduate Medical Education (ACGME) [23]. The ACGME recognizes physicians' role in addressing the social determinants of health and improving health disparities, and as such require education on navigating differences for graduate medical trainees. The specialties with the most organized geriatrics education—internal medicine, family medicine, and emergency medicine—also acknowledge this deficit in training and include cultural competency training in most curricula [24–27]. The AGS outlines parallel competencies for geriatrics fellows and practicing physicians [28, 29].

Many have expressed critique of cultural competency in medical education. Cultural competency focuses on individuals' beliefs and behaviors, and several of the related skills target interpersonal interactions [18]. The knowledge of culture is often prescriptive, overlooking the variation of beliefs and practices within social groups [18]. Moreover, cultural competency deemphasizes the systemic forces that shape and constrain individual action [18]. As a result, there has been a shift in medical education from cultural competency to structural competency to promote health equity. *Structural competency*, as defined by Metzl and Hansen (2014), is:

> the trained ability to discern how a host of issues defined clinically as symptoms, attitudes, or diseases (e.g., depression, hypertension, obesity, smoking, medication "non-compliance," trauma, psychosis) also represent the downstream implications of a number of upstream decisions about such matters as health care and food delivery systems, zoning laws, urban and rural infrastructures, medicalization, or even about the very definitions of illness and health [18].

This shift has only recently been introduced in geriatrics—spurred by the murder of George Floyd in 2020 and the resulting calls for antiracist action from medical institutions [30]. In 2021, the AGS put forth a multi-year initiative to combat structural racism and ageism, including reexamining the aforementioned cultural competency curriculum [31]. The AGS also introduced a health equity theme in the *Minimum Competencies in Geriatrics for Medical Students* [32]. However, similar language has not yet been introduced in competencies for graduate and continuing geriatrics medical education.

The current medical education paradigm for teaching issues of DEI falls short. To the authors' knowledge, there are few organized health equity themes within geriatrics educational components in medical schools beyond cultural competency. Longitudinal health equity curricula have been shown to increase medical students' knowledge of the social determinants of health and confidence in working with marginalized populations [33, 34]. However, this has not yet been applied to geriatrics medical education. Beyond increasing awareness of issues related to DEI, geriatrics medical education must also train faculty and learners in the skills necessary to address health inequities and their unique manifestations in older adulthood.

The following sections outline best practices for integrating issues of DEI into geriatrics curricula as well as highlight special considerations for educators when developing these educational activities. These best practices are compiled from existing literature in medical education, with a particular focus on antiracist practice. Although much of the medical education literature focuses on UME, these principles can be applied to geriatrics curricula for all levels of learners.

Best Practices for DEI Geriatrics Curriculum: Shift from Cultural Competence to Health Equity

Issues of DEI should be integrated through geriatrics curriculum—from didactic teaching on the biological underpinnings of health and disease, clinical medicine, and public health to clinical skills to experiential learning. Specific examples of how to adapt existing educational activities to integrate health equity themes are found in Table 18.2.

Table 18.2 Approach to addressing diversity, equity, and inclusion in geriatrics medical education

	Old curricular perspective		New curricular perspective		
Educational activity	Cultural competency approach	Cultural competency example	Health equity approach	Health equity example	Best practice resource
Didactics on health disparities	Educate learners about health disparities among older adults, emphasizing interpersonal and behavioral causes for different identity groups	"Lesbian and bisexual women are less likely to have routine screening mammograms than heterosexual women, due to lack of perceived importance of screening and reluctance to access health services"	Educate learners about health disparities among older adults and their origins, emphasizing systemic drivers of disparities as well as the cumulative effects of intersecting disparities throughout life course	"Lesbian and bisexual women are less likely to have routine screening mammograms than heterosexual women, due to the relative lack of access to health services resulting from the historical exclusion of these groups in employment and society in general and ongoing stigma and bias encountered in clinical settings"	*Health Disparities Beginning in Childhood: A Life Course Perspective* [13]
Clinical cases	Include identifiers of sexual orientation, race, place of origin, and/or primary language in patient presentations to highlight prevalent conditions or experiences within that population	"S. T. Is a 76-year-old native American IV drug user who presents with elevated liver transaminases" (patient has delayed presentation of hepatitis C)	Include identifiers in patient presentations only when relevant, avoiding stereotypes and misleading heuristics	"S. T. Is a 76-year-old with a history of substance use disorder who presents with elevated liver transaminases" (patient has medication side effect in the context of polypharmacy)	*Race and Culture Guide for Editors of Teaching Cases* [35]
Clinical skills	Solicit patients' cultural beliefs and practices surrounding health and illness	Inquire about diet, suggesting modifications of cultural foods to make them healthier	Solicit patients' explanatory model of health and illness, asking directly about social determinants of health	Inquire about diet and barriers to healthy eating, such as food and housing insecurity, proximity to grocery store, access to transportation, etc.	Screening tools such as PRAPARE [36] or Centers for Medicare & Medicaid Health-Related Social Needs Screening Tool [37]

	Old curricular perspective		New curricular perspective		
Educational activity	Cultural competency approach	Cultural competency example	Health equity approach	Health equity example	Best practice resource
Experiential learning	Guest speakers from a particular identity group are invited to speak about their experience aging in their culture	Elderly immigrant patients come to the classroom to share their experience with aging in home countries and in US	Longitudinal community partnerships with diverse older adult communities including community service, clinical care, and community-led advocacy	Year-long program in which learners are assigned to community health centers serving marginalized communities for clinical rotations and nonclinical volunteering	*Faculty Toolkit for Service-Learning in Higher Education* [38]

Teaching About Health Disparities in Geriatric Populations

Integration of DEI themes in geriatrics medical education begins in the preclinical curriculum of medical school and extends into didactics in graduate medical training and beyond. Presenting epidemiological data on health disparities without context, using race interchangeably with genetic ancestry, and hosting one-time "diversity" lectures are common in medical school curricula [39]. This approach to DEI, however, devalues this education, implicitly conveying that these issues are ancillary to clinical medicine and that health professionals do not have a responsibility to combat these problems. Moreover, the lack of interrogation of disparities in geriatric populations flattens complex health and social issues into a narrative of aging, ignoring the diversity of lived experiences in older populations.

Health disparities should be taught as cumulative effects of inequities throughout the lifespan and should be throughout the curriculum accompanying relevant clinical topics. Educators should use frameworks such as the aforementioned Life Course Theory to discuss the origins of health disparities, noting structural and historical forces and the embodiment of stress through allostatic load that lead to differential health outcomes in geriatric populations. Educators should also incorporate the concept of *intersectionality*—a term coined by Kimberlé Crenshaw in 1989—to discuss how inequities across multiple axes interact and uniquely manifest in individuals' health [40]. Medical mythology and imprecise language should be explicitly deconstructed and corrected. Specifically, race-based algorithms—like calculators for heart failure mortality risk, osteoporosis, and estimated glomerular filtration rate—that impact decision-making for the care of older adults should be eliminated from medical education and clinical use. Such "corrections" based on race and ethnicity often underestimate risk or severity of disease for Black and Latinx patients, guiding clinicians toward less aggressive diagnostics and treatments for these patients [41].

Representing Diversity in Clinical Cases

Educators must also practice inclusivity in case representations, diversifying the patients and clinical settings presented. Images, videos, and audio that accompany clinical teaching cases should feature persons of various racial and ethnic backgrounds, people with limited English proficiency, individuals with disabilities, and people of various gender expressions, among a host of other identities, without these aspects of identity as the primary issue of the case [42]. *Race and Culture Guide for Editors of Teaching Cases* is a tool for educators that outlines how to incorporate aspects of patients' identities and social determinants of health in clinical cases [35]. Examples of inclusion in clinical cases include featuring dermatological conditions on people of various skin tones [42], describing social histories reflecting the diverse nature of social networks (such as grandparents as the primary caretakers of their grandchildren, individuals with chosen rather than biological families, older adults living in residential communities or congregate care settings, etc.), and noting patients' preferred pronouns. *Aquifer Geriatrics*, a collection of online case-based modules on various geriatrics topics as the AGS national online geriatrics curriculum, provides examples of the integration of DEI and social determinants of health issues into teaching cases [43]. A sample clinical vignette can be found in Box 18.1.

Box 18.1: Sample Vignette for Clinical Teaching Cases [Modified from Aquifer Geriatrics]

Your first patient is a 72-year-old male, Mr. John Hernandez. His prior primary care physician in the practice recently retired, and this is his first appointment with you. As with his previous visits, he reports being generally healthy and reports no specific concerns. On the pre-visit questionnaire that he filled out in the waiting room, however, he indicated that he has lost about 6.8 kg (15 lbs) in the past six months. He reports that he has not had much of an appetite lately but has not noticed any other changes to his health.

- *Past medical history:* Hypertension, diabetes mellitus type 2, and hyperlipidemia. No prior surgeries or recent hospitalizations.
- *Medications:* Hydrochlorothiazide, simvastatin, metformin, and aspirin. He takes no other over-the-counter (OTC) medications or supplements.
- *Social history:* Mr. Hernandez is a retired professor of history. He is divorced with two children, is a former smoker (20 pack-years; quit over 16 years ago), and drinks alcohol occasionally. He reports no history of recreational drug use.
- *Functional history*: Independently performs all of his ADLs but has recently required some help with his grocery shopping and chores around the house.
- *Physical exam:* He weighs 61.2 kg (135 lbs), BMI = 19.4. In general, he appears thin but well-groomed. The complete physical exam revealed mild bitemporal muscle wasting, reduced muscle mass all extremities, strength 4/5 in all extremities, heavy arm support to stand up but gait steady and average speed without any device.
- *Labs:* Complete blood count (CBC), comprehensive metabolic profile (CMP), and thyroid stimulating hormone (TSH) are normal.

You are concerned about depression in this patient. You administer the Patient Health Questionnaire (PHQ-9), which screens positive for depression. He does not have any suicidal thoughts. You decide to ask him more about his life. Upon further questioning, he reveals that his divorce from his wife 25 years ago was difficult for his adult children, and they have stopped speaking to him. When you ask about social supports, he shares that he has a few friends, and his roommate, Joe, has been very supportive to him. You ask him about romantic relationships, and he discloses that he is in a romantic relationship with his roommate. How would you proceed to ask about this relationship and its potential effects on how Mr. Hernandez has been feeling recently?

Patient presentations should avoid identity-based heuristics, such as the association of glaucoma with Black race and macular degeneration with White race. Patient presentations framed in this way rely on representativeness bias (a cognitive bias that categorizes cases based on how closely they match the perceived "prototype" of that category) and can reinforce stereotypes of marginalized groups. Ideally, cases should be developed in inclusive teams that contain people with similar backgrounds or lived experiences, or—if these members are not present—in consultation with individuals who can speak to the lived experiences of the patients in the cases and voice concerns about inaccurate or stereotyped characterizations. Producing teaching materials in this manner not only helps to safeguard against inaccurate representations but also aligns with the principles of community-academic partnerships (CAPs), which will be described in more detail later in the chapter.

Developing Clinical Skills

Clinical practice requires effectively conducting histories and physical exams, developing differential diagnoses, prioritizing problems, proposing diagnostic and therapeutic interventions, and communicating health information to patients. As such, trainees and practicing physicians must learn to perform these skills with a variety of patients and in a variety of clinical settings. Trainees should be able to communicate with patients using interpreters. They should also be comfortable screening for social determinants of health using validated tools [36, 37, 44, 45]. When taking clinical histories, trainees should solicit individuals' explanatory model in addition to cultural beliefs and practices surrounding illness and health. They should ask about historical events that may impact patients' health or healthcare behaviors (such as the War on Drugs, the HIV-AIDS epidemic, the forced sterilization of individuals with intellectual disabilities), using a trauma-informed care approach. Educators should discourage the omission of particular parts of the history for geriatric patients, especially questions related to sexuality (which reinforces the invisibility of LGBTQ+ older adults and perpetuates the stereotype that older adults are uncomfortable discussing sexual activity or are asexual) [46], education and occupation (which assumes that older adults have lower educational attainment and health literacy), and substance use (which assume that older adults do not use drugs or misuse medications). A summary of suggested phrases when talking to patients can be found in Box 18.2.

Box 18.2: Taking a Geriatrics History with a Diversity, Equity, and Inclusion Focus: Suggested Phrases

Explanatory Model

- What do you think is going on?
- What are you most concerned about?

Cultural Beliefs and Practices

- You shared with me that you identify as [a member of a certain group]. Are there particular beliefs or practices that you participate in that would be helpful for me to know?
- Do you see any other people about your health besides a doctor?
- Do you use things other than prescribed medication for your health (like vitamins, herbs, supplements, teas, etc.)?

Gender Identity

- I want to make sure that I am addressing you correctly. What name do you go by?
- What pronouns do you use? For example, I use [personal pronouns].

Sexual Orientation

- Are you in a romantic relationship? Who is/are your partner(s)?
- Do you consider yourself gay, straight, bisexual, or something else?

Trauma

- Many people live through experiences, including historical events, that they consider traumatic and can affect their health or the way they interact with the healthcare system. Have you experienced something like that?
- Have you ever been treated differently or discriminated against based on who you are?
- What things would make you more comfortable when you come to [a provider or clinical setting]?

Education and Occupation

- Do you have a high school degree?
- What is the highest level of schooling you have completed?
- Are you currently working? What did you do for work in the past?
- How do you spend your day?

Social Determinants of Health[1]

- Are there things in your life that make it difficult to come to the doctor or get your medications?
- What are some things that we can do to help you [achieve health goals/reduce barriers]?

---

[1] Health professionals should use validated tools for screening for specific social determinants of health.

These clinical skills can be developed using several methods, including standardized patients, clinical clerkships, dedicated geriatrics rotations, or community-based experiential learning. With each of these methods, care should be taken to expose learners to diverse patient populations, with particular attention to those populations prevalent in the communities in which the medical institutions serve. For example, as a part of their longitudinal geriatrics clerkship, students at the Herbert Wertheim College of Medicine are placed in a primary care practice providing integrated care tailored to the needs of the predominately Cuban immigrant geriatric population that it serves [47]. This setting both exposed students to the local community and allowed them to cultivate crucial skills such as using interpreters, screening for social determinants of health, and navigating complex care needs. Some topics, such as providing gender-affirming care to transgender older adults, may be better suited for standardized patient encounters. Learners may not be exposed to these issues in the communities in which they are training given their relatively low prevalence in the general population, and standardized encounters provide a venue to practice clinical skills and reflect on the experience from both a provider and patient perspective. In these situations, it is important that patient scripts and presentations are thoroughly vetted and do not include stereotyped characterizations of identities.

Learning Through Experience

Themes related to DEI can also be learned outside of classroom or clinical settings. Experiential learning—including community service and other community-based activities—integrates engagement with curricular topics with reflective exercises to make meaning of experiences and apply them to trainees' work. Experiential learning has been widely incorporated into geriatrics medical education. Many medical institutions already include volunteer work, home or site visits, and community health projects in their geriatrics curriculum (Table 18.3)

Table 18.3 Examples of experiential learning in geriatrics education

Institution	Program setting	Program description
Herbert Wertheim College of Medicine	Community-based organization in Miami-Dade County, Florida	Medical students partner with local community members through the green family foundation neighborhood HELP to conduct home visits and community-based healthcare planning and promotion projects [47]
University of California Irvine School of Medicine	Home-based sites in Orange County, California	Students are paired with older adults for the first 3 years of medical school, completing learning modules conducted through home visits [48]
University of North Carolina School of Medicine at Chapel Hill	Community-based sites in Chapel Hill, North Carolina	Students are assigned longitudinally to community sites in which they conduct needs assessment and develop health education projects to address an identified need for older adults living in that community [49]

[47–49]. Experiential learning is an ideal method of teaching about health disparities and interventions to mitigate them. In addition to the benefits previously outlined, this educational strategy narrows the power differential often experienced by providers and patients in clinical settings. Learners leave their authority role, and community members are positioned as experts in their community and health. Learning outside of academic or clinical environments also helps trainees deconstruct the "us versus them" mentality between the medical community and patients, promoting a collaborative relationship between healthcare institutions and the communities they serve.

Experiential learning can integrate DEI themes through several avenues. Representatives from communities may be invited to speak to learners about their experience or to teach concepts as expert consultants. Narrative medicine—such as patient storytelling, art and literature, or other creative works—have been shown to improve communication, increase understanding of cultural diversity and the experience of illness, and strength empathy [50]. Narrative medicine can be integrated as a reflective practice to engage with themes introduced in other parts of the geriatrics curriculum. Learners can also conduct community-based participatory research projects in geriatrics-related topics, which serves the dual role of exposing trainees to geriatrics research and partnering with local communities to build programming or create solutions. Working with marginalized communities through service or volunteer work can also allow learners to discuss and reflect on DEI topics while cultivating social engagement. Experiential learning in these ways is best achieved through longitudinal relationships with older adults and longstanding CAPs.

Competency in advocacy is also a vital skill for healthcare professionals. Efforts exist to train medical students and residents in advocacy at every level—including patient, community, state, national, and global advocacy [51–53]. Experiential learning allows learners to apply didactic training in advocacy and activism to real-world issues affecting geriatric populations. Learners can work in existing community partnerships and advocacy groups to tackle health-related issues or create new ways to fulfill a community need. Sidney Kimmel Medical College at Thomas Jefferson University offers a 1-month advocacy elective for medical students and residents through the Department of Pediatrics [52]. During this elective, trainees address issues related to child health through community organizing, direct patient advocacy, and legislative action. Practical skills related to effective patient communication, oral and written advocacy work (i.e., testimonies, white papers, op-eds), and coalition-building are taught through didactics, clinical care, and community engagement. This program has been successful at raising awareness of physicians' role in addressing the social determinants of health in the broader public sphere, fostering sustainable CAPs, and implementing effective change [52]. Similar curricula in advocacy can be applied to geriatric medical education, particularly for vulnerable populations of older adults. Partnerships with organizations that advocate for issues important to older adults on the local, state, and national level provide an avenue for training healthcare professionals in the skills needed to enact structural changes to improve health for these groups and a starting point for the development of more robust advocacy curricula in geriatrics medical education [54].

Recruiting a Diverse Geriatrics Workforce

In addition to integrating DEI into geriatrics curricula, medical institutions play a role in promoting a diverse geriatrics workforce. The Institute of Medicine has long recognized the importance of workforce diversity in combatting health disparities [19]. Workforce diversity's influence on health inequities occurs through several mechanisms. Health professionals that come from groups that are under-represented in medicine (URiM) are more likely to care for underserved populations, increasing access to healthcare for these communities [55]. Workforce diversity expands the focus of research efforts, as URiM faculty are more likely to pursue scholarly work in DEI issues [17]. Additionally, diversity in educational settings improves the awareness of and sensitivity to DEI issues for all learners [55]. Because of these benefits, both the LCME and the ACGME advocate for the recruitment and retention of diverse trainees and faculty [20, 23].

The field of geriatrics has not yet achieved a diversity reflective of the US population. According to the 2020 US Census, approximately 20% of the US population identify as Black, Native American, Hawaiian, or Pacific Islander and 18% identify as Hispanic or Latinx [56]. In contrast, only 15.5% of practicing geriatricians are from these URiM backgrounds. One program to increase the number of URiM trainees that enter the specialty is the Johns Hopkins Geriatrics Summer Scholars Program [57]. This program exposes medical students to topics within geriatrics and aging, provides mentorship from URiM faculty members, and gives students research experience in geriatrics. Many of the program attendees subsequently participated in aging and geriatrics clinical and research fellowships, presented at AGS national meetings, and endorsed plans to pursue a career in geriatrics in the future [57]. Pipeline programs such as this should be implemented at institutions to expose and encourage URiM groups in careers in geriatrics.

Beyond pipeline programming, systemic change is also necessary to achieve a diverse geriatrics workforce. Substantial structural barriers still exist to URiM trainees entering the field of geriatrics. Lack of faculty role models and lack of emphasis on health inequities may lead trainees to self-select out of the specialty. Low-income and URiM students often graduate from medical school with substantial debt and as a result may select specialties with higher earning potentials [55]. At the institutional level, steps must be taken to ensure that the learning and clinical environment is inclusive. Such measures include comprehensive integration of DEI themes into all institutional activities (as this chapter outlines), dedicated support systems for URiM students, trainees, and faculty, and long-term planning and evaluation of outcomes related to DEI. Exposure to geriatrics is not sufficient to attract trainees to the field; institutions must also invest in trainees' success in professional school, early career, and beyond.

Special Considerations for Educators

Community-Academic Partnerships

Community involvement is vital to the education of trainees. Most educational activities outlined in this chapter require the participation of individuals outside of the healthcare sphere. In a systematic review of community-based medical education, Hunt et al. (2011) found that few programs were designed with community input or tracked community outcomes in addition to learner outcomes [58]. Moreover, most educational programs had goals directed toward the learner but did not mention collaboration or mutual benefit for communities [58]. There is a long history of the exploitation of marginalized groups in medical education and innovation—particularly those who are low-income, disabled, non-White, and have limited English proficiency [59]. Given these findings, the process by which individuals are recruited to participate, integrated into program development, and compensated for their work must be interrogated.

Academic medical centers, in addition to producing the majority of healthcare research and training health professionals, care for over a third of the US uninsured population [60]. This makes academic medical centers not only sources of innovation but safety nets for communities, both of which utilize public funds. Academic medical institutions have a responsibility to develop innovations and teach trainees in ways that benefit the communities they serve. CAPs are the mechanisms by which community members are involved in the workings of medical institutions in a mutually beneficial manner. A CAP approach necessitates that community members be involved in creating institutional missions, identifying community needs and priorities, allocating funding, designing and implementing programs, and evaluating impact [60]. An additional goal of these partnerships is to build capacity within communities so that programs are sustainable and adaptable to changes over time. When applied to medical education, CAPs involve establishing learning objectives and methods reflective of community needs and assets, involving community members in curricular development and implementation, and providing mechanisms for community evaluation of educational programs. CAPs are bidirectional, built on the mutual recognition of expertise and equal partnership in action. As such, community partners must be adequately acknowledged and compensated for their time and efforts in educating health professionals.

Faculty Development

The dearth of diversity within the faculty of most medical institutions hinders the implementation of DEI educational activities. Historically, the vast majority of educational, scholarly, clinical, and administrative work related to DEI are done by the few faculty members or trainees who identify with marginalized groups, commonly called the *minority tax* [17]. Moreover, these activities are seldom supported by the larger institutional infrastructure. Given the substantial upheaval of geriatric medical education that must be accomplished to achieve the incorporation of DEI themes, it is untenable to rely on the work of a handful of individuals and unrealistic to expect that the few faculty members who hold marginalized identities would have adequate time or resources to meaningfully address these issues. To integrate DEI themes in an ethical and sustainable way, all faculty members must contribute to this work.

The first step to achieving this is creating a common expectation for faculty. On an institutional level, leadership should convey the importance of these topics and the expectation that all faculty members should be competent in teaching them. All faculty members—including clinical and nonclinical faculty—should be encouraged to participate in bias and antiracism trainings. Such trainings can be modeled on published workshops for faculty on implicit bias, microaggressions, and structural racism. The goal of these trainings is to provide a foundational knowledge of DEI issues and familiarize faculty with a common language for discussing these concepts. The Society for General Internal Medicine offers a "train the trainer" resource that provides practical information for educators responsible for teaching DEI curricula [61]. Included in this resource are data on specific health disparities, terminology and definitions, teaching exercises, and examples of health equity educational activities. This toolkit can be used by faculty members when creating or revising learning activities.

Evidence suggests that trainings in unconscious bias and diversity alone do not lead to behavior change [62]. Given this, such trainings should be implemented as a part of a multi-intervention strategy to combat inequities within institutions. Interventions such as recruiting, retaining, and promoting a diversity faculty, mentorship and career development programs for women and URiM faculty, and mechanisms of reporting and investigating instances of bias and discrimination among faculty should also be implemented [62]. Intervention outcomes must also be tracked and disseminated so that institutions can monitor the effects of their efforts and identify areas of improvement.

Protecting the Learner

Although this chapter focuses primarily on DEI issues in older adult populations, the experience of learners from marginalized backgrounds must also be considered. As learners engage in educational activities, they may encounter identity-based bias, discrimination, and stigma from faculty, staff, patients, and community members. The University of California Irvine School of Medicine (UC Irvine SOM) faced this issue in their geriatric curriculum. Medical students from a diversity of backgrounds were placed in pairs and assigned senior partners who were almost exclusively White, English-speaking older adults. Issues arose, such as a male senior who conversed with the older, male learner and ignored the younger, female learner and a senior who made Islamophobic and xenophobic comments to a student of Middle Eastern descent [48].

Because of their role, learners may hesitate to address these incidents themselves or report them to the institution. As such, educators should regularly monitor and provide mechanisms for recourse when such instances arise. In the case of UC Irvine SOM, the students were reassigned to different senior partners [48]. However, simply removing learners from discriminatory environments may not be sufficient. Additional methods, such as providing dedicated time for skills-based discussions of bias and discrimination commonly faced by learners, holding debriefing sessions after instances occur, and creating anonymous systems for reporting incidents can help learners who may encounter prejudice in educational settings cope and build resiliency [63, 64].

Finally, medical institutions must ensure equity in assessment, specifically with trainee evaluations. Research has consistently demonstrated that White medical students obtain higher grades [65] and more favorable narrative evaluations [66] than their URiM colleagues. Furthermore, female trainees are subject to gender-biased language in their evaluations [66, 67]. These evaluations lead to differential achievement between groups, with non-White medical students less likely to receive honors in clerkships and be inducted into honors society like Alpha Omega Alpha [68]. These achievements have direct implications on students' specialty choice, residency selection, and career opportunities. In light of this, it is imperative that there are institutional safeguards to combat bias in grading [69]. Evaluators should use standardized feedback and evaluation guides to mitigate bias. Data on evaluations should be tracked longitudinally by the institution and stratified at a minimum by race, ethnicity, gender identity, and sexual orientation. Furthermore, trainees should have the ability to review and contest evaluations that they feel are discriminatory, mischaracterized, or retaliatory in nature. Mechanisms should be in place to investigate any instance of discrimination and correct any wrongdoing. These policies can mitigate the effects of bias that pervades the evaluation process in medical training.

Conclusion

This chapter outlined the ways in which geriatrics medical education can provide learners with a framework for approaching health inequities among older adults. Through a variety of methods including didactics, clinical exposure, and experiential learning, learners of all levels can engage with DEI issues and apply these skills to their future practice. Educators can also encourage URiM learners in their interest in geriatrics through establishing pipeline programs. To enact these changes, however, educators must foster sustainable partnerships with communities of older adults, train faculty to be proficient in teaching DEI themes, and provide safeguards for learners. As this chapter demonstrates, medical education is one crucial intervention to combat health disparities among older adults, but a multifaceted approach in which other drivers of inequities are also addressed is needed. Comprehensive geriatric medical education must empower learners with the knowledge and skills to promote equity for older adults at all levels.

References

1. Administration on Aging. 2020 Profile of older Americans. Washington, DC: Administration for Community Living; 2021. p. 21. https://acl.gov/sites/default/files/Aging%20and%20Disability%20in%20America/2020ProfileOlderAmericans.Final_.pdf.
2. The Williams Institute, UCLA School of Law. LGBT Data & Demographics (Interactive). 2019 [cited 2021 Jul 20]. https://williamsinstitute.law.ucla.edu/visualization/lgbt-stats/?topic=LGBT&sortBy=percentage&sortDirection=descending#ranking.
3. Tse SC. Racial/ethnic differences in influenza and pneumococcal vaccination rates among older adults in New York City and Los Angeles and Orange counties. Prev Chronic Dis. 2018 [cited 2021 Jul 16];15. https://www.cdc.gov/pcd/issues/2018/18_0101.htm.
4. Fuchs JR, Fuchs JW, Tietz SE, Lum HD. Older adults with limited English proficiency need equitable COVID-19 vaccine access. J Am Geriatr Soc. 2021;69:888–91.
5. Ashana DC, D'Arcangelo N, Gazarian PK, Gupta A, Perez S, Reich AJ, et al. "Don't talk to them about goals of care": understanding disparities in advance care planning. J Gerontol A Biol Sci Med Sci. 2021;77:glab091.
6. Jones T, Luth EA, Lin S-Y, Brody AA. Advance care planning, palliative care, and end-of-life care interventions for racial and ethnic underrepresented groups: A systematic review. J Pain Symptom Manag. 2021;62:e248–60.
7. Katz SJ, Kabeto M, Langa KM. Gender disparities in the receipt of home care for elderly people with disability in the United States. JAMA. 2000;284:3022–7.
8. Fredriksen-Goldsen KI, Kim H-J, Barkan SE, Muraco A, Hoy-Ellis CP. Health disparities among lesbian, gay, and bisexual older adults: results from a population-based study. Am J Public Health. 2013;103:1802–9.
9. Arias E, Betzaida T-V, Ahmad F, Kochanek K. Provisional life expectancy estimates for 2020. National Center for Health Statistics (U.S.); 2021. https://stacks.cdc.gov/view/cdc/107201.
10. Fredriksen-Goldsen KI, Cook-Daniels L, Kim H-J, Erosheva EA, Emlet CA, Hoy-Ellis CP, et al. Physical and mental health of transgender older adults: an at-risk and underserved population. The Gerontologist. 2014;54:488–500.
11. US Department of Health and Human Services Officer of Disease Prevention and Health Promotion. Social determinants of health literature summaries. Healthy People 2030. 2021 [cited 2021 Sep 5]. https://health.gov/healthypeople/objectives-and-data/social-determinants-health/literature-summaries.
12. Carl V, Hill P, Pérez-Stable EJ, Anderson NB, Bernard MA. The National Institute on Aging health disparities research framework. Ethn Dis. 2015;25:245–54.
13. Braveman P, Barclay C. Health disparities beginning in childhood: a life-course perspective. Pediatrics. 2009;124:S163–75.
14. Jones NL, Gilman SE, Cheng TL, Drury SS, Hill CV, Geronimus AT. Life course approaches to the causes of health disparities. Am J Public Health. 2019;109:S48–55.
15. Fredriksen-Goldsen KI, Simoni JM, Kim H-J, Lehavot K, Walters KL, Yang J, et al. The health equity promotion model: reconceptualization of lesbian, gay, bisexual, and transgender (LGBT) health disparities. Am J Orthopsychiatry. 2014;84:653.
16. American Board of Medical Specialties. ABMS Board Certification Report (2019–2020). 2020 p. 60. https://www.abms.org/wp-content/uploads/2020/11/ABMS-Board-Certification-Report-2019-2020.pdf.
17. Rodríguez JE, Campbell KM, Pololi LH. Addressing disparities in academic medicine: what of the minority tax? BMC Med Educ. 2015;15:6.

18. Metzl JM, Hansen H. Structural competency: theorizing a new medical engagement with stigma and inequality. Soc Sci Med. 2014;103:126–33.
19. Smedley BD, Stith AY, Nelson AR, editors. Unequal treatment: confronting racial and ethnic disparities in health care. Washington, DC: National Academies Press; 2003 [cited 2021 Jun 25]. http://www.ncbi.nlm.nih.gov/books/NBK220358/.
20. Liaison Committee on Medical Education. LCME® functions and structure of a medical school: standards for Accreditation of Medical Education Programs Leading to the MD Degree. 2021. https://lcme.org/publications/.
21. Severance JS, Yeo G. Ethnogeriatric education: a collaborative project of geriatric education centers. Gerontol Geriatr Educ. 2006;26:87–99.
22. Periyakoil V. Ethno med: ethnic-specific geriatric Care in the United States. ECampus Geriatr. 2010. https://geriatrics.stanford.edu/ethnomed.html.
23. Accreditation Council for Graduate Medical Education. Common program requirements; 2020. p. 52. https://www.acgme.org/Portals/0/PFAssets/ProgramRequirements/CPRResidency2020.pdf.
24. Hesselink G, Demirbas M, Rikkert MO, Schoon Y. Geriatric education programs for emergency department professionals: a systematic review. J Am Geriatr Soc. 2019;67:2402–9.
25. Hogan TM, Losman ED, Carpenter CR, Sauvigne K, Irmiter C, Emanuel L, et al. Development of geriatric competencies for emergency medicine residents using an expert consensus process. Acad Emerg Med. 2010;17:316–24.
26. Levine SA, Chao SH, Caruso LB, Jackson AH, Russell ML, Young ME, et al. Chief resident immersion training in the care of older adults: a successful national replication of an interspecialty educational intervention. Acad Med J Assoc Am Med Coll. 2018;93:1341–7.
27. Streiter S, Loewenthal J, Berry S, Schwartz AW. Better together: promoting geriatrics education across residency specialties with a pilot peer teaching exchange. J Am Geriatr Soc. 2019;67:E1–3.
28. American Geriatrics Society Ethnogeriatrics Committee. Achieving high-quality multicultural geriatric care. J Am Geriatr Soc. 2016;64:255–60.
29. Parks SM, Harper GM, Fernandez H, Sauvigne K, Leipzig RM. American Geriatrics Society/Association of Directors of Geriatric Academic Programs curricular milestones for graduating geriatric fellows. J Am Geriatr Soc. 2014;62:930–5.
30. Argueza BR, Saenz SR, McBride D. From diversity and inclusion to antiracism in medical training institutions. Acad Med. 2021;96:798–801.
31. Lundebjerg NE, Medina-Walpole AM. Future forward: AGS initiative addressing intersection of structural racism and ageism in health care. J Am Geriatr Soc. 2021;69:892–5.
32. Lundebjerg N, Drootin M, Leipzig R, Sehgal M, Schwartz A, Granville L, et al. Minimum geriatric competencies for medical students. American Geriatrics Society; 2021. https://adgap.americangeriatrics.org/sites/default/files/media/files/AGS%20Medical%20Student%20Geriatric%205Ms%20Competencies.pdf.
33. Denizard-Thompson N, Palakshappa D, Vallevand A, Kundu D, Brooks A, DiGiacobbe G, et al. Association of a Health Equity Curriculum with medical students' knowledge of social determinants of health and confidence in working with underserved populations. JAMA Netw Open. 2021;4:e210297.
34. Gonzalez CM, Fox AD, Marantz PR. The evolution of an elective in health disparities and advocacy: description of instructional strategies and program evaluation. Acad Med J Assoc Am Med Coll. 2015;90:1636–40.
35. Krishnan A, Rabinowitz M, Ziminsky A, Scott SM, Chretien KC. Addressing race, culture, and structural inequality in medical education: a guide for revising teaching cases. Acad Med. 2019;94:550–5.
36. National Association of community health centers. PRAPARE. 2019 [cited 2021 Jul 18]. https://www.nachc.org/research-and-data/prapare/.
37. Centers for Medicare & Medicaid Services Center for Medicare and Medicaid Innovation. The Accountable Health Communities Health-Related Social Needs Screening Tool. 2017 [cited 2021 Jul 18]. https://innovation.cms.gov/files/worksheets/ahcm-screeningtool.pdf.

38. Community campus partnerships for health. Faculty toolkit for service-learning in higher education. Scotts Valley: National Service-Learning Clearinghouse; 2007. p. 169. https://www.vanderbilt.edu/oacs/wp-content/uploads/sites/140/faculty-toolkit-for-service-learning.pdf.
39. Tsai J, Ucik L, Baldwin N, Hasslinger C, George P. Race matters? Examining and rethinking race portrayal in preclinical medical education. Acad Med. 2016;91:916–20.
40. Crenshaw K. Demarginalizing the intersection of race and sex: a black feminist critique of antidiscrimination doctrine, feminist theory and antiracist politics. Univ Chic Leg Forum. 1989;1989:31.
41. Vyas DA, Eisenstein LG, Jones DS. Hidden in plain sight — reconsidering the use of race correction in clinical algorithms. N Engl J Med. Massachusetts Medical Society; 2020 [cited 2021 Jun 23]. https://www.nejm.org/doi/10.1056/NEJMms2004740.
42. Nolen L. How medical education is missing the bull's-eye. N Engl J Med. Massachusetts Medical Society; 2020 [cited 2021 Jun 16]. https://www.nejm.org/doi/10.1056/NEJMp1915891.
43. Sehgal M, Syed Q, Callahan KE, Powers BB, Eleazer GP, Gleason LL, et al. Introducing aquifer geriatrics, the American Geriatrics Society national online curriculum. J Am Geriatr Soc. 2019;67:811–7.
44. Bourgois P, Holmes SM, Sue K, Quesada J. Structural vulnerability: operationalizing the concept to address health disparities in clinical care. Acad Med. 2017;92:299–307.
45. Cohen A, Lehmann L, Russell L. Systematic screening of veterans for health-related social needs: an ethical imperative. U.S. Department of Veterans Affairs; 2020. https://confluence.hl7.org/display/FHIR/CMS2021-07+Military+and+Veteran+SDOH?preview=/116458199/120094739/ACORN_(Assessing_Circumstances__Offering_Resources_for_Needs)_Screening_Tool__CMS_Connectathon_updated_citations_(071521).pdf.
46. Crisp C, Wayland S, Gordon T. Older gay, lesbian, and bisexual adults: tools for age-competent and gay affirmative practice. J Gay Lesbian Soc Serv. 2008;20:5–29.
47. Martinez IL, Mora JC. A community-based approach for integrating geriatrics and gerontology into undergraduate medical education. Gerontol Geriatr Educ. 2012;33:152–65.
48. Fitzpatrick C, Musser A, Mosqueda L, Boker J, Prislin M. Student senior partnership program: University of California Irvine School of Medicine. Gerontol Geriatr Educ. 2006;27:25–35.
49. Laks J, Wilson LA, Khandelwal C, Footman E, Jamison M, Roberts E. Service-Learning in Communities of Elders (SLICE): development and evaluation of an introductory geriatrics course for medical students. Teach Learn Med. 2016;28:210–8.
50. Milota MM, van Thiel GJMW, van Delden JJM. Narrative medicine as a medical education tool: a systematic review. Med Teach. 2019;41:802–10.
51. Daya S, Choi N, Harrison JD, Lai CJ. Advocacy in action: medical student reflections of an experiential curriculum. Clin Teach. 2021;18:168–73.
52. Chung EK, Kahn S, Altshuler M, Lane JL, Plumb J. The JeffSTARS advocacy and community partnership elective: a closer look at child health advocacy in action. MedEdPORTAL. 2016;12:10526.
53. Howell BA, Kristal RB, Whitmire LR, Gentry M, Rabin TL, Rosenbaum J. A systematic review of advocacy curricula in graduate medical education. J Gen Intern Med. 2019;34:2592–601.
54. Petriceks AH, Kumar A, Schwartz AW. The urgency of now: opportunities for advocacy among geriatrics health professionals and trainees. J Am Geriatr Soc. 2021;69:2445–8.
55. Institute of Medicine, Smedley BD, Stith Butler A, Bristow LR, editors. In the Nation's compelling interest: ensuring diversity in the health-care workforce. Washington, DC: National Academies Press (US); 2004 [cited 2021 Mar 19]. http://www.ncbi.nlm.nih.gov/books/NBK216009/.
56. United States Census Bureau. 2020 Census redistricting data (public law 94–171) summary file. Washington, DC; 2021. https://www.census.gov/library/visualizations/interactive/race-and-ethnicity-in-the-united-state-2010-and-2020-census.html.
57. Simpson CF, Durso SC, Fried LP, Bailey T, Boyd CM, Burton J. The Johns Hopkins geriatric summer scholars program: a model to increase diversity in geriatric medicine. J Am Geriatr Soc. 2005;53:1607–12.

58. Hunt JB, Bonham C, Jones L. Understanding the goals of service learning and community-based medical education: a systematic review. Acad Med. 2011;86:246–51.
59. Nuriddin A, Mooney G, White AIR. Reckoning with histories of medical racism and violence in the USA. Lancet. 2020;396:949–51.
60. Smitherman HCJ, Baker RS, Wilson MR. Socially accountable academic health centers: pursuing a quadripartite mission. Acad Med. 2019;94:176–81.
61. Bussey-Jones J, Blackman D, Fernández A, Fernández L, Horowitz C, Lee M, et al. A train the trainer guide: health disparities education. Washington, DC: Society of General Internal Medicine; 2008.
62. Dobbin F, Kalev A. Why doesn't diversity training work? The challenge for industry and academia. Anthropol Now. 2018;10:48–55.
63. Sofia SR, Titilayo A, Jordan S, Spencer D, Avik C, Daniele Ö. Building a tool kit for medical and dental students: addressing microaggressions and discrimination on the wards. MedEdPORTAL. Association of American Medical Colleges; 2020 [cited 2021 Jun 27];16. https://www.mededportal.org/doi/10.15766/mep_2374-8265.10893.
64. Sue DW, Alsaidi S, Awad MN, Glaeser E, Calle CZ, Mendez N. Disarming racial microaggressions: microintervention strategies for targets, White allies, and bystanders. Am Psychol. 2019;74:128–42.
65. Low D, Pollack SW, Liao ZC, Maestas R, Kirven LE, Eacker AM, et al. Racial/ethnic disparities in clinical grading in medical school. Teach Learn Med. 2019;31:487–96.
66. Ross DA, Boatright D, Nunez-Smith M, Jordan A, Chekroud A, Moore EZ. Differences in words used to describe racial and gender groups in medical student performance evaluations, vol. 12. PLoS One; 2017. p. e0181659.
67. Klein R, Julian KA, Snyder ED, Koch J, Ufere NN, Volerman A, et al. Gender bias in resident assessment in graduate medical education: review of the literature. J Gen Intern Med. 2019;34:712–9.
68. Teherani A, Hauer KE, Fernandez A, King TEJ, Lucey C. How small differences in assessed clinical performance amplify to large differences in grades and awards: a Cascade with serious consequences for students underrepresented in medicine. Acad Med. 2018;93:1286–92.
69. Onumah CM, Lai CJ, Levine D, Ismail N, Pincavage AT, Osman NY. Aiming for equity in clerkship grading: recommendations for reducing the effects of structural and individual bias. Am J Med. 2021;134:1175–1183.e4.

Chapter 19
Teaching Person-Centered Care in Geriatrics

Karen Chahal, Shaleen Thakur, and Susan Nathan

What Is Person-Centered Care?

In recent years there has been momentum in healthcare, and specifically geriatrics, to move toward a person-centered care approach to healthcare. This cultural shift was itself a movement away from the biopsychosocial approach that was the dominant conceptualization of the provision of healthcare starting in the late 1970s and early 1980s that recognized biological, psychological, and social factors that contribute to the health or illness of a person [1]. Before the biopsychosocial model, the dominant framework for the practice of modern western medicine focused on health solely in terms of biological factors. The biopsychosocial model was the beginning of a shift toward focusing on the individual as a whole to empower healthcare systems to consider an individual's needs and preferences beyond a patient's biological factors.

To understand this evolution, we must first understand the culture shift within the medical community that led to the introduction and adoption of the patient-centered care framework into the common vernacular. In 2001 the Institute of Medicine

K. Chahal (✉)
Beth Israel Deaconess Medical Center, Harvard Medical School, Boston, MA, USA
e-mail: kchahal@bidmc.harvard.edu

S. Thakur
Wake Forest School of Medicine, Winston-Salem, NC, USA
e-mail: sthakur@wakehealth.edu

S. Nathan
VA Boston Healthcare System, Harvard Medical School, Boston, MA, USA
e-mail: susan.nathan@va.gov

A. W. Schwartz (ed.), *Medical Education in Geriatrics*,
https://doi.org/10.1007/978-3-031-32499-4_19

published a report entitled *Crossing the Quality Chasm: A New Health System for the twenty-first Century,* in which six core components of a highly functioning healthcare system were outlined. One of those features was that an effective healthcare system must be patient-centered, defined as "providing care that is respectful of, and responsive to, individual patient preferences, needs and values, and ensuring that patient values guide all clinical decisions" [2].

The word "patient" indicates someone receiving medical, surgical, or other forms of treatment for a disorder or illness. To reduce the person to the role of patient is to pathologize the person receiving care. In substituting "person" for "patient" we go beyond this reductive definition and view first, the whole person, and subsequently the impact of their suffering, disease, or treatment on their person as a whole, and this dictates our care plans [3]. Quite broadly stated, the main goal of patient-centered healthcare is a functional life for the patient, while person-centeredness attempts to develop a meaningful life for the patient [3].

In this person-centered model the aim of the healthcare provider is to support an individual's choice and autonomy in their healthcare decisions by taking into consideration a person's values, preferences, and needs to tailor the medical plan to support these considerations [4]. In 2015, the American Geriatrics Society, in collaboration with the SCAN Foundation and research and clinical team from the Keck School of Medicine University of Southern California, established an expert panel in hopes of better defining essential elements of person-centered care and to establish a more definitive definition of this approach, specifically in relation to older adults with chronic conditions and/or functional limitations. Their definition is as follows:

> *"Person-centered care" means that individuals' values and preferences are elicited and, once expressed, guide all aspects of their health care, supporting their realistic health and life goals. Person-centered care is achieved through a dynamic relationship among individuals, others who are important to them, and all relevant providers. This collaboration informs decision-making to the extent that the individual desires* [4]

By switching the term "patient" for "person" it is implied that medical practitioners shift away from the traditional health/illness model of evaluation of the patient to a broader, holistic view of the patient as a person to include an individual's personally held beliefs, views, needs, and desires. Older adults are more likely than their younger counterparts to have complex care needs that affect their daily living, which makes this population especially suited for this shift in paradigm [5].

In 2018, researchers in Sweden published findings from a systematic review where they compared patient-centered care studies versus person-centered care studies in order to identify potentially common themes and important differences between the two [3]. They found common themes to be: empathy, respect, engagement, building relationships, enhancing communication, engaging in shared decision-making, having a holistic and individualized focus, and coordinating care [3]. A notable difference was that person-centered care evokes an important goal of "living a meaningful life": 90% of person-centered studies documented this, versus just 9% of patient-centered studies. This was in contrast to the concept of "living a functional life" where they found 91% of patient-centered studies focused on this, while 9% of person-centered studies focused on this aspect [3].

Person-Centered Care and the Geriatrics 5Ms Framework

In 2017, Tinetti, Huang, and Molnar debuted the geriatrics 5Ms—mobility, medications, mind, multicomplexity, and what matters most to patients—as a way to organize, communicate, and explain the domains of geriatric medical care. This model is both explanatory and organizational to guide clinicians' approach to the older patient and their unique needs as they age [6, 7]. In reviewing the geriatrics 5Ms through a person-centered approach, these are some considerations:

Mobility: This domain refers to a person's ability to mobilize themselves in their daily life and to assess their functional capacity to perform tasks of daily living as defined as instrumental activities of daily living (IADLs) and activities of daily living (ADLs). Mobility aides are also considered in this aspect of care. As a person-centered model, this domain includes consideration of how a mobility aide or assist device improves a person's quality of life, i.e. does using a walker help or hinder the person in safely and independently transferring out of bed in the morning and going to the bathroom on their own? Is the person able to incorporate mobility aides (i.e. walker, cane, rollator) into their daily routine without these aides adding more stress or being cumbersome during their desired activities? In reviewing the activities of daily living, one should also ask: what are the aims for this person?

In order to teach a person-centered approach to mobility we would encourage learners to go beyond simply documenting mobility to asking broader questions about how mobility impacts their lives. Such as:

- "I see you use a walker at home. Does the walker make you feel more independent?"
- "Does having a walker make getting around easier or do you find it to be cumbersome? Do you feel safer with your walker or without it?"

This type of questioning allows for more conversation with the patient and allows an easier dialogue between patient and health care provider. It establishes rapport while eliciting key information about a person's struggles, triumphs, and goals.

Medications: In reviewing medications, it is important to consider the amount of medications a person has been prescribed (i.e. polypharmacy, pill burden), the potential side effects of these medications, as well as drug–drug interactions that may impact their cognition, mobility, quality of life, and how the person is able to manage these medications at home. Do they organize the medications themselves? How do they remember to take these medications and how often do they miss a dose? Once key information is gathered we encourage the learner to go beyond the facts and inquire more about how the medications make a person feel. Such as asking:

- "I see you are prescribed 12 pills a day. Do you ever find it difficult to swallow all your medications?"
- "I see you are prescribed Drug X for this condition. How does the medication make you feel? "
- "I see you take Drug Y three times a day. I imagine that can be a difficult schedule for anyone - how do you manage that schedule?"
- "What medications have you found that impacted your life in a positive way?"

Mind: It is common for older adults to be concerned or worried about memory loss as they age. Geriatricians are trained to evaluate and consider abnormal forms of memory loss and how they may impact a person, and their loved ones. In order to teach a more person-centered approach, we suggest the learner be encouraged to ask the patient about their memory, and any worries about their memory, and how this may impact their day-to-day activities. And, if the patient permits, it is also helpful for the learner to ask about how potential memory loss may be impacting their loved ones or caretakers. Incorporating perspectives from a patient's care team broadens a clinician's understanding of the person as a whole, and can lead to more precisely tailored treatment and/or support planning. In understanding a person's baseline cognitive status, clinicians are better able to tailor pharmacological therapies and non-pharmacological therapies appropriately. For instance, a person with a mild cognitive impairment may be able to utilize a walking aide to improve their mobility, while a person of the same age with advanced dementia may not be able to use an aide due to their lack of executive planning, safety awareness, and short term memory. Major neurocognitive disorders (i.e. Alzheimer's, Vascular Dementia, etc) severely impact a person's own sense of self and identify and also for those around them. If an abnormal memory loss is identified in an older adult, healthcare providers should rely heavily on a person's values and belief systems when devising an overall healthcare plan that will support both patient and their loved ones through this chronic and irreversible diagnosis.

Multicomplexity: The multicomplexity "M" speaks to the interwoven nature of a person's medications, medical conditions, social determinants of health and function along with their personal values and goals—these interplay together to form a person-centered plan of action for their healthcare. This is where we contemplate a person's identities and what they mean to them. Individuals rarely have one singular identity to which they ascribe all of themselves - it is more common that an individual has a myriad of identities that come together to make a person unique. Asking a person about their sexual identity, gender-preference and gender identity, race, education, socioeconomic status, marital/relationship status and belief or non-belief in spirituality will greatly inform a healthcare provider to the person as a whole and complex individual. Understanding and showing interest in a person's identities and preferences will lead to better rapport and trust and the information gathered will contribute to a tailored approach to any healthcare challenge an individual may be facing. It is also an important time to consider a person's accessibility to equitable healthcare and understand their social determinants of health. For more on this important topic, please refer to Chap. 18.

Matters Most: When asking a patient about what matters most to them, we inherently move away from viewing them as a "patient" and rather focus on the patient as a person. Exploring and identifying goals may be as broad as "I want to live long enough to see my grandchildren live healthy lives," or as specific as "I want to live long enough to see my roses bloom in my garden next month." Some questions to elicit these goals might include: In the future, how do you want to be there for your loved ones? What does your ideal day look like? When you think of your future, what do you still want to accomplish? A person's stated goal may be as seemingly simple as "I want to be able to stay at our vacation home every summer." By asking what matters most to someone, we are afforded valuable insight into what motivates them to stay connected to their health care team, their health care plan, and how we can accommodate them holistically. For more on patient priorities care please refer to Chap. 20.

A Person Centered Approach to the Social History

In medical school, physicians-in-training are taught to take a thorough history of present illness as part of a new evaluation of each patient. Included in this assessment is a Social History. Often, this part of the evaluation is sparse and diluted down to document the history of potentially harmful habits such as alcohol use, tobacco use, and illicit drug use. This focused social history is centered on a disease-based approach, given that these behaviors may impact a person's disease or disease risk. The social history may include demographic information such as marital status, number of children, type of housing or current/former occupation, and language preference, but there is wide variability in what may or may not be included in a social history.

In taking a person-centered approach to healthcare, trainees should be encouraged to revive the social history and elevate it in the full assessment of a patient. There is now more understanding, supported by growing literature and published studies, regarding the various social, educational, environmental and economic factors that contribute to an individual's access to or lack of access to equitable healthcare, referred to collectively as Social Determinants of Health (SDOH). The SDOH vantage point into a person's background helps place their story and history front and center translating into a more meaningful evaluation, assessment and plan [8]. Geriatrics educators should incorporate this approach in their visits to model for trainees they work with.

One example of a successful incorporation of elevating the social history in clinical practice is the My Life, My Story (MLMS) program which originated within the Veterans Health Administration (VHA) [9]. This program was developed out of the tradition of life story work (LSW), a teaching method that has been employed in geriatric education in which a trainee interviews an older adult about their background from childhood to older adulthood and documents these findings from their interview in narrative form. LSW promotes intergenerational interaction, teaching lifespan developmental principles and reduces ageism and stigma by the nature of the exercise itself for both patient and provider [10]. MLMS was developed in 2015 at the William S. Middleton VA and has spread to 67 VA medical centers across the USA, and beyond the VA to other non-VA medical centers. In this program, interviewers perform a semi-structured life story interview guided by standard questions and construct a 1000 word first-person narrative. The veteran has the opportunity to review the story and with the veteran's permission the story is entered into the electronic medical record as a resource for the healthcare team [9].

One study of MLMS at VA Boston found that trainees who participated as writer/interviewers felt this experience was a good use of their time. It allowed them to understand the whole person, allowed the interviewer to show empathy, build relationships and trainees found value in this exercise as a specific contrast to usual medical care. One trainee participant noted in anonymous post-experience feedback that: *We can sometimes forget that our patients are more than their medical/psychiatric conditions. They are whole people with a lifetime of history that is influencing how they are coping with their condition and interacting with their providers. I think that the project allows us as providers to remember this and might also be a reminder to the patient that they are more than their medical conditions* [9]. To ensure that trainees are able to incorporate MLMS into their educational experience, we can look to formats suggested by the faculty implementation guide, dependent on the trainee's clinical setting, and rotation duration: (1) Inpatient Setting 1—all in one session during a blocked off afternoon/evening with all aspects completed in one sitting with the patient; (2) Inpatient Setting 2—in segments over the course of a few days, doing the interview on one day, writing the interview the next, and then the read back the next; (3) Outpatient Setting 1—all in one visit, similar to Inpatient Setting 1; (4) Outpatient Setting 2—at various time points, questions asked with the patient at one visit with the read back occurring at following visits, great for a longitudinal experience; (5) Outpatient Setting 3—one question at a time at each clinical encounter, also great for a longitudinal experience for the learner [9].

The My Life, My Story program [9], while framed as a patient-centered care intervention, illustrates the use of narrative, first-person interview and veteran life story, to be incorporated directly into the clinical rotation experience of an interprofessional group of trainees doing rotations throughout a VA medical center. The action of placing that veteran's life story, in their own words and containing content they deem important to include, in contrast to the traditional social history as mentioned above, is one concrete tool to teach person-centered care and the relevant supporting documents including trainee and faculty implementation guide are freely accessible on the internet [11]. As summarized by a trainee comment: *Firstly, a patient is more than their diagnosis; they are a person with a past and a life and feelings. Knowing their background may make it easier for the team to empathize with them or understand their current behavior better* [9].

Strategies to Teach Person-Centered Care

Person-centered care has the potential to improve the quality of care as well as experiences and outcomes of care in terms of an individual's interactions with their healthcare providers by asking "'What matters to you?' as well as 'What is the matter?'" [12]. There are still challenges with how to operationalize this concept and overcome barriers of implementing these changes. Ultimately, there must be a shift in cultures to enact this complex task—instilling a new culture around engagement with a person to safeguard these values and attitudes [3].

When approaching a patient from a "person-centered" approach it is important to gain the knowledge and input from these interdisciplinary teams when formulating an assessment and plan of action. Enhancing attitudes toward team-based healthcare and improving interaction among these interdisciplinary providers improves understanding and care in a person-centered approach [13].

Geriatrics is a team-based discipline that incorporates expertise from many professions working in tandem including the physician, physical and occupational therapists, nurses, care coordinators or managers, social workers, health care attendants, pharmacists, cognitive and behavioral specialists, and other healthcare specialists. In addition, incorporating an older person's primary caregiver or caregivers is paramount to exploring the feasibility of existing care plans and how best to incorporate meaningful changes.

In the hopes of focusing on the person and their values a fundamental change in the structure of a healthcare system would need to be addressed. In a 2017 study entitled "How to practice person-centered care: A conceptual framework" the authors identify three pillars of organizational structure that need to be addressed. The largest piece is addressing the structure of an organization by creating a culture surrounding person-centered care as a goal and value of the healthcare system, such as creating a mission statement and educational opportunities for healthcare providers around this topic. In addition, the system would need to be supportive of those individual healthcare providers committed to person-centered care with regular feedback mechanisms in place to work on quality improvement and monitor progress, challenges, and potential barriers. The second level of this work is in the process of a healthcare system by cultivating communication, rewarding and encouraging respectful and compassionate care, and integrating care across disciplines for the individual. The third pillar is based on outcome measures such as ensuring access to this kind of care for all patients within the system and monitoring patient-reported outcomes to gauge success and challenges [14].

In one study conducted at the Michael E. DeBakey Veterans Affairs Medical Center the investigators implemented a Patient Priorities Care (PPC) framework, the aim of which is to align patient priorities with the care they receive, in a geriatrics outpatient clinic (note, PPC is further discussed in Chap. 20). In the intervention cohort a dedicated clinician facilitator performed an intake focused on identifying a person's healthcare priorities and then document the results of this intake in the electronic medical records where their primary care providers could easily access this information, versus the usual care. In the cohort where this intervention occurred, they found that those who had fewer prescription medications had more referrals to community services and supports and more priorities-aligned self-management tasks to their care plan [15].

Given the vast benefits to patients seen through PCC programs such as the VA's Whole Health (https://www.va.gov/wholehealth/), educators should emphasize and integrate the PCC approach in their teachings to trainees. We can look to utilizing standardized patient exercises as seen in the *VICTORS* study [16] and developing 90-min workshops introducing trainees to a patient's experience through a video, a first-person memoir of said experience, and then an exercise to practice using PCC language in the patient's EMR as demonstrated in the workshop presented at AADPRT in March 2016 [17]. Such activities would help set trainees up for success in utilizing person-centered care in every one of their clinical encounters.

Teaching Person-Centered Care While Teaching Geriatrics Education: Necessary and Feasible

Effective care of an older adult in a healthcare context requires high level interprofessional collaboration, careful consideration of the intersections of biologic, social, and environment factors and always at the core demands a recognition of the rich lived experience that older adult brings with them to this current moment in time. Placing each unique person central to this nuanced and intricate web of care that many of our patients may require enhances the likelihood that their personhood remains an integral part of their care despite facing potential diminution of some of those core elements to the external observer. The healthcare system can create barriers to provision of such care, whether in the form of time constraints or algorithms that are not designed to capture the needs and experience of older adults. Despite these challenges it remains necessary and is feasible to imbue trainees in geriatrics with concrete skills to provide person-centered care. Teaching these skills may be integrated in the already nuanced teaching provided to learners in geriatric settings. By coming to each patient encounter with curiosity about the uniqueness of that individual person as our touchstone, this cultural shift can continue to move forward.

References

1. Engel GL. The clinical application of the biopsychosocial model. Am J Psychiatry. 1980;13(7):535–44.
2. Institute of Medicine (US) Committee on Quality of Health Care in America. Crossing the quality chasm: a new health system for the 21st century. Washington, DC: National Academies Press (US); 2001. PMID: 25057539.

3. Håkansson Eklund J, Holmström IK, Kumlin T, Kaminsky E, Skoglund K, Höglander J, et al. "Same same or different?" A review of reviews of person-centered and patient-centered care. Patient Educ Couns. 2019;102(1):3–11.
4. Person-centered care: a definition and essential elements. J Am Geriatr Soc. 2015;64(1):15–8.
5. Kogan AC, Wilber K, Mosqueda L. Person-centered care for older adults with chronic conditions and functional impairment: a systematic literature review. J Am Geriatr Soc. 2015;64(1):e1.
6. Tinetti M, Huang A, Molnar F. The geriatrics 5m's: a new way of communicating what we do. J Am Geriatr Soc. 2017;65(9):2115.
7. Phillips SC, Hawley CE, Triantafylidis LK, Schwartz AW. Geriatrics 5Ms for primary care workshop. MedEdPORTAL. 2019;15(1):10814.
8. Pooler J, Srinivasan M. Social determinants of health and the aging population. AARP Foundation and IMPAQ International; 2018.
9. Nathan S, Fiore LL, Saunders S, Vilbrun-Bruno PA-CSO, Hinrichs KLM, Ruopp MD, et al. My life, my story: teaching patient centered care competencies for older adults through life story work. Gerontol Geriatr Educ. 2019;43:1–14.
10. Life story work. Dementia UK; 8 April 2021. https://www.dementiauk.org/life-story-work/. Accessed 19 April 2022.
11. https://www.va.gov/boston-health-care/work-with-us/internships-and-fellowships/my-life-my-story/. Accessed 12 June 2022.
12. Barry MJ, Edgman-Levitan S. Shared decision making — the pinnacle of patient-centered care. N Engl J Med. 2012;366(9):780–1. https://doi.org/10.1056/nejmp1109283.
13. Williams B, Remington T, Foulk M. Teaching interdisciplinary geriatrics team care. Acad Med. 2002;77(9):935.
14. Santana MJ, Manalili K, Jolley RJ, Zelinsky S, Quan H, Lu M. How to practice person-centred care: a conceptual framework. Health Expect. 2017;21(2):429–40.
15. Freytag J, Dindo L, Catic A, Johnson AL, Bush Amspoker A, Gravier A, et al. Feasibility of clinicians aligning health care with patient priorities in geriatrics ambulatory care. J Am Geriatr Soc. 2020;68(9):2112–6.
16. Lypson ML, Ravindranath D, Ross PT, Pfeiffer P, Griggs JJ, Buckler S, Whitman L, Tremblay A, Weiner S, Fitzgerald JT. Veteran interactive cases to reinforce service (victors): standardized patient assessment of veteran-centered care. MedEdPORTAL. 2016; https://doi.org/10.15766/mep_2374-8265.10326.
17. Stagno S, Crapanzano K, Schwartz A. Keeping the patient at the center: teaching about elements of patient-centered care. MedEdPORTAL. 2016;12:10500. https://doi.org/10.15766/mep_2374-8265.10500.

Chapter 20
Teaching Communication and Goals of Care in Geriatrics

Angela G. Catic

Introduction

Communication skills, crucial to providing high-quality, patient-centered care, are recognized as essential in geriatrics education [1, 2]. However, the care of older adults can be associated with a number of communication challenges secondary to increasing medical complexity, cognitive impairment, sensory impairment, low health literacy, and frequent involvement of surrogate decision makers. It is imperative to recognize and address these challenges as poor communication is associated with a variety of undesirable outcomes including decreased mediation adherence, clinical outcomes, and patient/family satisfaction [3, 4]. Fortunately, research has determined that communication skills can be codified that providers can learn them with training, and, most importantly, that acquiring improved communication skills improves clinical outcomes [5]. Implementing education among geriatrics trainees and providers regarding methods to enhance communication, both during ongoing or current care and at the end-of-life, is critical to optimizing the care of older adults. In addition, individuals working in geriatrics must be aware of health literacy challenges commonly faced by older adults and how these can most effectively be addressed. Generalized and structured communication strategies are available and can be effectively incorporated into geriatric focused education (Chart 20.1).

A. G. Catic (✉)
Michael E. DeBakey VA Medical Center, Baylor College of Medicine, Houston, TX, USA
e-mail: acatic@bcm.edu

A. W. Schwartz (ed.), *Medical Education in Geriatrics*,
https://doi.org/10.1007/978-3-031-32499-4_20

Chart 20.1 Selected communication models relevant to geriatric medical education

Communication model	Focus	Patient outcomes	Educational outcomes
Patient Priorities Care [30]	Shared decision-making framework to align healthcare decision-making and care with patient health priorities	• Decrease in treatment burden	• Interactive, case-based virtual education for interprofessional learners
		• Decreased undesired care	• High satisfaction and confidence for skills related to patient aligned decision-making
		• Increased documentation of health priorities	• Identification of need for practice change
SPIKES Model [38]	Communication model for breaking bad news	• Varying degrees of compliance with steps of the model	• Literature regarding in-person and virtual education
		• Identification of the summary portion and privacy as critical to successful conversation	• Positive results in ability to use the model during role-playing and simulated encounters
Geritalk [46]	Communication skills training program focused on patients with serious illness	• Increased use of communication skills during family meetings	• Literature regarding in-person and virtual education
			• Increased learner self-assessed preparedness for specific communication challenges
Serious Illness Care Program [48, 51]	Multicomponent, structured communication intervention program for patients with serious illness	• Decreased symptoms of anxiety and depression among patients	• Multimodality instruction with reflection, didactic, and role-playing
		• Significant percentage of patients reported receiving the right amount of information at the right time	• Best practices available
		• Clinicians reported program was feasible and led to enhanced patient care	

Chart 20.1 (continued)

Communication model	Focus	Patient outcomes	Educational outcomes
Veterans Health Administration Life-Sustaining Treatment Initiative [53]	Standardization of communication around end-of-life decisions, including elicitation, documentation, and implementation of veterans' goals of care and life-sustaining treatment decisions	• Completion of life-sustaining treatment decision documentation in >100,000 veterans during first 7 months of initiative	• Variety of education materials with primary focus on train-the-trainer model
		• Association with patient-centered, quality care	• Profession specific skills training programs

General Communication Skills

Until relatively recently, most clinicians did not receive specific instruction on communication but were expected to learn how to communicate with patients and family members during medical practice. However, research has determined that clinicians who do not receive communication training have variable skills and do not reliably improve with time or experience [6]. For optimal communication, a number of skills beyond simply gathering information must be considered including creating and sustaining a therapeutic relationship; adapting communication to meet individual patient needs; facilitation of shared decision-making; and negotiating patient-centered treatment plans [7]. To most effectively teach communication skills, it is critical that instructors be trained in teaching and assessing communication skills using specific communication frameworks (i.e. Patient Priorities Care, Geritalk, etc.). Communication skills should be introduced early in medical education and, ideally, continued through all years of training and practice to ensure increasing skills over time and permanent understanding. Literature suggests that communication skill programs which employ practical or experimental components, including simulation, self-reflection through video recordings, and role-playing, are more effective than those that rely more heavily on didactics [8]. Thoughtful feedback from skilled communicators, both in formal communication training and during clinical encounters, allows for longitudinal improvement of communication skills among trainees and practicing clinicians.

Health Literacy in Older Adults

Health literacy, which can be understood as the cognitive and social skills necessary to gain access to, understand, and use information to manage health conditions, is determined by a variety of personal, situational, cultural, and healthcare system factors [9, 10]. Health literacy can be classified into three different categories which denote the impact that skill differences may have on healthcare decisions and actions [11].

1. **Functional health literacy** consists of basic-level skills which allow individuals to obtain relevant health information and apply this to a range of prescribed actions.
2. **Interactive health literacy** refers to more advanced skills by which individuals are not only able to obtain health information but are facile with different forms of communication, can apply information to changing circumstances, and can engage with others to process information and make decisions. Individuals with interactive health literacy are more successfully able to access healthcare information which is interactive and available through structured communication channels such as interactive websites and mobile apps.
3. Individuals with the most advanced health literacy skills, termed **critical health literacy**, can obtain and use information to have greater control of situations impacting their health. Examples of critical health literacy skills include evaluating information regarding personal health risks; understanding social, environmental, and economic determinants of health; and engaging in collective action to improve healthcare policy.

Compared to younger individuals, older adults are more likely to have health literacy which is "below basic," with only 3% of individuals age 65 years or older demonstrating "proficient" health literacy [12]. Among older adults, 71% have difficulty using print materials, 80% demonstrate difficulty using forms or charts, and 68% have difficulty interpreting numbers and doing calculations [13].

Appropriate communication strategies can maximize health literacy in older adults. These are multifaceted and include avoiding medical jargon; providing focused information; repeating or providing information in multiple formats (i.e. verbal and written); and prioritizing in-person, face-to-face communication whenever possible. Written educational materials should be reviewed to ensure ease of understanding and readability. Visual aids, including simple illustrations, infographics, and videos, can be very useful in reinforcing verbal and written communication. Healthcare providers should ensure understanding by asking open-ended questions to review comprehension and using a "show back" technique to verify patients understanding of medical device use. Although the "teach-back" communication method is often employed to assess for patient understanding, this technique is less reliable in older adults who suffer from executive dysfunction since they may be able to repeat instructions but unable to implement complex medical tasks at home [14, 15]. In these situations, it is crucial to involved caregivers in communication to ensure important healthcare instructions are understood and carried out.

The ability to access and use e-health tools, digital resources designed to help individuals find health information, make health-related decisions, and manage their health are important components of health literacy. Most e-health tools are accessed via the Intranet. The ability to access and use them effectively is significantly influenced by technical skills (i.e. comfort with the Internet, ability to navigate websites) and cognitive function. Among older adults, reasoning, working memory, and perceptual speed are significant predictors of the ability to perform effective health-related Internet searches [16]. Appropriate communication from healthcare providers can help to bridge the digital divide faced by many older adults. This includes providing clear written instructions regarding how to access specific online resources, recommending resources with content geared specifically to older adults, and having staff who can demonstrate e-health tools to patients and caregivers. Specific recommendations for assisting older adults and their caregivers with technology are available through The Gerontological Society of America and include assisting Internet-savvy older adults in finding reputable online sources of medical information and support and how to collaboratively use technology during in-person visits [17].

Multiple programs are available which focus on education regarding health literacy and communication. While many focus on pediatrics or general health literacy, the "Geriatric Health Literacy Workshop for Medical Students and Residents" is a 2.5 h hands-on educational experience focused on the unique health literacy dynamics of older adults. It includes brief didactic, role-playing using "teach-back cases," and use of the Suitability of Assessment of Materials (SAM) tool to review patient educational materials [18, 19]. Additional instructional resources regarding health literacy in older adults are available on The Portal of Geriatrics Online Education, including a recorded professional development didactic on the topic and a health literacy kit "Health Literacy and Patient Safety: Help Patients Understand" through the AMA Foundation [20].

Incorporating standardized patients in health literacy education is an innovative method to enhance the engagement of learners with a topic which is traditionally taught via didactic. In a 4-week family medicine clerkship at the Wake Forest School of Medicine, third-year medical students participate in five case-based seminars regarding recognition of problems and solutions associated with low health literacy [21]. Specific seminar topics included common ground, health literacy, implicit bias, mindfulness training, and diabetes care. The students then participate in 20-min standardized patient encounters that include a focused interview, exam, treatment plan, and completion of a SOAP note. This is followed by 2 weeks of team-based clinical teaching followed by a repeat standardized patient encounter. Health literacy competency for the standardized patient encounters is evaluated using seven questions from the US Health Resources and Services Administration (HRSA) health literacy website [22]. These included identifying "red flags" and risk factors for limited health literacy; using newest vital sign scores to tailor dialogue with patient; tailoring information given to the patient to address their health literacy level and cultural background; presenting manageable amounts of information in plain language; summarizing patient education and follow-up plan based on patient's level of understanding; utilizing the interactive techniques to verify patient understanding of the information given; and adjusting instructional methods appropriate to the patient's level of understanding based on teach-back. In analysis of the program, students demonstrated significant improvement in the use of the health literacy checklist between the standardized patient encounters. This model provides a framework for interactive, iterative health-literacy education which can be adapted to diverse clinical settings and learner groups.

Current Care Communication

Although end-of-life communication skills are generally introduced in medical school and training continues through fellowship and beyond, typically during palliative medicine rotations or focused continuing medical education offerings, instruction regarding optimizing communication during routine care is less common. Shared decision-making, including the Patient Priorities Care framework, is an important tool to improving current care communication.

Shared Decision-Making

Shared decision-making (SDM), a process through which medical providers present options and review risks/benefits and patients discuss their preferences and values, enables everyone involved to have increased understanding of all relevant factors and reach a nuanced decision [23]. Literature on SDM has found it to be associated improved patient outcomes including increased knowledge, more accurate perception of risk, increased consistency between values and decisions, increased satisfaction with the decision-making process, and less decisional conflict [24, 25]. SDM is particularly relevant in geriatrics given the high degree of medical complexity, heterogeneity of patient values, and limited evidence base due to minimal inclusion of medical complex, functionally impaired older adults in studies. SDM can be optimized by robust generalized communication training and implementation of patient decision aids. Patient decision aids, tools that provide evidence-based, objective information including risks/benefits of treatment options, can increase patient participation in decision-making and increase the likelihood that the treatment decision aligns with patient values [26]. Decision aids, some of which are intended for patient use and others to be used by the patient and medical provider, include videos, written materials, web-based tools, and apps. In selecting patient decision aids for use by or with older adults, their individual health literacy needs and any cognitive impairment should be considered.

Teaching SDM is an important role for geriatric educators. For healthcare providers to skillfully facilitate shared decision-making encounters, they must be comfortable serving as a decision facilitator, accommodate for any communication challenges with the older adults, and incorporate caregivers as appropriate [27]. The Communication Skills Training and Research ("Comskil") Laboratory at Memorial Sloan Kettering Cancer Center was created to train healthcare providers in communication skills, including development of a *Geriatric Shared Decision-Making* module developed to train oncology providers to communicate with older adults and their caregivers in a manner which promotes shared decision-making [28]. The module consisted of a brief didactic focused on communication and SDM strategies; a video modeling the key strategies and skills of SDM; and a substantial period of time engaging in experiential role play. Eight strategies for SDM, with related skills and process tasks, were taught and evaluated. Results were significant for high healthcare provider satisfaction with the module and increased self-efficacy in using communication skills for geriatric SDM. A subset of participants engaged in standardized patient assessment which demonstrated improvement in declaring an agenda, inviting an agenda, and checking preferences.

Patient Priorities Care

Secondary to provider uncertainty and lack of evidence to guide care in older adults with multiple chronic conditions, patients frequently receive care that is burdensome, fragmented, siloed, and may not be consistent with what matters most to them. In response, Patient Priorities Care (PPC), a SDM framework that aligns healthcare decision-making and care by all clinicians with patient health priorities, was developed (Fig. 20.1) [29, 30]. At the core of the PPC process is the identification of patient health priorities. Through conversations with a facilitator or using a self-directed website, patients have the opportunity to consider their core values or what matters most [31]. Value categories to consider include connection, managing health, functioning, and enjoying life. Once core values are identified, they are used

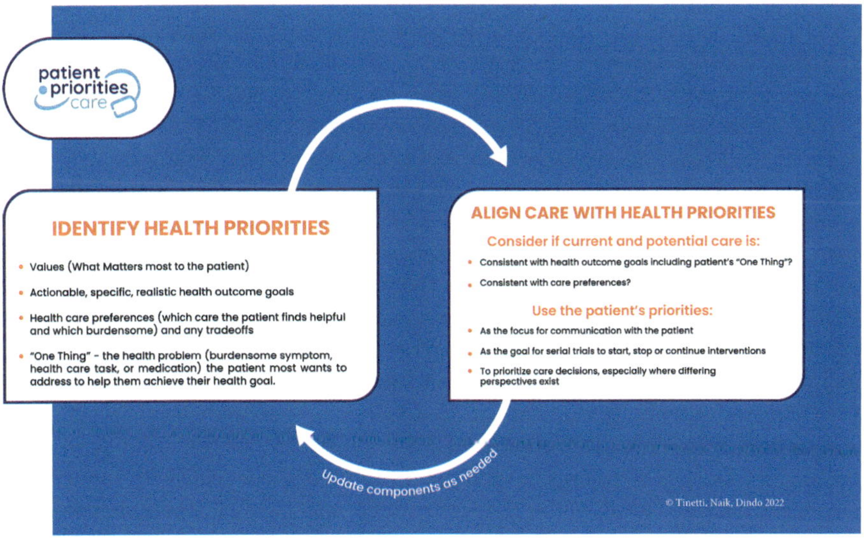

Fig. 20.1 Patient priorities care flowchart. (Printed with permission from Dr. Mary Tinetti and Dr. Aanand Naik)

to formulate one or two realistic, meaningful health outcome goals. Formulating goals that are specific and actionable is critical to ensuring they can be monitored over time as a barometer of care plan success. During the care alignment portion of PPC, clinicians work with patients to identify at least one healthcare activity that is helping with and one that is interfering with them achieving the identified goal. By considering tradeoffs of current and potential medical interventions, including medications, self-management tasks, supportive services, medical appointments, testing, and procedures, care is aligned with the patient's priorities and health trajectory. Strategies which can be employed in this process include using the patient's priorities as the focus of communication and decision-making; implementing serial trials to determine optimal interventions; and aligning decision-making among clinicians with the patient's priorities when there are differing perspectives or recommendations. When engaging in PPC communication, it is important to realize that these strategies are not sequential or mutually exclusive. Typically, they will be used in combination. The PPC Decision Guidance tool provides details about using the strategies as well as advice for troubleshooting common challenges which arise during the process of aligning decisions with health priorities. It is important to revisit the elicitation of values and goals with subsequent realignment of care after patients experience a significant medical or life events.

Implementation of the PPC framework is associated with improved patient and provider outcomes. In a nonrandomized clinical trial including 163 adults aged 65 years or older with three or more chronic conditions, the PPC cohort had a 5-point greater decrease on the Treatment Burden Questionnaire score compared to individuals in the usual care group [32]. Considering healthcare tasks and interventions, PPC participants were more likely to have medication stopped (adjusted odds ratio [APR], 2.05), were less likely to have diagnostic tests ordered (AOR, 0.22), and had fewer self-management tasks added (AOR, 0.59). Subjects in the PPC group were also much more likely to have documentation by the provider regarding discussion or decision-making regarding health priorities (66.3% in the PPC versus 0% in the usual care group). A retrospective chart review of older veterans with multiple medical conditions receiving PPC versus usual care demonstrated similar findings including consistent documentation of patient priorities and evidence of appropriate care alignment including the addition of fewer medications ($P = 0.05$), more referrals to community services and supports ($P = 0.03$), and the addition of more priorities aligned self-management tasks ($P = 0.005$) in patients receiving PPC versus usual care [33]. Clinicians engaging in PPC also perceived several benefits including more patient centered, less burdensome care; increased patient knowledge and activation; improved communication focused on patient priorities; enhanced patient provider relationships; and improved clinical workflow [34].

Interactive, case-based virtual education in patient priorities aligned care, focused on the PPC framework, has successfully been conducted for interprofessional learners including geriatric medicine fellows, geriatric psychiatry fellows, palliative care fellows, internal medicine residents, geriatric pharmacy students, and practicing providers [35]. A post-session survey of participants was significant for high satisfaction and increased confidence for all skills related to patient aligned decision-making including identifying the values of patients; identifying the health-care preferences of patients; developing specific and measurable goals based on patients' values; assessing how patients' priorities align with current care; communicating available treatment options based on patient priorities; collaborating with patients on shared goals for care; and making treatment recommendations to accomplish shared goals. The majority of respondents identified a need for practice changes after the session with primary themes including "identifying what matters most and patient care preferences," "developing specific and measurable health outcome goals," and "communicating treatment choices in alignment with patient priorities."

End-of-Life Care Communication

As is the case in current care communication, effective communication at the end-of-life is associated with improved outcomes. These include improved patient satisfaction, optimal transition to hospice care, and increased caregiver satisfaction [36]. Unfortunately, there are multiple barriers to effective end-of-life communication including uncertainty regarding when to initiate conversations due to uncertain clinical trajectories, lack of clarity between providers regarding who should engage in end-of-life conversations, discomfort in engaging in end-of-life communication, and disagreement between patients and caregivers regarding goals of care [37]. Communication models and focused communication skills training programs to address end-of-life care, as well as breaking bad news, include SPIKES, Geritalk, the Serious Illness Care Program, and the Veterans Health Administration Life-Sustaining Treatment Initiative [38–41].

SPIKES: A Communication Tool for Breaking Bad News

Breaking bad news, while not always a component of end-of-life communication, is a frequent occurrence as older adults experience acute life-threatening illness or life-limiting progression of chronic illness. The SPIKES protocol, developed for breaking bad news in oncology patients, has been widely disseminated to enhance difficult conversations in other areas of medicine [38]. SPIKES is an acronym which describes sequential steps in breaking bad news: setting up, perception, invitation, knowledge, emotions, and strategy and summary. Implementation of SPIKES, in conjunction with experiential teaching methods such as role play, has been associated with increased confidence among graduate medical education trainees and faculty in breaking bad news using the protocol. In a survey of 226 oncology patients in whom the SPIKES protocol was implemented during disclosure of a malignancy diagnosis, subjects noted varying levels of compliance with the protocol: Setting up (70.6%), Perception (27.7%), Invitation (30.4%), Knowledge (72.8%), Emotions

(75.3%), and Strategy and Summary (56.9%) [42]. Subjects agreed that the Summary portion is critical to success of the overall conversation and significant improvement could be made in this communication. The authors note that more attention should be given to this final step as patients will not perceive the interaction as having gone well if they do not understand the follow-up plan. Ensuring privacy during the conversation was also noted to highly influence subject perception of the conversation ($p < 0.01$).

The SPIKES protocol is commonly included in educational activities on breaking bad news. While this has traditionally occurred during in-person sessions, innovations have been added to allow for virtual instruction during the COVID-19 pandemic. In-person education on SPIKES typically includes application of the model to prepared cases and engaging in role-playing or standardized patient encounters. At the University of Texas Health Science Center, a 12-h curriculum, which included use of the SPIKES protocol for breaking bad news, was implemented for fourth-year medical students participating in a palliative care elective [43]. Students used the SPIKES protocol to respond to a sequential case scenario in which they played the role of the fictious patient's primary care provider. Following their initial responses, students were informed regarding the actual trajectory of the patient on whom the case was based and were provided with an opportunity to revise what they would do for the patient. The students demonstrated an ability to use the SPIKES protocol but were noted to use strategic ambiguity and curative talk when the protocol did not align with the reality of the diagnosis or the communication goal of the student. This highlights the need for ongoing mentorship of trainees as they learn to break bad news and for incorporation of an interprofessional approach. One virtual educational module to teach SPIKES to nursing students consisted of a multifaceted educational experience which included a narrated PowerPoint, an article on breaking bad news, a communication challenge activity, and a tele-simulation activity with simulated patients [44]. The interaction between the nursing student and standardized patient was observed by nursing peers and instructors. Following the simulated encounter, a debriefing was held where the nursing student and standardized patient shared their experience and feeling regarding the encounter with a focus on performance of each step of the SPIKES protocol.

Geritalk: Effective Communication with Older Adults and Their Families

Geritalk, a communication skills training program, was developed in response to lack of formal communication curricula in many geriatric fellowship programs and reports by trainees that communication education was inadequate [39]. Based on the evidence-based, interactive teaching methods of Oncotalk, Geritalk sought to improve the communication skills of fellows during interactions with patients with serious illness and their families [45]. When conducted in-person, Geritalk consists of a 2-day retreat which includes large-group overview sessions and small-group skills practice. The large-group instruction focuses on specific communication tasks including basic communication skills, giving bad news, negotiating goals of care, and forgoing life-sustaining treatment. Following these presentations, participants engage in small-group sessions where they have an opportunity to practice the recently presented skills and receive feedback for faculty and other participants. At the conclusion of the retreat, participants identify two communication skills they wish to practice over the coming month. The impact of Geritalk was assessed through three anonymous surveys including baseline assessment, process measures, and outcome measures. The course resulted in a significant increase in self-assessed preparedness for specific communication challenges, including expressing empathy, conducting a family conference, and discussing various treatment options. Additionally, participants reported a high frequency of deliberate skills practice, including expressing empathy, avoiding jargon, exploring with open-ended questions, and asking family members what the patient would have wanted, following completion of the course. Among fellows who had completed the Geritalk course, subsequent evaluation of performance during family meetings found a greater than 20% improvement in the use of applicable skills, assessed using a real-time Family Meeting Communication Assessment Tool (FaMCAT) [46].

Secondary to the onset of the COVID-19 pandemic in 2020, there was an increased need for communication skills training and a shift to virtual instruction. In response, the Geritalk course was redesigned to occur via a virtual format over 4 days [47]. Compared to prior outcomes of in-person Geritalk instruction, participants reported comparable and significant improvement in mean self-reported preparedness in all surveyed communication skills including giving bad news; conducting a family conference; expressing empathy; discussing various treatment options, including comfort care; discussing discontinuation of life-sustaining treatments; discussing religious or spiritual issues; and eliciting concerns at the end-of-life.

Serious Illness Care Program

The Serious Illness Care Program (SICP), a multicomponent, structured communication intervention, was developed to improve conversations regarding values and goals in patients with serious illness [40]. While initially developed for oncology providers, the program is extremely relevant to geriatric care as areas of focus include optimizing alignment between patient goals and medical care as well as enhancing quality of life throughout late stage illness. In addition to including many aspects common to communication guides for breaking bad news (i.e., understanding, information preferences, prognosis), the SICP structures conversations using a seven-item Serious Illness Conversation Guide (SICG) which includes discussion of patient goals, fears/worries, function, tradeoffs, and family. SICP and the SICG were evaluated using a prospective, cluster-randomized controlled trial. Enrollees included oncology physicians, nurse practitioners, physician assistants, and ambulatory oncology patients with their surrogates. Clinicians underwent a 2.5 h training program to develop competencies including a number of communications skills: use of silence, facilitating patient talk; acknowledging and responding to patient/family emotion; eliciting patient concerns; assessing patient receptivity; recognizing appropriate time for exploration and for making a recommendation; identifying key challenges in using the SICG and strategies for addressing them; and use of follow-up questions to further explore unclear or limited patient responses. Initial assessment of the intervention was null for the co-primary outcomes of goal-concordant care and peacefulness at the end-of-life and the secondary outcome of therapeutic alliance [48]. However, significant improvement was noted in symptoms of depression and anxiety among patients in the intervention group.

A secondary analysis from the initial trail was performed to evaluate patient and clinician experience using the SICG [49]. Seventy-nine percent of patients who had a SICG discussion with their physician responded to the survey. Of the respondents, 79% described the conversation as somewhat (16%), very much (42%), or extremely worthwhile (21%). With communication guided by the SICG, 64% of patients reported receiving the right amount of information from the discussion and 64% stated that the conversation was held at the right time. Ninety-five percent of clinicians who engaged in a SICG discussion completed a survey regarding their experience. Overall, they reported that the method was feasible to use with 87% somewhat or strongly agreeing that the guide allows for discussion in a timely manner and 77% somewhat or strongly agreeing that it was easy to use. In addition, compared to usual care, physicians reported that use of the SICG led to enhanced clinical care of the patient (95%) and that they learned something surprising about the patient (90%). Among providers engaging in conversations using the SICG, 70% note a slight or great increase in satisfaction with their role in patient care.

A follow-up of the SICP was conducted with 23 clinicians (19 general internists, 3 nurse practitioners, and 1 social worker), who were not involved in the original development or evaluation, to assess their experience 1 year after the program was implemented [50]. Goals of the study included evaluating which elements of SICP implementation (1) Supported changes in provider behavior, (2) Shifted the focus of goals of care conversations beyond code status, and (3) Influenced clinicians professional and personally. Participants reported that several elements of the program provided structure and supported behavioral change including having a unit champion, engagement of an interprofessional team, ensuring easy access to copies of the guide, and use of a template in the electronic medical record to documented conversations. Respondents noted changing what was asked and creating space for conversation; facilitating understanding of patient illness and altering clinician agendas were all important in shifting the conversation focus away from code status to include a more comprehensive discussion of goals of care. Finally, clinicians reported that the SICP increased their comfort with having conversations about serious illness, brought meaning to their work while reducing moral distress, and allowed for individualization of care to support patient wishes.

At Partners Healthcare, >2000 interprofessional clinicians have been trained using an adaptation of the SICG and a set of educational best practices has been developed regarding how to teach this effectively using facilitated small-group roll-playing [51]. Instructional sessions last 2.5–3 h and are divided into an hour-long large group session followed by the role-playing exercise. The large group session includes a guided reflection on the trainees experiences with serious illness communication, a review of data supporting serious illness conversations, orientation to and demonstration of the SICG, and practice using the SICG during a scripted drill. The small-group role play includes three to six learners, one to two communication facilitators, and a standardized patient. Each learner has an opportunity to engage in the role play and received feedback. In addition to describing the instructional program used at their institution, Daubman and colleagues review best practices educators can incorporate when teaching this material at their own institutions including how to foster a safe learning environment, how to explicitly teach structed communication, and adapting to different skill levels among participants.

Veterans Health Administration Life-Sustaining Treatment Initiative

The Veteran Health Administration (VHA) National Center for Ethics in Health Care implemented the Life-Sustaining Treatment Decision Initiative (LSTDI) across the VA National Health System to establish standards for the elicitation, documentation, and implementation of veterans' goals of care and life-sustaining treatment decisions [41]. The LSTDI is a multi-pronged initiative which includes engagement and buy-in from leadership; comprehensive, interprofessional staff education and communication skills training regarding conducting and documented goals of care conversations; a standardized life-sustaining treatment template and order sent within the electronic medical record; use of technology to identify and monitor implementation of the LSTDI in high-risk veterans; and a program to evaluate outcomes of the LTSDI. The staff education and training component of the LSTDI focuses on knowledge and skill attainment to plan for, conduct, and document goals of care conversations across locations of care. A variety of educational materials were created to support the LSTDI including written materials, videos, online modules, podcasts, and simulations. A train-the-trainer model is a key component of the LSTDI, with a focus on enhancing communication skills during goals of care conversations. Trainers are identified by their home facility, attend a 2.5 day course, and then disseminate the training using nationally standardized curricula. The train-the-trainer programs were developed in partnership with VitalTalk. [52] The skills training program for physicians, advanced practice nurses, and physician assistants include five interactive modules on delivering serious news, assess patient's understanding of their illness and prognosis, eliciting goals and values, discussing goals of care and life-sustaining treatment decisions, and communicating treatment recommendations based on patient priorities. The skills training program for nurses, social workers, psychologists, and chaplains focuses on exploring patient values and responding to their emotions. Initial review of the LSTDI demonstrated that documentation was completed for 108,145 veterans during the first 7 months of the initiative. The initiative is ongoing and recent data has found an association between the presence of a system-wide, standardized approach to eliciting and documenting goals of care and patient-centered, quality care [53].

Conclusion

Effective communication skills, during current care encounters, when breaking bad news, and at the end-of-life, are critical to optimizing patient outcomes and satisfaction among older adults. Traditionally, instruction on optimizing communication has not been included in formal medical education but this is changing with increasing recognition that these skills can and must be taught to all providers, from those in undergraduate medical education to practicing providers. When teaching communication skills in geriatrics, particular attention to understanding challenges related to health literacy in older adults and techniques to address these must be included. Instructional resources, including the "Geriatric Health Literacy Workshop for Medical Students and Residents" and the "Health Literacy and Patient Safety: Help Patients Understand" kit, are useful in addressing this topic [18, 20]. In recent years, there has been increased understanding regarding the importance of SDM in improving patient outcomes. SDM is particularly important given that many older adults suffer from multiple chronic illnesses, have functional challenges, and may vary widely in what they desire from their medical care. Patient Priorities Care, a SDM framework which aligns health decisions with patient priorities, is associated with improved patient and provider outcomes [29]. In addition, evidence suggests that PPC can be successfully taught to interprofessional learners using interactive, case-based instruction [35]. Instruction regarding the SPIKES model, Geritalk, the Serious Illness Care Program, and the Veterans Health Administration Life-Sustaining Treatment Initiative have demonstrated desired outcomes among patients and learners [38–41]. Continued development and assessment of communication frameworks specific to the needs of older adults and scholarship on how to best instruct learners in these methods is critical to ensuring patient-priority aligned decision-making in geriatrics.

References

1. American Geriatrics Society. Geriatrics competencies for medical students. 2021. ADGAP - Association of Directors of Geriatrics Academic Programs. americangeriatrics.org. Accessed 1 Sept 2021.
2. The Accreditation Council for Graduate Medical Education. Geriatric medicine milestones. 2021. GeriatricMedicineMilestones2.0.pdf (acgme.org). Accessed 1 Sept 2021.
3. Stenihauser KF, Chistakis NA, Clip EC, et al. Factors considered important at the end of life by patients, family, physicians, and other care providers. JAMA. 2000;284(19):2476–82.

4. Hancock K, Clayton JM, Parker SM, et al. Discrepant perceptions about end-of-life communication: a systematic review. J Pain Symptom Manag. 2007;34(2):190–200.
5. Back AL, Fromme EK, Meier DE. Training clinicians with communication skills needed to match medical treatment to patient values. J Am Geriatr Soc. 2019;67(S2):435–41.
6. Fallowfield L, Jenkins V. Effective communication skills are the key to good cancer care. Eur J Cancer. 1999;35(11):1592–7.
7. Tan XH, Foo MA, Lim SLH, et al. Teaching and assessing communication skills in the postgraduate medical setting: a systematic scoping review. BCM Med Educ. 2021;21(1):483.
8. MacDonald-Wicks L, Levett-Jones T. Effective teaching of communication to health professional undergraduate and postgraduate students: a systematic review. JBI Libr System Rev. 2012;10(28 Suppl):1–12.
9. Nutbeam D. Health literacy as a public health goal: a challenge for contemporary health education and communication strategies into the 21st century. Health Promot Int. 2000;15(3):259–67.
10. Rheault H, Coyer F, Jones L, Bonner A. Health literacy in indigenous people with chronic disease living in remote Australia. BCM Health Serv Res. 2019;19(1):1–10.
11. Nutbeam D, Lloyd JE. Understanding and responding to health literacy as a social determinant of health. Ann Rev Public Health. 2021;42:159–73.
12. Centers for Disease Control and Prevention. Improving health literacy for older adults: expert panel report 2009. Atlanta: U.S. Department of Health and Human Services; 2009. cdc.gov. Accessed 13 Sept 2021.
13. National Center for Education Statistics. National assessment of adult literacy. 2003. National Assessment of Adult Literacy (NAAL) - Health Literacy (ed.gov). Accessed 13 Sept 2021.
14. Pugh KG, Kiely DK, Milberg WP, Lipsitz LA. Selective impairments of fronto-executive cognitive function in African Americans with cardiovascular risk factors. J Am Geriatr Soc. 2003;51(10):1439–44.
15. Agarwal KS, Bhimaraj A, Xu J, et al. Decreasing heart failure readmissions among older patients with cognitive impairment by engaging caregivers. J Cardiovasc Nurs. 2020;35(3):253–61.
16. Sharit J, Hernandez MA, Czaja SJ, Pirolli P. Investigating the role of knowledge and cognitive abilities in older adult information seeking on the web. ACM Trans Comput Hum Interact. 2008;15(1):3.
17. The Gerontological Society of America. Communicating with older adults: an evidence-based review of what really works. 2012. ku.edu. Accessed 31 Jan 2022
18. Farrell TW. Review of a geriatric health literacy workshop for medical students and residents. J Am Geriatr Soc. 2011;59(12):2347–9.
19. Doak CD, Doak LG, Root JH. Teaching patients with low literacy skills, vol. 96. 2nd ed. Philadelphia: J.B. Lippincott; 1996. p. 16M.
20. Weiss BD. Health literacy and patient safety: help patients understand manual for clinicians. 2nd ed. AMA Foundation. 2007. New Health Literacy Kit.pdf (pogoe.org). Accessed 31 Jan 2022
21. Marion GS, Hairston JM, Davis ST, Kirk JK. Using standardized patient assessments to evaluate a health literacy curriculum. Fam Med. 2018 Jan;50(1):52–7.
22. US Department of Health and Human Services. Health Literacy. HRSA. Health Literacy | Official web site of the U.S. Health Resources & Services Administration (hrsa.gov). Accessed 1 Feb 2022.
23. Barry MJ, Edgman-Levitan S. Shared decision making- the pinnacle of patient-centered care. N Engl J Med. 2012;366(9):780–1.
24. Scalia P, Durand MA, Berkowitz JL, et al. The impact and utility of encounter patient decision aids: systematic review, meta-analysis and narrative synthesis. Patient Educ Couns. 2019;102:817–41.
25. Stacy D, Legare F, Lewis K, eta l. Decision aids for people facing health treatment or screening decisions. Cochrane Database Syst Rev. 2017;4:CD001431.
26. Ankolekar A, Dekker A, Fijten R, Berlanga A. The benefits and challenges of using patient decision aids to support shared decision making in health care. JCO Clin Cancer Inform. 2018;2:10–0.

27. Bradley JG, Zia MJ, Hamilton N. Patient preferences for control in medical decision making: a scenario-based approach. Fam Med. 1996;28(7):496–501.
28. Shen MJ, Manna R, Banerjee SC, et al. Incorporating shared decision making into communication with older adults with cancer and their caregivers: development and evaluation of a geriatric shared decision-making communication skills training module. Patient Educ Couns. 2020;103(11):2328–34.
29. Tinetti ME, Esterson J, Ferris R, et al. Patient priority-directed decision making and care for older adults with multiple chronic conditions. Clin Geriatr Med. 2016;32(2):261–75.
30. Patient Priorities Care. 2019. https://patientprioritiescare.org. Accessed 2 Aug 2021.
31. Identifying my health priorities. https://myhealthpriorities.org. Accessed 15 Sept 2021.
32. Tinetti ME, Naik AD, Dindo L, et al. Association of patient priorities-aligned decision-making with patient outcomes and ambulatory health care burden among older adults with multiple chronic conditions: a nonrandomized clinical trial. JAMA Intern Med. 2019;179(12):1688–97.
33. Freytag J, Dindo L, Catic A, Johnson AL, et al. Feasibility of clinicians aligning health care with patient priorities in geriatrics ambulatory care. J Am Geriatr Soc. 2020;68(9):2112–6.
34. Ouellet GM, Kiwak E, Costello DM, et al. Clinician perspectives on incorporating patients' values-based health priorities in decision-making. JAGS. 2020;69(1):267–9.
35. Ouellet JA, Mecca MC, Tinetti ME, et al. Education outcomes of a multisite, virtual, interprofessional training in patient priorities aligned care. J Am Geriatr Soc. 2022;70(1):E5–7.
36. Ko E, Fuentes D. End-of-life communication between providers and family caregivers of home hospice patients in a rural US-Mexico border community: caregivers' retrospective perspectives. Am J Hosp Palliat Care. 2020;37(5):329–35.
37. Im J, Mak S, Upshur R, et al. "Whatever happens, happens" challenges of end-of-life communication from the perspective of older adults and family caregivers: a qualitative study. BMC Palliat Care. 2019;18(1):113.
38. Baile WF, Buckman RL, Glober G, et al. SPIKES-a six-step protocol for delivering bad news: application to the patient with cancer. Oncologist. 2000;5(4):302–11.
39. Kelley AS, Back AL, Arnold RM, et al. Geritalk: communication skills training for geriatric and palliative medicine fellows. J Am Geriatr Soc. 2012;60(2):332–7.
40. Bernacki R, Hutchings M, Vick J, et al. Development of the Serious Illness Care Program: a randomized controlled trial of a palliative care communication intervention. BMJ Open. 2015;5(10):e009032.
41. Foglia MB, Lowery J, Sharpe VA, et al. A comprehensive approach for eliciting, documenting, and honoring patient wishes for care near the end f of life: the Veterans Health Administration's Life-Sustaining Treatment Decisions Initiative. Jt Comm J Qual Patient Saf. 2019;45(1):47–56.
42. Marschollek P, Bakowska K, Bakowski W, et al. Oncologists and breaking bad news- from the informed patients' point of view. The evaluation of the SPIKES protocol implementation. J Cancer Educ. 2019;34(2):375–80.
43. Goldsmith J, Wittenberg-Lyles E, Shaunfield S, Sanchez-Reilly S. Palliative care communication curriculum: what can students learn from an unfolding case? Am J Hosp Palliat Care. 2011;28(4):236–41.
44. Kurji Z, Aijaz A, Aijaz A, et al. Telesimulation innovation on the teaching of SPIKES model on sharing bad news. Asia Pac J Oncol Nurs. 2021;8(6):623–7.
45. Back AL, Arnold RM, Baile WF, et al. Efficacy of communication skills training for giving bad news and discussing transitions to palliative care. Arch Intern Med. 2007;167(5):453–60.
46. Gelfman LP, Lindenberger E, Fernandez H, et al. The effectiveness of the Geritalk communication skills course: a real-time assessment of skill acquisition and deliberate practice. J Pain Symptom Manag. 2014;48(4):738–44.
47. Frydman JL, Gellman LP, Lindenberger EC, et al. Virtual Geritalk: improving serious illness communication of clinicians who care for older adults. J Pain Symptom Manage. 2021;62(3):206–12.
48. Bernacki R, Paladino J, Neville BA. Effect of the serious illness care program in outpatient oncology: a cluster randomized clinical trial. JAMA Intern Med. 2019;179(6):751–9.

49. Paladino J, Koritsanszky L, Nisotel L, et al. Patient and clinician experience of a serious illness conversation guide in oncology: a descriptive analysis. Cancer Med. 2020;9(13):4550–60.
50. Lagrotteria A, Swinton M, Simon J, et al. Clinicians' perspective after implementation of the serious illness care program: a qualitative study. JAMA Netw Open. 2021;4(8):e2121517.
51. Daubman BR, Bernacki R, Stoltenberg M, et al. Best practices for teaching clinicians to use a serious illness conversation guide. Palliat Med Rep. 2020;1(1):135–42.
52. VitalTalk. Home page. Home - VitalTalk. Accessed 3 Feb 2022.
53. Batten A, Cohen JH, Foglia MB, Alfandre D. Associations between the veteran health administration's life-sustaining treatment decisions initiative and quality of care at the end of life. J Palliat Med. 2022;25:1057.

Chapter 21
Creating a Positive Feedback Culture in Geriatrics Education

Natalie Young and Anna Chang

Creating a positive feedback culture is an essential skill for clinician educators teaching the care of older persons. The goal of effective feedback is to help learners improve performance. While feedback is integral to earning, its main purpose is not to test the learner or evaluate the program. Effective feedback encourages learning and enhances the learners' attitudes, knowledge, and skills while narrowing the gap between actual and desired performance. Research over the last decades point out that feedback conversations are more than one-way information downloads, but rather are complex interpersonal interactions influenced by sociocultural factors including the relationship between learner and teacher, perceptions of credibility, learner receptivity, the learning environment, and institutional culture [1]. These newer definitions of effective feedback highlight the importance of learner self-assessment, behavior change, and professional growth [2].

If educators in geriatric medicine and its associated health professions can create a positive feedback culture embedded in the growth mindset for all its undergraduate, graduate, and interprofessional trainees, entire generations of health care providers can possess expertise needed to provide the highest standards of care for all older persons. This chapter begins with the growth mindset as a framework and offers recommendations for the educator as a professional role model in helping learners with clear expectations, reflective self-assessment, and create learning goals. It then discusses the feedback setting, the role of the interprofessional team, and a consideration of feedback across differences. Specific to the care of older persons, the chapter concludes with a structured example of specific skills and behaviors for focus that can be applied by busy clinicians, educators, and learners.

N. Young (✉) · A. Chang
University of California, San Francisco School of Medicine, San Francisco, CA, USA
e-mail: Natalie.young@ucsf.edu; anna.chang@ucsf.edu

A. W. Schwartz (ed.), *Medical Education in Geriatrics*,
https://doi.org/10.1007/978-3-031-32499-4_21

A Framework: The Growth Mindset

With a growth mindset, the definition of success is the result of hard work; prioritizing learning and improvement from conflict or failure [3]. In contrast, learners with a fixed mindset might define success as a trait determined by innate ability. Learners with a fixed mindset tend to reject constructive feedback as evidence of failure and as a negative statement of their abilities rather than an opportunity for improvement. A learning culture founded in a growth mindset is one where feedback is valued, expected, and actively sought. Creating a learning environment that fosters the growth mindset is important to effective feedback and learning in all educational contexts, including in the care of older adults.

A number of strategies in four domains can help enhance the growth mindset [1] (Fig. 21.1). First, the teacher (or feedback provider) can serve as a role model, observe learner performance, and offer opportunities for reflection and debrief. Second, the learner (or feedback receiver) can be taught to seek feedback and to own the development of their own learning action plans. Third, the relationship between educator and learner can become one that is founded on a strong educational alliance of trust, and both together can actively create opportunities for learning and improvement. And finally, the learning environment can emphasize the importance of continuous improvement and seek to balance autonomy with supervision to enhance professional growth. With these principles in mind, the educator and learner can co-create an environment where every encounter with a real or simulated older person becomes an engaging and rich learning opportunity.

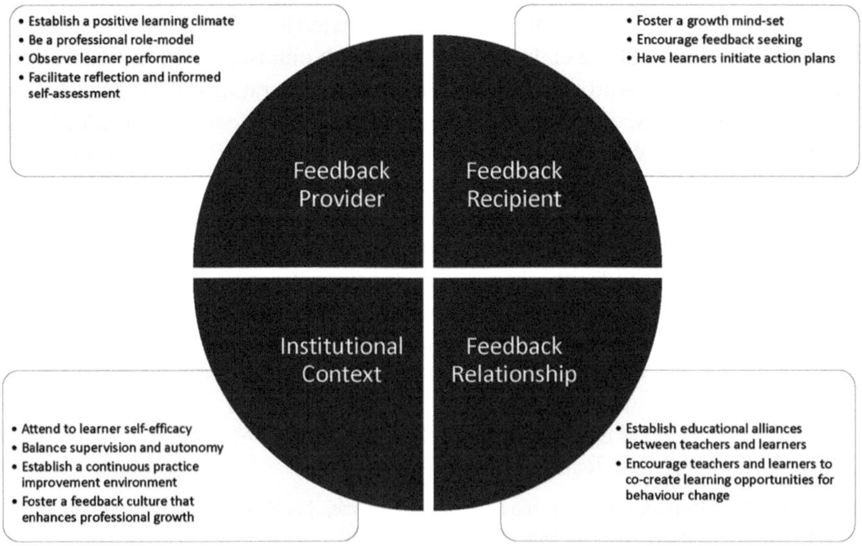

Fig. 21.1 Establishing a feedback culture with a growth mind-set: strategies from multiple perspectives

The Educator as Professional Role Model

The educator has an important role in framing the educational relationship and the learning environment with the growth mindset as a foundation in order to establish a strong educational alliance [4]. Similar to a physician–patient therapeutic alliance, an effective educational alliance includes shared goals of an optimal learning environment and an active multi-directional learning community that consists of the educator, the learner, and others on the team. An educator can role model by demonstrating respect for all and welcoming multiple perspectives as feedback of educational effectiveness or input into patient care plans, including that of the learner, patient, family, health care surrogate, and interprofessional team members. Further, an educator can demonstrate a readiness to admit and correct missteps and model a culture of continuous practice improvement. This perspective of continuous improvement of the community of practice enables supervisors and trainees to both offer and receive feedback [5]. When the educator seeks and offers feedback in a context of a trusting learning relationship, the feedback has the potential of influencing memorable learning and lasting behavioral change.

The Feedback Process

Step 1: Setting Expectations and Learning Goals

It is important to set expectations early that feedback will be a normal, frequent part of the educational relationship, whether it spans the course of a half day or several months. As a part of expectation setting, it is important to agree upon learning objectives and clear criteria against which performance will be assessed [6, 7]. When possible, learning objectives should be explicitly linked to broader curricular goals. Medical student geriatrics competencies serve as an important guide for key knowledge and skills at the undergraduate medical education level [8, 9]. The Accreditation Council for Graduate Medical Education (ACGME) establishes curricular milestones for residency and fellowship training programs and often includes specific aims for the care of older persons. For example, all family medicine residency trainees are expected to perform a comprehensive geriatric assessment by the end of training (Fig. 21.2). The ACGME defines different sub-competencies as a trainee works toward mastery of this milestone, including a description of behaviors [10].

We also recommend routinely asking the trainee at the start of each learning session to share their own learning goals or areas of focus. Often, educators are in contact with learners episodically in the midst of the learner's longitudinal learning trajectory that may encompass different rotations, different practice settings, and different teachers or preceptors. Thus, it can be helpful to start with establishing what the learner has already observed and practiced, and what gaps remain. Learners

Patient Care 1: Comprehensive Geriatric Assessment				
Level 1	Level 2	Level 3	Level 4	Level 5
Identifies domains of a comprehensive geriatric assessment, including medical, psychosocial, and functional elements	Performs a comprehensive geriatric assessment, eliciting information from ancillary sources, including the patient, family, caregivers, and interdisciplinary team	Formulates a care plan that integrates findings from a comprehensive geriatric assessment focused on optimizing physical, psychosocial, and functional health	Implements a unified, patient-centered care plan that integrates all domains of the comprehensive geriatric assessment in collaboration with the interdisciplinary team and community partners	Implements a comprehensive geriatric assessment methodology for use with innovative models of care delivery, new care settings, and/or unique patient populations
Comments:				Not Yet Completed Level 1 Not Yet Assessable

Fig. 21.2 AGCME geriatric medicine milestones: family medicine

can also carry a particular question or skillset that is at the top of their minds based on their personal experience, their curricular journey, the sociopolitical context, or new developments in the field of aging that is highlighted in the media. Hearing the learners' own learning goals guides the educator's plan for observation and feedback and ensures that the learner leaves each learning session having addressed their most urgent queries and topics.

Step 2: Practice and Observation

While didactic sessions can be educational, we recommend for all educators to design opportunities for trainees to demonstrate their knowledge and skills, which can occur in the classroom, in simulation, or in real clinical settings. In the classroom setting, for example, students can be asked to role-play with each other or with the educator and state the questions that they would ask an older person in order to determine their functional status and level of independence in performing the instrumental activities of daily living. In simulation, learners can be asked to demonstrate their physical examination skills with a standardized patient in assessing gait or cognition. In real clinical settings, learners can be invited to initiate a family meeting, with pre-meeting and real-time support, to begin to demonstrate their complex communication skills in disclosing a serious diagnosis and addressing goals of care. When this opportunity is offered to a medical student, for example, they may choose to start the conversation and then hand it over to another clinician. If a learner is a fellow, however, they may have the experience to conduct the entire conversation. Thus, observing learners in action, at whatever setting or level, becomes the foundation of effective feedback.

In the field of geriatrics, there are numerous clinical, communication, and teamwork skills that benefit from observation and feedback. For example:

- *Clinical Skills*: Gait assessment, use of assistive devices, cognitive testing, comprehensive medication reconciliation, home safety assessment.
- *Communication Skills*: Advance care planning, goals of care conversations, disclosing a medical error, sharing difficult news.
- *Teamwork Skills*: Designing care plans taking into account multiple different inputs, conflict resolution as a member of an interprofessional team.

During the observation period, the educator should make note of specific behaviors related to the stated learning objectives to reinforce or correct as examples when providing feedback.

Step 3: Learner Self-Assessment and Reflection

Initiating feedback conversations with learner self-assessment can be invaluable. The educator can start with a general, open-ended question such as, "what do you think went well in that encounter?" Inviting the learner to start with self-reflection can help the educator better understand a learner's insight into their own strengths and weaknesses and provide opportunities for the educator to reinforce strengths and enhance self-efficacy. It is important to note that while it is helpful to routinely ask for learner self-assessment, there is evidence that learner self-assessment is not always accurate. For example, some high-performing learners may offer what sounds like harsh self-assessment statements, and some low-performing learners may lack insight into their own areas for further development [11]. While we recommend starting each feedback session with an opportunity for self-assessment, the learner's self-assessment can serve as only a starting place for conversation and not the sole basis for the content of the educator's feedback.

Step 4: Focus on Behaviors/Skills

When providing feedback, it is helpful to remind the learner that the goal of feedback is to improve and work toward stated learning goals. Feedback is most effective when focused on specific behaviors and skills [12]. For example, saying "I noticed that you maintained eye contact, nodded your head, and held the patient's hand when they were sharing their concerns which demonstrated active listening and made the patient feel supported in this moment" is more effective than "good job" by highlighting and reinforcing specific communication skills.

Receiving feedback can be difficult for some learners so when providing feedback it is critical to attend to the learner's emotional response to the situation and/or the feedback provided [13].

Step 5: Creation of an Action Plan

To summarize the feedback encounter, it can be helpful to create a learning action plan that includes commitment to behavior change and updated learning goals. When developing an action plan, consider using a SMART goals framework [14]:

- Specific: what will be accomplished? What actions will you take?
- Measurable: how will success be measured?
- Achievable: is the goal doable?
- Relevant: how does the goal align with broader goals?
- Time-Bound: what is the timeframe for accomplishing this goal?

For example, if the learner is developing competency in gait assessment, we could consider the following goal: "in my next three clinical encounters, I will observe the patient while ambulating and use a gait assessment checklist to evaluate for gait abnormalities. I will compare my observations with that of the team's physical therapist, when available."

Important Contexts

Feedback Setting

When providing feedback, it is important to try to choose the "right time, right person, right place" [15]. It is often helpful to provide formative feedback at the time of or shortly after an observation of the learners' performance. If possible, agree on a time in advance, minimize distractions, and ensure that the setting is private, quiet, and away from potential interruptions [6]. When establishing expectations and learning goals, consider setting expectations about when, where, and how feedback will be discussed.

There are times when feedback in a group is helpful also. For example, just after bedside rounds to see a patient together in which a learner took the lead to conduct the visit, the team, which may include the educator, interprofessional colleagues, and additional learners, may take 2 min to share observations and feedback. This could start with the educator asking the learner to share their own thoughts on how that went, and what they did well. Then the team might take turns sharing the effective components of what they observed and some additional suggestions to consider for the next encounter. This allows learners to participate in the feedback process and takes advantage of the most timely opportunity for feedback (before seeing the next patient). Beware that if this occurs in the hallway of an inpatient ward, this may not be the ideal setting to offer exceptionally constructive feedback on very sensitive topics.

Including Voices of Interprofessional Team

Providing competent, compassionate care to older adults requires a high-functioning interprofessional team. A 360° evaluation includes feedback from multiple sources including members of the interprofessional team, peers, and patients/caregivers [11]. One example is asking the team social worker to share insights on communication skills and ability to address emotional distress after a family meeting to review goals of care. Another example is asking the pharmacist to provide feedback on medication reconciliation or medication teaching. One can achieve this by creating a larger institutional culture based in a growth mindset that values frequent feedback, multiple voices, and actively engages in continuous practice improvement. With this strategy, the learner gains invaluable learning, and the learning community is strengthened with each conversation.

Learning Across Differences

Implicit bias occurs naturally as humans develop different social identities and lead us to generalize individual characteristics onto a group. Microaggressions, a term introduced in 1970 by Dr. Chester Pierce, are interactions that convey negative messages about a group [16]. In medical education in general, bias and microaggressions occur in multiple axes, such as patient to learner (and vice versa), faculty to learner (and vice versa), etc. Bias and microaggressions can be based on any characteristic: age, gender, race/ethnicity, and health profession, to name a few. Studies show that biases and microaggressions influence learner evaluations, decrease effective learning, and affect patient relationships [17, 18]. Thus, these important internal and shared experiences will inevitably become a core part of feedback conversations.

Scholars have begun to describe guidelines for educators to work toward creating a learning environment that advances health equity for patients as well as equity in medical education [19]. A starting place is to set the stage for including bias and microaggressions in routine teaching and feedback conversations. This can sound like: "To learn and care for patients effectively, we need to be able to discuss biases and microaggressions in our learning environment." A next step is to identify instances where bias or microaggressions may have affected the learning or care relationship. One example can be: "I felt uncomfortable when the patient spoke about our medical student's hair." The next step is to invite a conversation about this topic. For example, "I've been reflecting on the patient encounter. Can we find some time to check-in?" [20]. And the final step is to decide on follow-up needed. This can include further conversations with the learner, patient, or education program directors.

When offering a learner feedback, educators need to be mindful of their own implicit biases [21].

Studies have shown that adjectives used to describe men have an emphasis on standout ability (e.g. exceptional, intelligent), while words used to describe women emphasize effort and community (e.g. diligent, empathetic) [22]. Describing learner behaviors can be more effective. (e.g. "The learner's evaluation of the patient's cognition is thorough and accurate.") Furthermore, while professionalism has been a core competency in medical education, the very concept is being reconsidered as it can be seen as a framework that is used to maintain current dominant standards, such that dress or appearance associated with minority groups can be mistakenly considered unprofessional, thus solidifying a less inclusive culture in medicine [23].

A more in-depth discussion of diversity, equity, and inclusion in geriatrics education appears in Chap. 18.

An Example: Feedback in Action

A structured approach to providing feedback incorporating the principles of fostering a growth mindset can achieve more consistent, meaningful, and effective feedback [6, 7]. We propose the following structure based on the steps outlined above: step 1—identify learning goals, step 2—observation and practice, step 3—learner self-assessment and reflection, step 4—focus on behaviors, and step 5—create an action plan for behavior change. As you will note in the example, we repeat steps 3 and 4 using the learner self-assessment as an opportunity to reinforce behavior and identify areas for improvement (Table 21.1).

Table 21.1 An example of structured approach to feedback discussion in geriatric medicine. In this example, the teacher is an attending geriatrician, and the learner is an internal medicine resident. They are conducting a home visit for routine follow-up

Before the observation	
Step 1: Discuss learning objectives and clearly define feedback expectations	*Teacher*: "I want to invite you to take the lead on the encounter with Mrs. Xu today, and I will be observing and supporting as needed. We are seeing Mrs. Xu today for routine follow-up of her dementia. Before we start with the clinical encounter, would you share what are your personal learning goals for our time together?"
	Learner: "I find it really challenging to communicate with patients with dementia and knowing how to balance the focus on the patient versus the family's concerns"
	Teacher: "You highlight some really important issues in geriatrics—communication with patients with cognitive impairment. Are there particular skills you want to practice and for me to give feedback on?"
	Learner: "I want to work on making sure I speak to the patient and direct some questions to the patient instead of just to the family members"
	Teacher: "Wonderful, I will observe you balancing your time between the patient and family. Would it be ok if we set aside 10 minutes at the end of our session today to go over feedback? We can meet in the team conference room so we can have this conversation uninterrupted"
	Learner: "Sure!"

Table 21.1 (continued)

Observation	
Step 2: Observe encounter with attention to learner behaviors	Teacher makes note of specific behaviors linked to learner's goals. In this example, the teacher observes as the learner leads the interval medical history conversation with the patient and family
After the observation	
Step 3: Ask the learner to assess own performance	*Teacher*: "How do you think that went?"
	Learner: "I think that went ok, but I worry it took a really long time"
Step 3: Ask the learner to assess what went well	*Teacher*: "What do you think went well?"
	Learner: "I directed some of my questions to the patient"
Step 4: Share observations and recommendations	*Teacher*: "At the beginning of the day, you shared your learning goal was to balance communication with the patient and family. I noticed that you directed questions to the patient, including making eye contact and placing a hand respectfully on Mrs. Xu's wheelchair to make sure she was included in the conversation"
Repeat step 3: Ask the learner to identify areas for improvement	*Teacher*: "Is there anything you would do differently next time?"
	Learner: "I am worried that I spent a really long time with them, it took over 30 minutes to get the history!"
Repeat step 4: Share observations and recommendations	*Teacher*: "You mentioned a concern about time management today. I agree that in some settings, we may need to obtain the history in less than 30 minutes"
Step 5: Develop an action plan, beginning by asking the learner for their ideas	*Teacher*: "What is something you could do differently to help with time management?"
	Learner: "I wonder if I should try setting an agenda at the start of the visit"
	Teacher: "Yes, this can be a really helpful tool to frame the visit. I like to ask both the patient and family for their full list of concerns and then prioritize the plan for the day"
	Learner: "That sounds like something I can try!"
	Teacher: "Let's try to make this a SMART goal"
	Learner: "In my next two clinical encounters, I will use set an agenda at the beginning of the visit and monitor how much time I spend gathering history"

Summary

Effective feedback in geriatrics starts with a learning culture grounded in the growth mindset. The growth mindset allows for learning to be an iterative process in which success is based on hard work and not innate ability. Educators can serve as professional role models by actively seeing feedback and engaging in self-reflection. Clarity of learning objectives linked to the learner's personal goals and the broader curricular context is critical. Feedback is most effective when it is based on direct observation and linked to specific behaviors. Developing a structured approach that includes expectation setting, self-assessment, a focus on behaviors, and creation of an action plan can achieve more consistent, meaningful feedback. A positive feedback culture relies on educator–trainee relationships and a supportive institutional culture. With effective feedback as a tool, the next generation of physicians and health care providers can learn to care for older persons with skill.

References

1. Ramani S, Könings KD, Ginsburg S, van der Vleuten CPM. Twelve tips to promote a feedback culture with a growth mind-set: swinging the feedback pendulum from recipes to relationships. Med Teach. 2019;41(6):625–31.
2. Boud D, Dawson P. What feedback literate teachers do: an empirically-derived competency framework. Assess Eval High Educ. 2023;48(2):158–71.
3. Dweck CS. Mindset. Random House; 2006.
4. Telio S, Regehr G, Ajjawi R. Feedback and the educational alliance: examining credibility judgements and their consequences. Med Educ. 2016;50(9):933–42.
5. Lefroy J, Watling C, Teunissen PW, Brand P. Guidelines: the do's, don'ts and don't knows of feedback for clinical education. Perspect Med Educ. 2015;4(6):284–99.
6. Kelly E, Richards JB. Medical education: giving feedback to doctors in training. BMJ. 2019;366:l4523.
7. Reddy ST, Zegarek MH, Fromme HB, Ryan MS, Schumann SA, Harris IB. Barriers and facilitators to effective feedback: a qualitative analysis of data from multispecialty resident focus groups. J Grad Med Educ. 2015;7(2):214–9.
8. Sargeant J, Eva KW, Armson H, et al. Features of assessment learners use to make informed self-assessments of clinical performance. Med Educ. 2011;45(6):636–47.
9. AGS Publishes Updated AGS Minimum Geriatrics Competencies for Graduating Medical Students. Accessed June 23, 2021. https://www.americangeriatrics.org/media-center/news/ags-publishes-updated-ags-minimum-geriatrics-competencies-graduating-medical
10. Accessed July 30, 2024. https://www.acgme.org/globalassets/pdfs/milestones/geriatricmedicinemilestones.pdf
11. Warm EJ, Schauer D, Revis B, Boex JR. Multisource feedback in the ambulatory setting. J Grad Med Educ. 2010;2(2):269–77.
12. Cantillon P, Sargeant J. Giving feedback in clinical settings. BMJ. 2008;337(v10 2):a1961.
13. Thomas JD, Arnold RM. Giving feedback. J Palliat Med. 2011;14(2):233–9.
14. Chatterjee D, Corral J. How to write well-defined learning objectives. J Educ Perioper Med. 2017;19(4):E610.
15. Bing-You R, Hayes V, Palka T, Ford M, Trowbridge R. The art (and artifice) of seeking feedback: Clerkship students' approaches to asking for feedback. Acad Med. 2018;93(8):1218–26.
16. Ackerman-Barger K, Jacobs NN. The microaggressions triangle model: a humanistic approach to navigating microaggressions in health professions schools. Acad Med. 2020;95(12S Addressing Harmful Bias and Eliminating Discrimination in Health Professions Learning Environments):S28–S32.
17. Gilliam C, Russell CJ. Impact of racial microaggressions in the clinical learning environment and review of best practices to support learners. Curr Probl Pediatr Adolesc Health Care. 2021;51(10):101090.
18. Sandoval RS, Dunleavy S, Afolabi T, et al. Equity in medical education: addressing microaggressions and discrimination on the wards. Med Teach. Published online December. 2021;3:1–8.
19. Wheeler DJ, Zapata J, Davis D, Chou C. Twelve tips for responding to microaggressions and overt discrimination: When the patient offends the learner. Med Teach. 2019;41(10):1112–7.
20. Ehie O, Muse I, Hill L, Bastien A. Professionalism: microaggression in the healthcare setting. Curr Opin Anaesthesiol. 2021;34(2):131–6.
21. Klein R, Ufere NN, Rao SR, et al. Association of gender with learner assessment in graduate medical education. JAMA Netw Open. 2020;3(7):e2010888.
22. Hemmer PA, Karani R. Let's face it: we are biased, and it should not be that way. J Gen Intern Med. 2019;34(5):649–51.
23. Frye V, Camacho-Rivera M, Salas-Ramirez K, et al. Professionalism: the wrong tool to solve the right problem? Acad Med. 2020;95(6):860–3.

Chapter 22
Faculty Development for Teaching Geriatrics

Sharon A. Levine and Deborah S. Lee

Importance

As of 2021, there were 7123 board-certified geriatricians in the USA [1, 2]. Even if one geriatrician were to have a panel of 700 complicated patients, it is estimated that the USA would need 33,200 such specialists by 2025 [3]. Currently, there is a stagnation in the number of medical trainees pursuing geriatrics training, especially when adjusted for the aging of the US population. This lack is more notable in rural settings, where poverty and other social determinants of health make aging an even more vulnerable process [4]. Thus, it is imperative that the relatively few specialty-trained geriatricians disseminate their specialized skillsets to other clinicians, especially to those in teaching roles [5, 6]. As our patients grow older, there is tremendous opportunity to optimize their care through faculty development in the various medical and surgical specialties. Moreover, as geriatrics care develops into a more multidisciplinary team model, it is important to empower clinician-educators throughout the interprofessional team spectrum [7].

Teach-the-Teacher Models in Geriatrics

To date, there have been a handful of large-scale models in training clinician-educators (both geriatricians and/or non-geriatricians) in the art of becoming more effective teachers, especially in selected geriatrics topics. While no list is

S. A. Levine · D. S. Lee (✉)
Massachusetts General Hospital, Harvard Medical School, Boston, MA, USA
e-mail: slevine9@mgh.harvard.edu; dslee70@mgh.harvard.edu

A. W. Schwartz (ed.), *Medical Education in Geriatrics*,
https://doi.org/10.1007/978-3-031-32499-4_22

comprehensive, our goal is to describe some successful models of teach-the-teacher programs in geriatrics and to reflect on those factors that make these models successful and/or replicable (see Table 22.1 for summary of selected examples).

John A. Hartford Foundation: Funding Centers of Excellence in Geriatrics Education

Since 1997, the John A. Hartford Foundation has funded more than $25.5 million to the national Centers of Excellence (CoE) program, with the goal of increasing the visibility of academic geriatrics [8]. By 2004, it had already supported 163 geriatrics fellows, of whom 63% entered careers in academic geriatrics. It had also offered support to 222 faculty members, of which nearly 2/3 have remained in geriatrics and 82% in academics [9].

Boston University Center of Excellence: Empowering Non-geriatricians in Disseminating Geriatrics Knowledge

One specific example of a CoE is the Boston University Center of Excellence (BUCOE) in geriatrics, which was initially funded by the Hartford Foundation in 1997. It trained a total of 25 non-geriatric clinician-educator faculty members, who, in cohorts of four to six, participated in a weekly curriculum spanning 9 months [10]. Four modules were taught: (1) geriatrics content; (2) evidence-based medicine; (3) clinical teaching; and (4) health care systems. First, geriatrics content was taught in small groups with cases, with an evidence-based approach. Topics included geriatrics assessment/evaluation, falls, cross-cultural issues, geriatric syndromes, dementia, urinary incontinence, substance abuse, polypharmacy, depression, late-life psychosis, gynecology, cancer, and osteoporosis. Second, participants were taught to use evidence-based medicine to provide guidance on finding, filtering, and judging the data driving clinical decision-making. Third, clinical teaching skills were taught based on the clinical teaching curriculum developed by the Stanford Faculty Development Center [11]. Lastly, the module on health care systems taught on health care finances like private and public payment systems, including the fundamentals of Medicare and Medicaid funding. In addition, each participating faculty learner was required to participate in six precepted clinical sessions in various settings where older adults receive care, including home, nursing home, and geriatrics assessment clinic.

At the end of the 9-month curriculum, learners participated in self-reported questionnaires (with 83% response rate), as well as individual structured interviews (with 75% response rate). In the questionnaires, learners most highly ranked the clinical teaching module (mean 3.69 ± 0.56 SD on a 1–5 Likert scale), closely followed by geriatrics content (3.60 ± 0.44). Notable commentary from the seven-item

Table 22.1 Selected examples of teach-the-teacher programs in geriatrics

Program	Target audience	Duration	Impact
Boston University Center of excellence [10]	Non-geriatrician academic faculty	Weekly curriculum for 9 total months	Clinical teaching skills, geriatric content knowledge
Collaborative centers for research and education in the Care of Older Adults [12]	Non-geriatrician academic faculty	2 years	Culture change in geriatrics clinical care and teaching, working relationships between geriatricians and non-geriatricians
FD-AGE (faculty development to advance geriatrics education) [15, 16]	Geriatricians and non-geriatricians, medical students, post-graduate students, non-MD providers (often w/ specialty tracks depending on site of care)	3–5 days	Self-efficacy in teaching geriatrics, one self-selected teaching goal in 6-month follow-up
CRIT (chief resident immersion training) [19]	Chief medical and surgical residents	2.5 days	Objective geriatric content knowledge, teaching skills, teaching geriatrics
PAGE (program for advancing geriatrics education) [21]	Hospitalist attendings	10 h over 1 year	Increased inpatient geriatrics teaching, increased knowledge translation of geriatrics skills by residents
Geriatrics scholars program [22]	Community-based generalist clinicians	30 h over 3 years	Increased self-efficacy in geriatrics knowledge translation and geriatrics teaching
SGEC (Stanford geriatric education center) [23]	Health care educators from multiple professions	1 week	Dissemination of knowledge or implementation of community projects incorporating culturally sensitive care for the elderly

structured interview showed increased integration of geriatrics contents by learners into their own clinical teaching for medical students and residents. One example response was: “I loved the organization of the COE program. It helped me to design our curriculum in Family Medicine; I met people who have helped me structure home visits. It is a good model. It combined so many aspects of care for older people. The program continues to be useful to me in terms of curriculum development and teaching” [12]. A similar response commented: “I listen to students and residents much more. I can discuss geriatric patients better now with residents. I draw their attention to issues in a clinical setting. In precepting residents in continuity clinic, I now include geriatric topics.” Such a model illustrated how non-geriatricians could be taught important geriatrics topics, which could then be further disseminated in their various teaching roles [13].

Collaborative Centers for Research and Education in the Care of Older Adults: Connecting Geriatricians to General Internists

The Collaborative Centers for Research and Education in the Care of Older Adults were funded by the John A. Hartford Foundation and administered by the Society of General Internal Medicine. Ten academic institutions received individual grants of $91,000, with required cost sharing. Three key program strategies, implemented over 2 years (2003–2004), included: re-branding of a limited number of “star educator” faculty who could become local advocates and role models for enhancing geriatrics education; development of educational projects to foster change in geriatrics clinical practice and teaching; and development of new one-on-one working partnerships between general internists and geriatricians [12]. As standardized evaluation was not a requirement for funding, its effectiveness was gauged by qualitative data on “sustained culture change” in geriatrics clinical teaching and learning. One principal investigator at a funded institution reported: “Our faculty have loads of confidence about teaching geriatrics that they did not have before this project. … Geriatrics is much more on the radar screen now and will have sustainability over time.” While quantitative data is limited, this program highlighted a non-traditional approach to bring a more comprehensive “culture change” so that enhanced geriatrics care and teaching become an institutional priority [12].

Donald W. Reynolds Foundation: Supporting Medical School Geriatrics Education

From 2001 to its end in 2017, the Donald W. Reynolds Foundation supported cohorts of 10 medical schools with 4-year $2 million grants to develop faculty training in geriatrics. In part, the grants increased access to clinician-educator career pathways by funding a second year to existing 1-year fellowship programs in clinical geriatrics [14]. Moreover, indirect support was given to additional institutions by promotion of inter-institutional collaborations.

Faculty Development to Advance Geriatrics Education: Increasing Visibility of Academic Geriatrics Through Building of Inter-Institutional Collaborations

In 2004, the Reynolds Foundation initiated the Consortium for Faculty Development to Advance Geriatrics Education (FD-AGE), wherein senior geriatrics educators from Duke, Johns Hopkins, Mount Sinai in New York, and University of California at Los Angeles collaborated to optimize geriatrics training in additional medical institutions not given the initial Reynolds grants.

The FD-AGE created geriatrics mini-fellowships comprising three to 5-day intensive courses, often with specialized tracks for clinicians in ambulatory care, hospitalist care, skilled nursing care, home care, and palliative care [15]. These courses were extended to both geriatricians and non-geriatricians, medical students, post-graduate trainees, and non-MD providers nation-wide. Evaluation of 42 non-geriatrician clinician-educator faculty from 17 academic institutions did not show significant change in geriatrics knowledge and attitude after attending a 3-day mini-fellowship. Notably, though, these learners self-selected to participate in this course and demonstrated high geriatrics knowledge at baseline. In contrast, there was significant improvement in reported self-efficacy to teach geriatrics ($p < 0.001$). Moreover, a quarter (10 out of 42) of participants reported having achieved at least one self-selected teaching goal in 6-month follow-up [15]. This finding suggests the potential of short intensive courses to cultivate highly motivated faculty who then can move onto become champions for geriatrics at their own academic institutions.

In addition, the consortium offered on-site consultations to clinicians and institutional leaders at their own academic campuses. Goals included: improvement in teaching skills, increased access to model teaching programs/resources, guidance on curricular design and assessment, and building of mentorship networks. These on-site consultative visits included talks and workshops by visiting faculty, as well as Strengths, Weaknesses, Opportunities, Threats (SWOT) analyses of their geriatrics educational programs. From 2004 to 2010, the FD-AGE trained 82 fellows as clinician-educators, hosted 899 faculty scholars in mini-fellowships and intensive courses, and conducted 65 site visits [16].

Portal of Geriatrics Online Education: Sharing Educational Materials on an Online Platform

In addition, the Reynolds Foundation created the Portal of Geriatrics Online Education (POGOe) [17] in 2004, so that grantees could share information and educational materials. The POGOe, which ran until 2022, contained more than 950 geriatrics educational materials that include virtual and standardized patients, games, tutorials, case-based teaching, self-directed learning, and traditional lectures [18]. Up to 2016, grantees also gathered for annual in-person national conferences to consolidate longitudinal collaboration across institutions. This model demonstrates the important potential of promoting a culture of mentorship networks and inter-institutional collaboration, both of which can persist beyond the duration of a specific grant or fellowship.

Chief Resident Immersion Training (CRIT): Empowering Junior Clinician-Educators as Geriatrics Educators

As another example, the Reynolds Foundation initially funded the Boston Medical Center (BMC) in the innovative development of the Chief Resident Immersion Training (CRIT) program, which uniquely targets chief residents (CRs) from various medical and surgical specialties. Based on a needs assessment of rising CRs, this annual 2.5-day intensive program was developed as a weekend retreat to foster interspecialty collaboration for effective care of complex older patients. As CRs are in a unique teaching role as junior teaching faculty, the goal was to build their geriatrics knowledge base as well as to introduce fundamental teaching skills to help disseminate this information. Key geriatrics content included: (1) assessing decision-making abilities of older patients; (2) conducting a preoperative assessment of an older patient; (3) conducting a functional assessment of an older patient; (4) recognizing/managing dementia; recognizing/managing delirium; (5) reviewing medications for evidence of polypharmacy; (6) assessing the adequacy of the patient's social support/living arrangements; (7) creating a post-discharge management plan; (8) understanding implications of different insurance coverage for older patients; (9) knowledge of long-term care services including home-care services; (10) recognizing the value of and facilitating the interprofessional, collaborative team process; and (11) incorporating the principles of geriatric rehabilitation. Each module started with a small-group discussion, followed by a 15–25 min-long evidenced-based lecture and interactive session focusing on specific teaching skills like providing effective feedback, teaching the "reluctant learner," conflict resolution, and small-group facilitation. At the end of the 2.5-day program, CRIT faculty worked with participating CRs in subsequent one-on-one sessions to design an education or clinical action project of their choice.

Given promising data on increased knowledge as well as self-efficacy in key geriatrics topics, the BMC faculty partnered with the Association of Directors of Geriatric Academic Programs (ADGAP) to extend this program to 12 carefully selected medical institutions nationwide in a 54-month national demonstration project. Faculty from these campuses first attended the BMC CRIT program, before being guided in implementing similar programs at their own campuses.

At the end of the 54-month project, feedback was sought from a total of 295 CRs and 86 faculty mentors, representing 28 specialties participating in 21 CRIT reiterations [19]. Response rate with matchable pre- and post-knowledge tests was 99%. Overall, geriatrics knowledge improved. Out of 12 knowledge questions, CRs correctly answered 6.32 questions on the pre-test (standard deviation 1.73) and 8.39 on the post-test (SD, 1.55) ($p < 0.001$). In addition, the proportion of CRs teaching the 14 geriatrics topics increased by at least 50% 6 months after CRIT, with *a* > 100% increase in eight of the topics. Importantly, CRs reported improvement in specific teaching skills. For example, pre- to post-CRIT, 87–91% of participants credited CRIT "somewhat" or "a lot" for improving their confidence in skills like providing feedback ($p < 0.001$). And perhaps most critically, there was increased confidence in incorporating geriatrics knowledge into formal and informal teaching ($p < 0.001$). These findings held true even in a smaller institution with only one geriatrician, suggesting the reproducible potential of this teach-the-teacher model.

Eventually, through extended funding through a combination of the Reynolds, Hartford, and Hearst Foundations, the CRIT program was further replicated at 33 medical institutions from 2005 through 2014. Since the end of the Reynolds Foundation funding, certain individual institutions that have found CRIT helpful have been able to use data on its effectiveness to secure other funding for continued reiterations of this program. This brings up the importance of rigorously evaluating a program's effectiveness, as discrete funding sources are usually limited in time [20].

Reynolds Program for Advancing Geriatrics Education: Training Hospitalists to Teach Geriatric in the Inpatient Setting

The inpatient ward is a core site of clinical teaching. As such, the Reynolds Foundation also funded the Reynolds Program for Advancing Geriatrics Education (PAGE). This 10-h geriatrics curriculum targeted hospitalists in teaching roles and was co-taught by faculty representing both the Geriatrics and Hospital Medicine Divisions at the University of San Francisco. The curriculum took place at existing noon conferences over 1 year. The program's goals were to provide exportable teaching modules that hospitalists attending could use to teach their residents during inpatient rotations and to increase residents' use of 15 specific geriatrics skills. Teaching topics were finalized by a needs assessment given to hospitalists (2007) as well expert opinion on topics gaining significant national attention at the time. These topics included: home/community resources, delirium/dementia, minimizing medication problems, using prognostic indices to make decisions, general approach to older inpatients, falls, pressure ulcers, indwelling catheters/incontinence, and pain management.

On average, 14 hospitalists attended each noon conference session, with an average of 72% completing the post-session evaluation form. Of the 36 hospitalists that participated in at least one session, 13 (36%) completed a post-program online questionnaire and reported significantly increased self-efficacy in teaching residents geriatrics content ($p < 0.001$). Notably, session attendance was positively correlated with increased self-efficacy ($p < 0.01$), whereas teaching experience was not ($p = 0.88$). Of 56 residents at the teaching site, 23 (41%) completed the pre-survey and 24 (43%) the post-survey. They reported increased frequency of inpatient geriatrics teaching by hospitalist attendings who received the PAGE curriculum; this increase was also notably reported for attendings who did not receive the PAGE curriculum, but the magnitude of increase was greater in those who directly participated in PAGE. Residents also reported increased clinical practice of geriatrics skills ($p = 0.052$) in this order (most increased first): assessing polypharmacy, performing skin exams, prognostication, performing functional assessments, and examining foley catheter use [21]. This model demonstrates the potential of a time-limited curriculum targeting attendings with various degrees teaching experiences, in increasing geriatrics teaching as well as residents' knowledge translation.

Geriatric Scholars Program: Targeting Community-Based Clinicians as Geriatrics Teachers

While many of the bigger grants focused on work in academic institutions, certain programs have primarily targeted building of geriatrics knowledge among community-based clinicians, especially as community-based programs increasingly become sites of teaching for undergraduate medical education. In 2001, the Reynolds Foundation funded the Virginia Commonwealth University School of Medicine (VCU) in establishing the VCU/Reynold Partnership in Geriatrics Education. One of its key components was the Geriatrics Scholars Program, a 2-year continuing medical education (CME) course. The target population comprised internists and family physicians within a 70-mile radius of the medical center. Most were faculty in the clinical skills course that spans the first 2 years of medical school, with some preceptors of third year medical students in ambulatory clerkships. A needs assessment, answered by 121 (48%) of the initially targeted 250 physicians, identified that 96% of respondents indicated the need to increase their knowledge and skills in geriatrics. In terms of teaching format, respondents indicated preference for: a 1-day program (63%), evening seminar (50%), computer-based methods (32%), and 2 to 3-day conferences (28%). Self-identified desired content included: managing chronic health problems, preventive health, acute care, resources that support independent living, long-term care, end-of-life issues, and incorporating geriatrics into office-based teaching. The curriculum eventually incorporated additional topics identified as core competencies for medical students by the American Geriatrics Society and VCU.

Based on these responses, a 3-year geriatrics continuing medical education (CME) course was conducted, from 2002 to 2005. Based on the target learners' preferences, a myriad of formats were offered, including: a 1-day "Geriatrics in Primary Care" conference, two half-day programs on Saturday mornings, and 15 evening programs at which dinner was provided. Participants could personalize their selection of courses but had to complete 30 total hours of curriculum to be designated "Reynolds Geriatrics Scholars." Of 88 CME participants, 60 physicians completed 30 or more hours of education. In an anonymous exit survey, these 60 physicians reported greater self-efficacy not only in translating new geriatrics knowledge to patient care, but also in teaching important geriatrics topics like medication use, cognition, and functional assessment [22].

Stanford Geriatric Education Center (SGEC): Disseminating Geriatrics Knowledge to the Multi-Disciplinary Team

The Stanford Geriatric Education Center (SGEC) was funded by the Bureau of the Health Professions in the Health Resources and Services Administration starting in 1987. Its mission is "to improve the quality of health care and the quality of life of diverse older adults in the United States by educating health care professionals about the health and social service needs of older people, particularly the ethnic minority older adults and their families, with a special emphasis on the cultural context of these needs." In particular, it targets faculty development and curriculum resources, including professional health care training materials on issues related to ethnicity and aging [23].

Since its inception, the SGEC has sponsored and co-sponsored several hundred conferences, targeting multi-disciplinary team members including those in teaching roles. One specific example of a successful faculty development program by the SGEC was its Health Literacy and Ethnogeriatrics (HLE) Program, whose core curriculum took place over 3 years, from 2008 to 2010 [24]. Each annual cohort comprised 8–14 health care educators from various health professions. Spanning over 12 h, this curriculum covered eight 90-min modules presented over an intensive week. The modules included: (1) Exploring Health Literacy, Ethnogeriatrics, and Health Disparities; (2) Aging and Culture; (3) Health Literacy in Patient-Centered Care; (4) Creating Health Messages for Low Literacy Elders; (5) Patient- and Relationship-Centered Communication Strategies; (6) Working with Interpreters and Translators; (7) Improving Ethnogeriatric Health Care; and (8) Teaching Strategy Toolbox. Each session was highly interactive and was based on instructional methods developed by the Stanford Faculty Development Center in teaching clinical medical faculty: didactic presentations, case discussions, brainstorming exercises, role-play exercises, and goal setting in their clinical practice, teaching, and institution [25].

Thirty-four participants from 11 health professions participated in this curriculum. They comprised faculty members from 19 institutions from 12 states. Participants reported that over 57% of the curriculum content was new. Over 91% reported having either disseminated the HLE content knowledge through teaching seminars given at their home institutions and/or implementing HLE-related projects in their local communities [23].

Challenges and Future Directions for Faculty Development in Geriatrics

There are several notable challenges in faculty development for teaching geriatrics. First, we must recognize the lack of standardized expectations regarding geriatrics training during residency training. Whereas family medicine residencies sponsored by the Accreditation Council for Graduate Medical Education (ACGME) are required to dedicate 1 month to geriatrics training [26], a parallel requirement no longer exists for ACGME-sponsored internal medicine residencies [27]. Therefore, there is great variability in knowledge and clinical competencies among learners at a similar stage of medical training. Consequently, it can be challenging to develop a curriculum to keep most learners of all levels actively engaged and adequately challenged. Therefore, it is even more critical that curricula are constructed based on thoughtful needs assessments of the learners beforehand.

Second, we must recognize the heterogeneity among clinician-educators themselves. There is notable diversity when it comes to faculty members' setting of clinical practice, prior experience as teachers, and teaching contexts. In addition, the widely different nature of the various medical and surgical specialties in itself adds to the complexity of effective teach-the-teacher programs. One of the intentional strategies of the Reynold's Foundation's FD-AGE project was to offer mini-fellowships that were tailored to specific provider groups. For example, there were separate programs designed for hospitalists, outpatient providers, skilled nursing facility providers, home-care providers, and palliative care providers. Therefore, it is imperative to constantly evaluate and adapt existing teach-the-teacher curricula to be pragmatic for one's specific target audience.

Third, sustainability remains a challenge in refining and re-iterating teach-the-teacher programs after grant funding of initial curriculum development ends. Therefore, developing a plan for sustaining these programs with internal and/or other external funding sources is critical from the time of initial development.

Today, there is growing recognition for the need to empower clinician-educators, both geriatricians and non-geriatricians, with skillsets imperative in caring for older adults. While a few of the bigger-scale projects have been described in this chapter, there have notably been smaller, more institution-specific efforts with similar goals. A review of programs targeting clinicians in smaller non-academic settings have shown multi-faceted teaching methods (combination of written materials/toolkits, feedback, individualized educational visits, and/or small-group learning) to be most effective [28]. To not repeat but rather build further upon previous efforts, it is critical for clinician-educators to effectively share their experiences. For example, interactive workshops at annual professional meetings can serve as a valuable tool, especially as they also offer opportunity for ongoing mentorships across institutions. Electronic platforms like the POGOe or MedEdPortal [29] serve as another place wherein curricula and teaching tools can be widely shared.

Importantly, there has been a notable effort to create a unified geriatrics curriculum to encourage greater uptake by training programs. For example, Aquifer Geriatrics [30], a virtual geriatrics curriculum based on 27 cases, has been co-produced with the American Geriatrics Society and is being increasingly utilized by medical schools. Written by authors from 35 different institutions, it covers topics such as medication management, cognitive disorders, falls, health care planning, and hospitalizations for older people. Though a single geriatrics curriculum has power in standardizing a core skillset, there is, however, benefit in tailoring a skeleton curriculum to a specific target audience based on clinical setting and teaching context [31]. This is even more true in teach-the-teacher models, as a major goal of this model is integrating geriatrics into the various medical and surgical specialties where geriatrics teaching has traditionally not been incorporated.

In summary, empowering clinician-educators to disseminate geriatrics knowledge has proven to be a promising strategy in training the next generation of clinicians to better care for our older adults. To be effective, a clear understanding of learners' needs as well as their teaching contexts is crucial. Teach-the-teacher programs should be thoughtfully tailored to faculty in various medical and surgical specialties. Importantly, in addition to becoming more interspecialty, geriatrics is becoming increasingly dependent on the multi-disciplinary care team. Therefore, interspecialty and interprofessional adaptations of faculty development curricula will be essential for the ongoing advancement of geriatrics care.

References

1. ABMS Board Certification Report 2020–2021. American Board of Medical Specialties.
2. Geriatrics Workforce by the Numbers. American Geriatrics Society: Geriatrics Healthcare Professionals. https://www.americangeriatrics.org/geriatrics-profession/about-geriatrics/geriatrics-workforce-numbers.
3. National and regional projections of supply and demand for geriatricians: 2013–2015. Health Resources & Services Administration. 2017. https://bhw.hrsa.gov/sites/default/files/bureau-health-workforce/data-research/geriatrics-report-51817.pdf.
4. Scalzo P, Ferrucci L. Chapter 1: demography. In: Harper GM, Lyons WL, Potter JF, editors. Geriatrics review syllabus: a core curriculum in geriatric medicine. 10th ed. New York: American Geriatrics Society; 2019.
5. Eleazer GP, Laditka SB, Roberts E, Hirth VA, Wieland D. Geriatrics training and education for nongeriatrician faculty: the Dean's Faculty Scholars in Aging Program. J Am Geriatr Soc. 2005;53(10):1806–10.
6. Pinheiro SO, White HK, Buhr GT, Elbert-Avila K, Cohen HJ, Heflin MT. Advancing geriatrics education through a faculty development program for geriatrics-oriented clinician educators. J Am Geriatr Soc. 2015;63(12):2580–7.
7. Arora V, Meltzer D, Podrazik P. Faculty development programs in geriatrics. Arch Intern Med. 2008;168(19):2167.

8. Centers of Excellence in Geriatric Medicine and Training. The Hartford Foundation's continued commitment to geriatric medicine. The John A. Hartford Foundation: working to improve the health of older Americans. https://www.johnahartford.org/ar2005/11_continued_commitment.html.
9. Reuben DB, Lee M, Katz D, Warshaw G, Medina-Walpole A, Bragg E, Frank JC. Building academic geriatric capacity: an evaluation of the John A. Hartford Foundation Centers of Excellence initiative. J Am Geriatr Soc. 2004;52(8):1384–90.
10. Levine SA, Caruso LB, Vanderschmidt H, Silliman RA, Barry PP. Faculty development in geriatrics for clinician educators: a unique model for skills acquisition and academic achievement. J Am Geriatr Soc. 2005;53(3):516–21.
11. Skeff KM, Stratos GA, Berman J, et al. Improving clinical teaching: evaluation of a national dissemination program. Arch Intern Med. 1992;152:1156–61.
12. Williams BC, Weber V, Babbott SF, Kirk LM, Heflin MT, O'toole E, Schapira MM, Eckstrom E, Tulsky A, Wolf AM, Landefeld S. Faculty development for the 21st century: lessons from the Society of General Internal Medicine-Hartford Collaborative Centers for the Care of Older Adults. J Am Geriatr Soc. 2007;55(6):941–7.
13. Williams BC, Weber V, Babbott SF, et al. Faculty development for the 21st century: lessons from the society of general internal Medicine-Hartford collaborative centers for the care of older adults. J Am Geriatr Soc. 2007;55(6):941–7.
14. Donald W. Reynolds Foundation awards $20 million for geriatrics teaching. The Portal of Geriatrics Online Education. https://pogoe.org/content/549.
15. Christmas C, Park E, Schmaltz H, Gozu A, Durso SC. A model intensive course in geriatric teaching for non-geriatrician educators. J Gen Intern Med. 2008;23(7):1048–52.
16. Heflin MT, Bragg EJ, Fernandez H, Christmas C, Osterweil D, Sauvigné K, Warshaw G, Cohen HJ, Leipzig R, Reuben DB, Durso SC. The Donald W. Reynolds Consortium for Faculty Development to Advance Geriatrics Education (FD~AGE). Acad Med. 2012;87(5):618–26.
17. The portal of geriatrics online education: be a quicker, better geriatrics educator. https://pogoe.org/.
18. Ramaswamy R, Leipzig RM, Howe CL, Sauvigne K, Usiak C, Soriano RP. The portal of geriatrics online education: a 21st-century resource for teaching geriatrics. J Am Geriatr Soc. 2015;63(2):335–40.
19. Levine SA, Chao SH, Caruso LB, Jackson AH, Russell ML, Young ME, Brett B. Chief resident immersion training in the care of older adults: a successful national replication of an interspecialty educational intervention. Acad Med. 2018;93(9):1341–7.
20. Mazotti L, Moylan A, Murphy E, Harper GM, Johnston CB, Hauer KE. Advancing geriatrics education: an efficient faculty development program for academic hospitalists increases geriatric teaching. J Hosp Med. 2010;5(9):541–6.
21. Mazotti L, Moylan A, Murphy E, Harper GM, Johnston CB, Hauer KE. Advancing geriatrics education: an efficient faculty development program for academic hospitalists increases geriatric teaching. J Hosp Med. 2010;5(9):541–6.
22. Willett RM, Boling PA, Meyers ME, Hoban JD, Lawson SR, Schlesinger JB. Professional development in geriatrics for community-based generalist faculty. J Am Geriatr Soc. 2007;55(2):300–4.
23. Stanford Geriatric Education Center. Mission and goals. https://sgec.stanford.edu/mission.html.
24. Evans KH, Bereknyei S, Yeo G, Hikoyeda N, Tzuang M, Braddock CH III. The impact of a faculty development program in health literacy and ethnogeriatrics. Acad Med. 2014;89(12):1640–4.
25. Johansson J, Skeff K, Stratos G. Clinical teaching improvement: the transportability of the Stanford Faculty Development Program. Med Teach. 2009;31:e377–82.
26. ACGME Program requirements for graduate medical education in family medicine. July 2020. file:///Users/deborah/Desktop/120_FamilyMedicine_2020.pdf.

27. ACGME program requirements for graduate medical education in internal medicine. https://www.acgme.org/globalassets/pfassets/programrequirements/140_internalmedicine_2022v4.pdf. Accessed 14 Aug 2022.
28. Thomas DC, Johnston B, Dunn K, Sullivan GM, Brett B, Matzko M, Levine SA. Continuing medical education, continuing professional development, and knowledge translation: improving care of older patients by practicing physicians. J Am Geriatr Soc. 2006;54(10):1610–8.
29. MedEdPortal: The Journal of Teaching and Learning Resources. Association of American Medical Colleges. Mededportal.org.
30. Aquifer geriatrics: a case-based virtual course. https://aquifer.org/courses/aquifer-geriatrics/.
31. Kramer BJ, Creekmur B, Howe JL, et al. Veterans Affairs Geriatric Scholars Program: enhancing existing primary care clinician skills in caring for older veterans. J Am Geriatr Soc. 2016;64(11):2343–8.

Chapter 23
Assessment in Geriatric Medical Education

Lisa Strano-Paul

Many practicing physicians are involved in assessment of trainees. This is especially true of geriatricians since there is an ever-increasing number of geriatric patients, with a limited pool of health care providers with expertise in geriatrics. This shortage has resulted in a need to educate the next generation of providers. Many geriatric content experts have not been formally educated on assessment in medical education. This results in a lack of familiarity with the educational tools at their disposal and limits their ability to assess the effectiveness of their teaching endeavors. The purpose of this chapter is to introduce the reader to the various types of assessment tools that are available in medical education and discuss their strengths and weakness.

A common adage in education is that "assessment drives learning." When studied it has been demonstrated that regular assessment can increase retention, knowledge, and motivation to learn [1, 2]. In fact, assessment is an important aspect of both learning and teaching as it frames the goals and objectives of an educational curriculum as well as future certification [3]. In education and assessment, Accreditation Council for Graduate Medical Education (ACGME) has developed the six domains of competence: medical knowledge, patient care, professionalism, communication and interpersonal skills, practice-based learning and improvement, and systems-based practice [4]. In addition to the ACGME competencies geriatricians focus on the 5 M's competency domains. The 5 M's are Mind, Mobility, Medications, Multicomplexity, and Matters Most to Me [5].

In medical education the primary goals of assessment are to provide direction and motivation for future learning, protect the public by upholding professional standards, satisfy the public's expectation of self-regulation and choose applicants

L. Strano-Paul (✉)
Stony Brook School of Medicine, Stony Brook, NY, USA
e-mail: lisa.strano-paul@stonybrookmedicine.edu

A. W. Schwartz (ed.), *Medical Education in Geriatrics*,
https://doi.org/10.1007/978-3-031-32499-4_23

for advanced training. Assessment can be broadly defined in terms of formative or summative [6] (Fig. 23.1).

Summative assessment is utilized to determine what a learner knows at a particular point in time. It is used typically at the end an instructional unit or training period and it compared against a standard or benchmark. Summative assessments are outcome focused and are often high stake exams. They are useful for evaluation designed to measure program effectiveness at achieving learning objectives. Summative assessments, such as board certification or re-certification are utilized to provide professional self-regulation and accountability. Summative assessments may include feedback on performance but are typically not designed to provide sufficient feedback to promote ongoing education. Summative assessment strongly influences learning even in the absence of feedback, as students study what they expect to be tested on. It also affects curriculum as educators may be held to performance benchmarks as determined by the outcomes of summative assessment. Examples of summative assessment include National Board of Medical Examiners clinical subject exams and medical licensure exams.

Formative assessment is part of the educational process. The goal of formative assessment is to help students identify their strengths and weakness so that they can target areas to improve upon. Ongoing feedback to learners is an integral component of formative assessment. Key components of formative assessment include providing feedback that will reassure learners while promoting reflection and shaping values that guide future learning. Formative assessment can be ungraded or a low stake component of an evaluation. They are designed to provide a check-in point along the longitudinal pathway toward competency. Formative assessments are very useful for the educators as well since they provide a check point during the

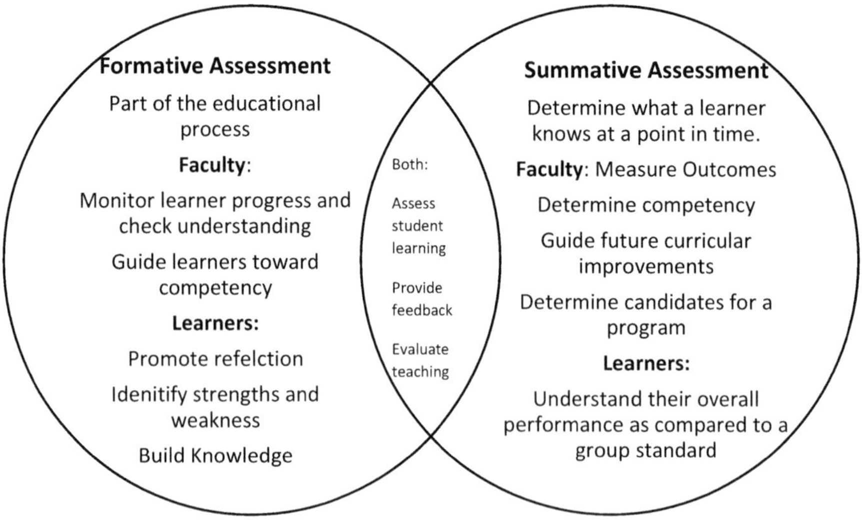

Fig. 23.1 Comparison of formative and summative assessment

educational process that may result in real time adjustment of an educational program to adapt to learners needs. One limitation of formative feedback may be that it does require active faculty participation and therefore can often take more time than a summative assessment such as a multiple choice exam. However formative assessments do not have to take an inordinate amount of time and can be varied to suit the demands of the educational program as well as faculty input.

Both formative and summative assessment are needed to determine competency. Epstein and Hunder have defined competency in medicine as "the habitual and judicious use of communication, knowledge, technical skills, clinical reasoning, emotions, values, and reflection in daily practice for the benefit of the individuals and communities being served" [7]. Competence is achieved longitudinally over time as trainees employ life-long learning skills to the practice of medicine with the goal of honing their skills. The development of competency is gained with deliberate practice, reflection, and the ability to respond to feedback [8–10]. The determination of competency is ideally assessed holistically with multiple observations and evaluations that correlate with the actual skills and knowledge required of a physician.

One should also consider the type of assessment which is best suited to the level of learner. The contextual format of Millers Pyramid provides an excellent framework for this determination [11, 12] (Fig. 23.2). As Miller stated in his original article "no single assessment method can provide all the data required for judgment of anything so complex as the delivery of professional services by a successful physician." He described a framework of a four part pyramidal structure for assessment of performance in medical education. Miller pointed out that assessment becomes more complex as you move up the pyramid. Miller placed "knows" as the foundation of his pyramid, recognizing the foundational importance of knowledge in the

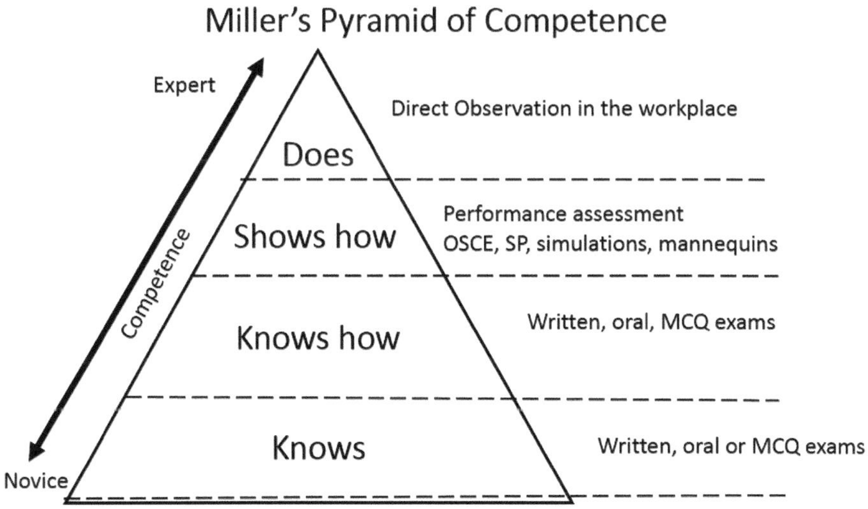

Fig. 23.2 Miller's pyramid of clinical competence. (Modified from Miller, G.E. The assessment of clinical skills/competence/performance. Acad. Med. 1990;65(9):s63–s67 [11])

practice of medicine. The assessment of knowledge is relatively straightforward and can be accomplished with computerized testing and MCQ. The next level is "Know How" which addresses how a trainee applies their knowledge to demonstrate their competency. Assessment at his level can involve written testing but must extend beyond the straightforward MCQ and include questions which encompass clinical reasoning or oral exams. The third level, "Shows How" is related to "performance." Here learners must demonstrate the application of knowledge and skills while being observed. Assessments that are useful in this stage are simulations and Objective Standardized Clinical Exercises (OSCE). At the top of the pyramid is "Does," representing how a learner functions in a clinical situation. Assessment at this level requires direct observation in a workplace setting. Ten Cate has extended Miller's Pyramid to include a fifth level which is "Trusted" [12]. The move toward competency-based educations (CBME) requires that a trainee can be entrusted to perform tasks independently without supervision or assistance, once a necessary level of competence has been demonstrated. Entrustment requires a complex set of assessments which include longitudinal observations in multiple different settings.

Professionalism and professional Identity formation are key elements in medical education. Cruess and Cruess et al. have addressed this key element in their adaptation of Miller's pyramid which includes "IS" as the fifth level [13]. The "IS" level refers to Professional Identity and requires a trainee to consistently demonstrate the attitudes, values, and behaviors expected of one who "think, act, and feel like a physician." These attitudes and values may be more elusive to capture and require ongoing observation in work-based setting for adequate assessment.

Assessment Types

Each method of assessment has its own unique strengths and weakness as well as a purpose in medical education. A fundamental aspect of assessment is that the best way to evaluate a learner is with multiple different types of assessments over the course of the educational program. In this section we will describe the various types of assessments and discuss the value and weaknesses inherent to each method. We will also discuss where each method fits in Miller's pyramid. Examples of assessment types in geriatric education can be found in Table 23.1.

Table 23.1 Examples of assessment types in geriatric medical education

Assessment type	Selected examples in geriatric medical education
Written Exam: Multiple-Choice Questions	UCLA Geriatric Knowledge Test for Primary Care Residents [14]
Written Exam: Short Answer	Aquifer Geriatrics https://aquifer.org/courses/aquifer-geriatrics/
Oral Exam	
Clinical simulations	Emergency Medicine Simulation Case: Septic Shock in the Geriatric Patient [15]
	78-Year-Old Female With Left Hip Fracture: Palliative Medicine in the Emergency Department Simulation Case [16]
	Brown Bag Simulation to Improve Medication Management in Older Adults [17]
	Unintentional Weight Loss in Older Adults: A Geriatric Interprofessional Simulation Case Series for Health Care Providers [18]
Objective Structured Clinical Exam (OSCE)	4Ms for Early Learners: A Skills-Based Geriatrics Curriculum for Second-Year Medical Students [19]
	Informed consent in the older adult: OSCEs for assessing fellows' ACGME and geriatric gastroenterology competencies [20]
Clinical Observations mini-CEX	Mini-Cog Clinical Evaluation Exercise (Mini-CEX) [21]
Self Assessment	Web-based Interactive Self-Assessment Learning Module: Falls and Dysmobility in Older Adults [22]
	Assessment of geriatric knowledge: an online tool for appraising entering APN students [23]

Written Exams

Written exams can have several different varieties including MCQ, matching, short answer, or essay exams. Written exams are best at assessing the base of Miller's pyramid, the knows or knows how. Although written exams can be formative or summative, the more typical use of written exams involves summative assessment. License exams or Board exams are typical examples of written assessments.

MCQ are straightforward to utilize and can allow for a large number of questions to assess a wide body of knowledge. Question banks which are standardized are also available and this allows for national comparison of educational programs. MCQ can be scored electronically which frees up faculty time and can be administered in a relatively short period of time. Questions can involve a clinical stem which requires a degree of clinical reasoning and be written in a way where added information may make a certain answer more or less likely. One inherent weakness of MCQ is that they are subject to cueing, which is when a learner recognizes a correct answer but could not have answered the question without options.

Short answer and essay exams are open ended and can require descriptions of clinical context which can promote more complex clinical reasoning and problem solving. A well-structured short answer or essay exam avoids cueing. These types of questions can be utilized to assess problem solving, diagnostic testing, and clinical reasoning skills. The limitation of short answer and essay written exams is that they are difficult to produce and time consuming to grade. There must be interrater reliability if more than one faculty member is involved in the grading process and there is a possibility of grader error. A well-structured rubric is an essential component of a robust short answer or essay exam.

Oral Examinations

Oral exams can be an effective mechanism for assessing clinical knowledge and allow learners to demonstrate that they "know how" to manage a clinical situation and can demonstrate clinical reasoning. Oral exams can be either formative or summative and have been utilized for high stakes situations such as licensure or board examinations. Limitations include that they are time consuming to develop and deliver. They may be subjective and race and sex based bias has also been a concern.

Clinical Simulations

Simulations require a learner to apply previously acquired knowledge and skills in a realistic setting which evaluates medical problem solving. These exams are higher up on Miller's pyramid as they require a learner to know how and show how. OSCEs can involve standardized patients or computer/mannequin simulation. OSCEs can be formative or summative assessments.

A standardized patient is an actor who is trained to portray a patient with a clinical condition. An OSCE can be designed to assess a learner across multiple domains above and beyond clinical knowledge. These include communication skills such as history-taking, interpersonal and communication skills, non-verbal language, and empathy. An OSCE can involve a singular case or be composed of multiple stations each with a different objective. They can either be graded by a faculty member or by the standardized patient. Each OSCE can be designed to meet required educational goals as needed for a specific program. Assessment for an OSCE is a specific checklist rating form which is tailored to educational goals and developed by content experts. The checklist may have both specific criterion relative to the case and common criterion used for all cases. Specific criteria include key elements of patient history, physical examination, and diagnosis or management. The common portion of the rating scale which is applicable to all cases assesses physician–patient interactions, such as communication skills, professionalism, and empathy. One limitation of the use of SP is the consistency of rater evaluation can vary between SPs and even the same SP may drift in their ratings over time. Regular review of SP grading can avoid this occurrence.

Simulation is another form of OSCEs and can include computer based, mannequin, or virtual reality simulations. In computer-based simulation the learner is given a case history and then they can manage the patient by asking questions, ordering tests, or reviewing additional data. The computer can be programed to unfold the scenario based on the choices the learner makes. Mannequin driven simulations can model the human body with high fidelity and provide realistic patient presentations of abnormal physical findings. They are useful for focusing on invasive procedures that require clinical skills, such as inserting a chest tube. Virtual reality devices can provide the learner with a real time sense of touch and are useful for teaching skills such as endoscopy.

Some limitations associated with all forms of clinical simulations are that they are expensive and time consuming to develop. The expense is increased further with the use of high-fidelity equipment. Scenarios should be developed in a realistic manner such that learners are not required to suspend belief to perform the assessment. As with most assessments regular review of case materials and technology has to be performed to assure the cases remain up to date.

Clinical Observations

One of the most common forms of assessment in clinical education is that of direct observation by a supervising faculty member, who is a physician or other health care provider. The supervising faculty member is trained in their specialty and works with the trainee over a period of time as they directly provide patient care. Direct observation enables a trainee to "show how" and "do" as they participate in patient care. Clearly defined standards are usually required to minimize the possibility of subjectivity. The expectations for workplace responsibility will vary with the level of training and these expectations are typically outlined in the competency-based framework of medical education. For clinical observations to be robust direct observation of skills and abilities while trainees are interacting with patients must occur.

Clinical observations typically include narrative assessments which may be either formative or summative. Narrative assessments are a very important component of clinical assessment as they often give granular insight into workplace performance. Narratives are a key component in the handoff of trainees as they advance through the medical education continuum. Many faculty are not well trained in this type of assessment and may construct narratives that are generic and lack meaning. Faculty development which focuses on the utilization of a competency-based framework can go a long way to improve narrative comment quality which will result in more meaningful, less subjective, or biased narratives.

Another form of clinical observation is the mini-clinical-evaluation exercise (mini-CEX) [24]. In a mini-CEX the learner is observed performing a defined task, such as a focused history and physical or a gait and balance assessment. The mini-CEX is usually a 10–20 min exercise and may include clinical reasoning and management discussion. The assessing faculty member rates the trainee utilizing a predetermined rubric and gives feedback to the trainee. The mini-CEX is designed to increase the frequency of direct observation and can be as reliable as an OSCE.

A limitation of both forms of clinical observation is that they are time consuming. Direct observation of clinical interactions is sometimes replaced with indirect supervision which relies on oral case reports or documentation in the electronic health record, which is then verified by the supervising faculty person. Since the mini-CEX is structured, it selects only the skills which are deemed important for direct observation. Since the trainee is observed the mini-CEX may not represent real time habitual behaviors or skills.

Other Forms of Assessment

Other forms of assessment include self-assessment, peer assessment, and even patient assessment. These are workplace observations that give insight into how a person "does."

Self-assessment is important in medical education as it fosters life-long habits of self-directed learning. Ultimately a provider will have to make judgements about their own capabilities, so it is important to develop the capacity for self-assessment. Many learners are not familiar or comfortable with self-assessment and may not fully understand what is expected from them. They can also be subject to self-deception, either overconfident in their skills and abilities or underestimate themselves as they hold themselves to higher standards. It is therefore important that the development of self-assessment skills be linked to performance-based criterion. Routine formative feedback on self-assessment is essential and can counteract inflated or undervalued self-assessment.

Peer assessment can be a powerful form of formative assessment and provide meaningful insight into attitudes and behaviors that are somewhat more challenging to assess. These include teamwork, responsibility, and professionalism. Confidentiality and buy-in from all involved are required and peer assessments may be subject to inaccuracies due to a general reluctance to give less than ideal feedback on a colleague's performance.

Patient feedback can be helpful and lend insight into a trainee's communication skills and ability to gain patient confidence. However, patients might not always be credible sources of information as they tend to rate providers highly. Patients who are very ill or have adverse outcomes may not be able to rate providers or have their impressions affected by their illness. Patients may also lack the understanding of the ideal standards of practice and may base their opinions on the congeniality of the provider. The ideal number of patient evaluations needed to form a valid opinion is also not clear but likely includes numerous surveys which can be difficult to obtain.

Longitudinal assessment is an important component of professional development. Competency-based medical education (CBME) requires the ongoing assessment of a learner's ability to gain skills over time. We all understand that a first-year medical student cannot be compared to a fourth year student who is about to graduate. Many of our assessments are time based and measure a trainee's ability at single point in the education. A core tenet of CBME is that individuals gain competence as they advance through training at variable rates. Expertise occurs when an individual demonstrates sufficient skill in a defined set of competencies, rather than at predetermined points during the training process. The competencies provide a framework for the determination of desired knowledge, skills, and outcomes of a training program and can determine assessment across the continuum of medical education. Examples of ongoing assessments include evaluation of performance with competency committees. Another mechanism for longitudinal assessment can be with progressive or unfolding case discussions or OSCEs.

The ideal assessment of any trainee should involve a variety of assessment methods as no single method of assessment is devoid of limitations. Both formative and summative assessments such be utilized. In designing an educational curriculum, assessment should be in the forefront to ensure alignment of learning objectives and outcomes. Multiple methods of assessment utilized longitudinally can provide data that is required to determine a trainee overall competence. Such varied assessments can also provide evidence for deficiencies in one or more area of expertise and provide the framework for remediation. Determining the frequency of assessments and if assessments should be formative or summative is challenging and must be customized to meet educational program requirements and outcomes. Assessment of attitudes and qualities which comprise professionalism and result in professional identity formation remain challenging and are an essential component to the Cruess and Cruess et al., "IS" level [13]. Assessment at this level requires longitudinal work-based evaluation which is formative and includes feedback to learners.

References

1. Larsen D, Butler A, Roediger H. Test-enhanced learning in medical education. Med Educ. 2008;42:959–66.
2. Wormald BW, Schoeman S, Somasunderman A, et al. Assessment drives learning: an unavoidable truth? Anat Sci Educ. 2009;2:199–204.

3. Norcini JJ. Peer assessment of competence. Med Educ. 2003;37:539–43.
4. Batalden P, Leach D, Swing S, Dreyfus H, Dreyfus S. General competencies and accreditation in graduate medical education. Health Aff (Millwood). 2002;21(5):103–11.
5. Molnar F, Frank C. Optimizing geriatric care with the GERIATRIC 5Ms. Can Fam Physician. 2019;65(1):39.
6. Epstein R. Assessment in medical education. N Engl J Med. 2007;356:387–96.
7. Epstein RM, Hundert EM. Defining and assessing professional competence. JAMA. 2002;287:226–35.
8. Ericsson KA. Deliberate practice and the acquisition and maintenance of expert performance in medicine and related domains. Acad Med. 2004;79(Suppl):S70–81.
9. Epstein RM. Mindful practice. JAMA. 1999;282:833–9.
10. Epstein RM. Mindful practice in action. II. Cultivating habits of mind. Fam Syst Health. 2003;21:11–7.
11. Miller GE. The assessment of clinical skills/competence/performance. Acad Med. 1990;65(9):s63–7.
12. Hecker K, Norris J, Coe J. Workplace-based assessment in a primary-care setting. J Vet Med Educ. 2012;39(3):229–34.
13. Ten Cate O, et al. Entrustment decision making: extending Miller's pyramid. Acad Med. 2021;96(2):199–204.
14. Dogbey GY. Critical synthesis package: UCLA geriatric knowledge test for primary care residents. *MedEdPORTAL*. 2015;11(1). doi:10.15766/mep_2374-8265.10130.
15. Collins M, Cooper D. Emergency medicine simulation case: Septic shock in the geriatric patient. *MedEdPORTAL*. 2011;7(1). doi:10.15766/mep_2374-8265.8372.
16. Van Vliet H, Thompson R, Ross J. 78-year-old female with left hip fracture: Palliative medicine in the emergency department simulation case. *MedEdPORTAL*. 2015;11(1). doi:10.15766/mep_2374-8265.10244.
17. Hawley CE, Triantafylidis LK, Phillips SC, Schwartz AW. Brown Bag Simulation to Improve Medication Management in Older Adults. *MedEdPORTAL*. 2019;15:10857.
18. Mulligan R, Gilmer-Scott M, Kouchel D, et al. Unintentional Weight Loss in Older Adults: A Geriatric Interprofessional Simulation Case Series for Health Care Providers. *MedEdPORTAL*. 2017;13:10631.
19. Goldberg GR, Solis G, John JT, Olvet DM, Kranz KA. 4Ms for Early Learners: A Skills-Based Geriatrics Curriculum for Second-Year Medical Students. *MedEdPORTAL*. Published online 2022. doi:10.15766/mep_2374-8265.11264.
20. Shah B, Miler R, Poles M, et al. Informed consent in the older adult: OSCEs for assessing fellows' ACGME and geriatric gastroenterology competencies. *Am J Gastroenterol*. 2011;106(9):1575–1579.
21. Mini-Cog Clinical Evaluation Exercise (Mini-CEX). Accessed August 14, 2022. https://pogoe.org/productid/21956.
22. Web-based Interactive Self-Assessment Learning Module 1: Falls and Dysmobility in Older Adults. Accessed August 14, 2022. https://pogoe.org/productid/20571.
23. Towner EM. Assessment of geriatric knowledge: an online tool for appraising entering APN students. *J Prof Nurs*. 2006;22(2):112-115.
24. Cruess R, Cruess S, Steinert Y. Acad Med. 2016;91(2):180–5.

Chapter 24
Online Resources to Support Teaching Geriatrics

Ravishankar Ramaswamy and Rebecca Masutani

Case
You are a geriatric medicine provider at a busy outpatient practice. Today, you also have a third-year medical student assigned to work with you in your very hectic clinic. You see an older adult with a history of frequent falls who presents after sustaining another fall in their home. Due to the busy nature of your clinic, you were unable to review the falls assessment in detail with the medical student, though they are clearly eager to learn. You wish to share helpful online resources with the student to help further their understanding of falls assessments in older adults.

Introduction

Online learning is described as access to learning experiences via the use of the Internet [1]. Within the past century, the progression of technology and the omnipresence of online multimedia platforms have transformed the field of medical education. Information once confined to physical books and manuals have become increasingly accessible through various online modalities, creating more innovative avenues for both teaching and learning. Indeed, the ease of obtaining medical information more efficiently via online resources seems to have allowed for more robust experiences for learners. Instead of solely relying on one textbook to guide their learning, individuals can now access multiple online resources with different levels of interactivity to supplement their education. In other words, technology has allowed for learners to move away from a one-size-fits-all pedagogical approach

R. Ramaswamy (✉) · R. Masutani
Icahn School of Medicine at Mount Sinai, New York, NY, USA
e-mail: Ravishankar.ramaswamy@mssm.edu; Rebecca.masutani@mssm.edu

A. W. Schwartz (ed.), *Medical Education in Geriatrics*,
https://doi.org/10.1007/978-3-031-32499-4_24

and instead created a rich, online forum whereby learners can now maximize their education by selecting modalities that best suit their own individualized learning styles and preferences [2–7]. Additionally, with the uncertainties of the coronavirus pandemic, we have also seen the benefit of providing online learning options to promote individual safety and encourage social distancing. Indeed, the increased availability of asynchronous learning and online resources brought on by the coronavirus pandemic allowed medical students to continue to engage in geriatric medical education [8, 9].

Traditional forms of teaching and learning involved lectures and formal presentations that typically last an hour and utilize technology like PowerPoint. However, they are not adaptive to learners who may have unique needs and learning gaps. Teaching by way of peer-reviewed online courses seems to offer the benefit of accessibility and adaptability that traditional formats cannot. An example of this is the "flipped classroom" approach whereby in-class lectures or instructions are replaced by independent and self-directed learning of core concepts beforehand, thereby allowing for higher-level discussion and application of learned material during class. While studies have shown mixed results on this approach, it generally leads to greater engagement among learners [10–12].

The additional benefit of peer-reviewed online courses is the standardization of the course material based on national competency frameworks, thereby reducing the variability of course content across lecturers and schools. In other words, learners can engage in online courses based on their own schedule and timeline and know that there will not be significant variation or content missed, as is sometimes the case with in-person lectures. See Table 24.1 for a list of potential benefits to using online resources while teaching geriatric medicine to learners.

Additionally, medical content has become increasingly available on various social media platforms comprised of blogs, networking sites, and virtual communities (e.g., Twitter, Facebook, YouTube, Instagram, TikTok). While much of the content created by individuals are variable and oftentimes, have not undergone rigorous peer-review and fact-checking processes as material published by established medical organizations, recent literature among various medical specialties suggests that

Table 24.1 How online resources can be useful in geriatrics

• Standardize competency-based medical education
• Provide geriatric-specific content in settings with limited number of geriatrician educators
• Provide educational content for different modalities of teaching (e.g., flipped classrooms)
• Supplement in-person learning and/or provider accessible educational content to learners with varying schedules
• Provide additional education for learners who require remediation
• Challenge advanced learners with enriched learning material
• Emphasize role and importance of interprofessional care in geriatric medicine
• Highlight various care settings for older adults (e.g., PACE, SNF) that may not be available at the site of clinical learning
• Encourage peer learning, mentorship, networking, and career development

social media can be an effective resource in health care education [13–16]. At the very least, it seems many look to social media to supplement the medical knowledge gleaned from textbooks and evidence-based sources [17–19].

This chapter will discuss online resources you can include in your teaching of geriatric medicine to learners at all stages. Please refer to Chap. 16 to read about synchronous online teaching and Chap. 17 for teaching via telemedicine.

Online Learning and Geriatric Medicine

Despite the trend of the aging demographic where 22% of the world's population will be older than 60 years of age by year 2050, there continues to be a shortage of geriatricians in the USA and globally [19–22]. Several factors, including disease chronicity and multicomplexity, make this a challenging field [23, 24]. Hence, it falls upon the relatively small pool of geriatrics-trained providers to teach learners, colleagues, and the community in order to better care for our aging population. The accessibility and availability of online resources offer the potential for effectively disseminating geriatric medical education to a range of health professions trainees and providers with varying levels of expertise and geographical locations.

Younger generations of learners are adept at using technology to enhance their education; technology-enhanced education allows for flexibility, interactivity, self-efficacy, and immediate feedback that appeals to these learners [25, 26]. Recognizing this need, many medical institutions have begun utilizing technology and web-based content to provide geriatric education to their learners [27–29].

Online Tools Available for Web-Based Learning of Geriatrics

While there are a multitude of online resources available to learners wishing to advance their knowledge in geriatric medicine, we highlight here those resources that are peer-reviewed and evidence-based. Given the thorough and intensive review process these web-based resources generally undergo, many of these modalities are associated with, if not fully endorsed, by national medical organizations and may fulfill core competencies for health professions trainees. Table 24.2 provides a list of available online geriatrics educational resources known to the authors at the time of publishing.

The American Geriatrics Society (AGS) offers many online resources, ranging from e-pamphlets to case-based modules to virtual toolkits [30]. In particular, the AGS endorses Aquifer Geriatrics as the national online curriculum for medical and health professions students. Aquifer Geriatrics consists of 27 online case-based modules for learners, as well as educators looking to complement their own pedagogical approach to teaching geriatric medicine [31]. These modules originated as the web-GEMs (Geriatrics Education Modules) and the Portal of Geriatrics Online

Table 24.2 Select online geriatric education resources

Aquifer Geriatrics[a]	www.aquifer.org	An online national curriculum of the American Geriatrics Society and Association of Directors of Geriatric Academic Programs that comprises case-based modules for health professions learners that are mapped to minimum geriatrics competencies for medical students. Includes self-assessment questions for the learner and the ability for the educator to assign and track case completion
NEJM Resident 360[a]	www.resident360.nejm.org/rotation-prep/geriatrics/	An online collection of resources geared toward medicine residents that includes a section specific to Geriatric Medicine, among other specialties
Center to Advance Palliative Care[a]	www.capc.org	A national organization dedicated to increasing the availability of palliative care by providing online toolkits, virtual courses, and webinars to healthcare professionals
Geriatrics Fast Facts	www.geriatricfastfacts.com	A series of easy-to-read 1–2 page reports on helpful geriatrics topics related to different medical specialties
Geriatrics Care Online	www.geriatricscareonline.com	An online collection of multiple resources, supported by the American Geriatrics Society, dedicated to geriatrics teaching
AGS Geriatrics Virtual Patient Cases[a]	www.edhub.ama-assn.org/ags-education	A compilation of virtual simulations of patient encounters, primarily geared toward healthcare professionals from surgical and related medical subspecialties
Academy Family Physician—Geriatric Care Modules[a]	www.aafp.org	A national organization that offers an online collection on geriatric care and related issues
ePrognosis	www.eprognosis.ucsf.edu	Offered through UCSF, a repository of geriatric prognostic indices that helps providers obtain information about patients' prognosis
GeriPal Podcast	www.geripal.org	A geriatrics and palliative care podcast for healthcare professionals offering a range of topics pertinent to both fields
GeriKit	https://apps.apple.com/us/app/gerikit/id1544200999	A downloadable phone application to help healthcare professionals facilitate geriatric evaluations/assessments
Vital Talk[a]	www.vitaltalk.org	Helpful resources include training videos, tip sheets, and pocket cards to advance communication skills among clinicians
Deprescribing.org	www.deprescribing.org	An online application and website for both patients and healthcare providers offering pamphlets and toolkits on deprescribing medications
Centers for Disease and Control Prevention, STEADI (Stopping Elderly Accidents, Deaths, and Injuries)	www.cdc.gov/steadi	Multiple online resources and toolkits available on the CDC website geared toward caring for older adults and specifically aiming to reduce fall risk among older patients, including patient education materials

[a]May require fee or institutional membership to access online resources
[b]Please note that this is not a comprehensive list of online geriatric educational resources available and is accurate to the best of the authors' knowledge at the time of publishing

Education (POGOe), the development of which was funded by grant support from the Donald W. Reynolds Foundation [32]. Aquifer Geriatrics was developed in an effort to standardize geriatric educational content, meet national core clinical competencies and ultimately, help address the shortage of geriatric medicine providers. And while many medical schools have thus incorporated these modules into their curriculum, the ease of accessibility of this web-based content has allowed for non-physician providers and specialists from other disciplines to further their understanding of geriatric medicine. Another benefit to these modules is the standardization of medical content available to learners with varying levels of geriatrics expertise. Indeed, the availability of online resources and the potential to widely disseminate said information among various healthcare providers align with the philosophy of inter-professionalism integral to the field of geriatrics.

Geriatric Fast Facts [33] is another helpful, quick online tool to consider for learners looking for concise information related to the care of older adults. This online resource captures 1–2 pages of high-yield and must-know facts related to multiple topics, which can also be filtered by medical specialty.

Other examples of entities offering structured modules on geriatric medicine are offered through the American Academy of Family Physicians website, Merck Manuals, and the New England Journal of Medicine Resident 360 website (Table 24.2). Many of these modules are organized by geriatric syndromes and are evidence-based, though notably may require a subscription in order to access the online resources.

Given the population of older adults living with serious illnesses, it is also very important for clinicians to consider advancing their knowledge and skills of palliative care. In particular, the Center to Advance Palliative Care (CAPC) is a nationally known organization that was established in 1999 and created to improve the care of individuals living with serious illnesses. While it may require online membership, the CAPC website offers online modules that can help further geriatric medicine providers' knowledge of pain and symptom management, as well as end-of-life discussions. Vitaltalk.org also offers online courses that purport to help clinicians navigate challenging conversations around serious illness. Notably, VitalTalk has partnered with the Veterans Affairs (VA) healthcare system as part of the VA Life-Sustaining Treatment Decisions Initiative, a national quality improvement project aiming to honor veteran patients' goals, values, and medical preferences [34].

Decision tools in geriatrics have also found their way onto the digital landscape in the forms of mobile apps and online calculators. When caring for older adults with multimorbidity, clinicians may benefit from using ePrognosis—a digital tool developed based off a systematic review investigating the quality and limitations of prognostic indices for older adults—to help guide provider–patient conversations around clinical decisions and advance care planning [35]. Similarly, Deprescribing.org is an online resource that offers tools to help providers deprescribe medications in a systematic algorithmic manner. The advantage to many of these online decision tools is that providers can share these tools with their patients and allow them to engage in shared-decision making. Furthermore, they may also serve as excellent teaching tools to help learners think more carefully about geriatric syndromes like polypharmacy.

Finally, the age of multimedia has allowed for new, innovative ways of conveying medical information. Social media tips are available online at the American Geriatrics Society website. Podcasts, tutorials on Twitter, YouTube videos are some of the ways clinicians have been adding to their medical knowledge and teaching geriatrics. Examples include the presence of online videos demonstrating how to conduct various clinical assessments, such as the Montreal Cognitive Assessment [36] and falls risk assessments, such as the *New England Journal of Medicine*'s Mobility Assessment in Older Adults resource [37]. Additionally, tutorials on Twitter, also known as "tweetorials," have become more popular ways to concisely share medical education and engage with the online medical community [38, 39].

The GeriPal podcast [40], in particular, offers episodes on wide-ranging topics related to geriatrics, palliative care, and hospice. These episodes may be particularly appealing to those who enjoy listening to podcasts on commutes to work, or those who simply enjoy learning by auditory means throughout various times of the day. At the Icahn School of Medicine at Mount Sinai, the geriatrics curriculum involves use of a flipped classroom format for teaching students about post-acute care and long-term care in the nursing home. In this instance, learners are asked to listen to podcasts before joining in for an expert-led discussion on nursing home care. This has resulted in robust discussions between students and educators, building on the knowledge from podcasts and providing opportunities for peer-to-peer teaching.

Challenges

The biggest challenge in the use of online resources for teaching of geriatrics asynchronously is ensuring the content matches the learning needs and knowledge gaps of the learner and remains applicable to their clinical experiences. This requires some initial time investment on the part of the educator to become aware of various resources in this chapter and elsewhere in this book to expand their toolkit.

It is important to recognize that online learning may not work well in isolation and lead to passive learning. Curriculum developers should appreciate the importance of embedding online resources in the context of experiential learning, a mix of synchronous and asynchronous learning, student–teacher and peer interactions, practice opportunities, and a learning community [41]. The educator adopts a role that is not limited to providing information, but to motivate and enrich the learning experience.

With social media platforms in particular, educators must be cautious about checking the accuracy of information disseminated, maintaining professionalism, and protecting patient and learner privacy and confidentiality. In general, we suggest that busy clinicians utilize curated online resources from well-known organizations, as described in Table 24.2. Finally, there exists a multitude of known barriers from the perspective of learners and educators to online learning that should be considered, including lack of technical skills, negative attitude about technology-enhanced education, limited faculty time, and lack of institutional support and resources [42, 43]. At the very least, institutions should continue to support the infrastructure needed to ensure these online medical education resources are reliable and comprised of up-to-date, evidence-based, peer-reviewed medical material. Similarly, with the multitude and variability of online educational material available, it may be helpful for educators and content creators to consider ensuring the content meets certain standards. In particular, Health.gov offers a health literacy online checklist that media content developers have used to ensure health-related content is appropriate for consumers; however, educators can consider using this in order to deliver efficacious pedagogical content via various online mediums (Table 24.3).

While many have accepted that the delivery and structure of medical education has changed in the context of our digital landscape, it is important to be aware of the challenges that arise with these emerging online learning modalities so that such challenges can be addressed ongoingly.

Table 24.3 Online health literacy checklist

Write actionable content
• Provide specific action steps
• Write in plain language
• Ensure content is accurate
Display content clearly
• Use meaningful headings
• Use readable font
• Make site accessible
• Use links effectively
Organize content
• Create simple homepage
• Create linear information paths
• Display search results clearly
Engage users
• Design intuitive graphics and tools
• Consider social media sharing options
Test
• Recruit users with limited literacy skills
• Identify logistical barriers
• Test the display of information on mobile devices

Adapted from [44]

Future Directions

The opportunities in providing online geriatric medical education are seemingly endless. Within the past few decades, the advent of online technology and multimedia has transformed previous paradigms of teaching and has allowed for more possibilities within education.

Within the field of medicine, we have seen benefits to transitioning to online education, particularly as this applies to distance learning for learners in rural regions or busy individuals hoping to align their personal schedules and professional goals.

Geriatrics has always been a team sport; however, the workforce limitations and physical distance between health professions learners were challenging to overcome. In the future, geriatrics online education has the potential to have a greater impact in interprofessional education, bringing teams closer to each other with the unified goal of patient-centered care of older adults. This needs more training and support of educators in the adoption of online resources in their curricula and reduces the digital divide between generations of teachers and learners. Augmented reality and virtual reality innovations can enhance learning experiences through interactivity and immersion. Also, there is room for more geriatrics questions and cases in online assessments like virtual patients.

The use of technology to deliver medical education offers exciting possibilities and seemingly endless opportunities. It remains to be seen how medical institutions will harness the use of technology to deliver medical content and largely, how they will continue to adapt within this age of digital multimedia to meet the needs of an ever-changing demographic of learners.

The geriatrics health care workforce shortage is real. Adopting online geriatrics education tools, wherever possible, can arm providers with essential tools and knowledge to care for an increasing population of older people.

Case Revisited

You review the list of online geriatric education resources (Table 24.2) and suggest the medical student complete the Aquifer Geriatrics module on falls in older adults. You also direct the student to the Centers for Disease Control and Prevention STEADI (Stopping Elderly Accidents, Deaths & Injuries) website, which offers toolkits and resources on falls risk screening and assessments [45]. Knowing that your patient has a history of polypharmacy, you suggest they also review the Deprescribing.org website to consider simplifying the patient's medication regimen and reducing their fall risk.

By the week's end, you dedicate time to meet with the medical student to discuss specific questions they may have and ask them to share with you a few takeaway points they learned from that specific module. A few years later, this medical student, now a resident physician, connects with you over e-mail and shares that they have been utilizing the *NEJM* Resident 360—Geriatric online resource while on their geriatric medicine rotations and have been listening to the GeriPal podcast on their commute to work. You are thrilled to hear that your former student is actively engaging in web-based geriatric educational resources and excited for newer geriatric-specific developments within the constantly evolving online medical education landscape.

Disclosure Dr. Ramaswamy serves as consortium member and assessment lead at Aquifer Geriatrics.

References

1. Moore JL, Dickson-Deane C, Galyen K. e-Learning, online learning, and distance learning environments: are they the same? Internet High Educ. 2011;14:129–35.
2. Hernandez JE, Vasan N, Huff S, Melovitz-Vasan C. Learning styles/preferences among medical students: kinesthetic learner's multimodal approach to learning anatomy. Med Sci Educ. 2020;30:1633–8.
3. Buşan A-M. Learning styles of medical students - implications in education. Curr Health Sci J. 2014;40:104–10.
4. Samarakoon L, Fernando T, Rodrigo C. Learning styles and approaches to learning among medical undergraduates and postgraduates. BMC Med Educ. 2013;13:42.
5. Kim RH, Kurtzman SH, Collier AN, Shabahang MM. The learning preferences of applicants who interview for general surgery residency: a multiinstitutional study. J Surg Educ. 2016;73:e136–41.
6. Wilkinson T, Boohan M, Stevenson M. Does learning style influence academic performance in different forms of assessment? J Anat. 2014;224:304–8.
7. Abouzeid E, Fouad S, Wasfy NF, Alkhadragy R, Hefny M, Kamal D. Influence of personality traits and learning styles on undergraduate medical students' academic achievement. Adv Med Educ Pract. 2021;12:769–77.
8. Ramaswamy R, Shah AA, Denson KM, Sehgal M, Syed Q, Powers BB, Schwartz AW, Leipzig RM, Gleason LJ. Teaching geriatrics during the COVID-19 pandemic: aquifer geriatrics to the rescue. J Am Geriatr Soc. 2021;69:1740–2.
9. Rodriguez V, Rivera V, Goldhirsch S, Ramaswamy R. Using Medicare Annual Wellness Visits and telehealth to enhance ambulatory geriatrics education among medical students. Gerontol Geriatr Educ. 2021;43:584.
10. Chen F, Lui AM, Martinelli SM. A systematic review of the effectiveness of flipped classrooms in medical education. Med Educ. 2017;51:585–97.
11. Hew KF, Lo CK. Flipped classroom improves student learning in health professions education: a meta-analysis. BMC Med Educ. 2018;18:1–12.
12. Riddell J, Jhun P, Fung C-C, et al. Does the flipped classroom improve learning in graduate medical education? J Grad Med Educ. 2017;9:491–6.
13. Cheston CC, Flickinger TE, Chisolm MS. Social media use in medical education: a systematic review. Acad Med. 2013;88:893–901.
14. Hollinderbäumer A, Hartz T, Ückert F. Education 2.0 - how has social media and Web 2.0 been integrated into medical education? A systematical literature review. GMS Z Med Ausbild. 2013;30:Doc14.
15. Wang AT, Sandhu NP, Wittich CM, Mandrekar JN, Beckman TJ. Using social media to improve continuing medical education: a survey of course participants. Mayo Clin Proc. 2012;87:1162–70.

16. Scott N, Goode D. The use of social media (some) as a learning tool in healthcare education: an integrative review of the literature. Nurse Educ Today. 2020;87:104357.
17. Bahner DP, Adkins E, Patel N, Donley C, Nagel R, Kman NE. How we use social media to supplement a novel curriculum in medical education. Med Teach. 2012;34:439–44.
18. Bergl P, Muntz M. Using social media to enhance health professional education. Clin Teach. 2016;13:399–404.
19. Shah V, Kotsenas AL. Social media tips to enhance medical education. Acad Radiol. 2017;24:747–52.
20. Lester PE, Dharmarajan TS, Weinstein E. The looming geriatrician shortage: ramifications and solutions. J Aging Health. 2020;32:1052–62.
21. Geriatrics Workforce by the Numbers_0.pdf.
22. Projected-Future-Need-for-Geriatricians_1.pdf.
23. Meiboom AA, de Vries H, Hertogh CMPM, Scheele F. Why medical students do not choose a career in geriatrics: a systematic review. BMC Med Educ. 2015;15:101.
24. Bagri AS, Tiberius R. Medical student perspectives on geriatrics and geriatric education. J Am Geriatr Soc. 2010;58:1994–9.
25. Law M, Rapoport MJ, Seitz D, Davidson M, Madan R, Wiens A. Evaluation of a National Online Educational Program in geriatric psychiatry. Acad Psychiatry. 2016;40:923–7.
26. Swagerty D, Studenski S, Laird R, Rigler S. A case-oriented web-based curriculum in geriatrics for third-year medical students. J Am Geriatr Soc. 2000;48:1507–12.
27. Hajjar IM, Ruiz JG, Teasdale TA, Mintzer MJ. The use of the internet in geriatrics education: results of a National Survey of Medical Geriatrics Academic Programs. Gerontol Geriatr Educ. 2007;27:85–95.
28. Gainor SJ, Goins RT, Miller LA. Using online modules in a multi-modality teaching system: a high-touch, high-tech approach to geriatric education. Gerontol Geriatr Educ. 2004;24:45–59.
29. St Hill H, Edwards N. Interdisciplinary gerontology education online: a developmental process model. Gerontol Geriatr Educ. 2004;24:23–44.
30. GeriatricsCareOnline.Org.
31. Sehgal M, Syed Q, Callahan KE, Powers BB, Eleazer GP, Gleason LL, Ramaswamy R, Sauvigne K, Leipzig RM, Shah A. Introducing aquifer geriatrics, the American Geriatrics Society National Online Curriculum. J Am Geriatr Soc. 2019;67:811–7.
32. Ramaswamy R, Leipzig RM, Howe CL, Sauvigne K, Usiak C, Soriano RP. The portal of geriatrics online education: a 21st-century resource for teaching geriatrics. J Am Geriatr Soc. 2015;63:335–40.
33. Geriatric Fast Facts.
34. The VA Life-Sustaining Treatment Decisions Initiative - National Center for Ethics in Health Care. https://www.ethics.va.gov/LSTDI.asp. Accessed 30 May 2022.
35. Yourman LC, Lee SJ, Schonberg MA, Widera EW, Smith AK. Prognostic indices for older adults: a systematic review. JAMA. 2012;307:182–92.
36. MoCA - Cognitive assessment. https://www.mocatest.org/. Accessed 30 May 2022.
37. James K, Schwartz AW, Orkaby AR. Mobility assessment in older adults. N Engl J Med. 2021;385:e22.
38. Breu AC, Abrams HR, Manning KD, Cooper AZ. Tweetorials for medical educators. J Grad Med Educ. 2021;13:723–5.
39. Breu AC. Why is a cow? Curiosity, tweetorials, and the return to why. N Engl J Med. 2019;381:1097–8.
40. GeriPal PodCast | A geriatrics and palliative care podcast for every healthcare professional. https://geripal.org/geripal-podcast/. Accessed 30 May 2022.
41. Rhim HC, Han H. Teaching online: foundational concepts of online learning and practical guidelines. Korean J Med Educ. 2020;32:175–83.
42. Muilenburg, Berge - Student barriers to online learning A factor anal.pdf; 2005.
43. O'Doherty D, Dromey M, Lougheed J, Hannigan A, Last J, McGrath D. Barriers and solutions to online learning in medical education – an integrative review. BMC Med Educ. 2018;18:130.
44. Health.gov, https://health.gov/healthliteracyonline/checklist/.
45. Centers for Disease Control and Prevention STEADI (Stopping Elderly Accidents, Deaths & Injuries). https://www.cdc.gov/steadi/index.html.

Index

A. W. Schwartz (ed.), *Medical Education in Geriatrics*,
https://doi.org/10.1007/978-3-031-32499-4

GPSR Compliance

The European Union's (EU) General Product Safety Regulation (GPSR) is a set of rules that requires consumer products to be safe and our obligations to ensure this.

If you have any concerns about our products, you can contact us on ProductSafety@springernature.com

In case Publisher is established outside the EU, the EU authorized representative is:

Springer Nature Customer Service Center GmbH
Europaplatz 3
69115 Heidelberg, Germany

Batch number: 10732076

Printed by Printforce, the Netherlands